P9-EEK-937

M. Katz
5 Whitney Ct.
Menlo Park, CA 94025-6648

SKIN PERMEATION

Fundamentals and Application

Edited by
Joel L. Zatz, PhD

Published by
Allured Publishing Corp.
Wheaton, IL

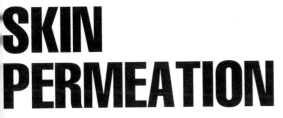

Allured Publishing Corporation
P.O. Box 318, Wheaton, IL 60189

Preface

Literature on absorption of drugs and other substances into and through the skin has grown amazingly in the past few years. This book is written for researchers who are just getting involved in the area of skin permeation, as well as individuals who need a review of recent developments. The emphasis here is on ideas and techniques that will be of immediate use to readers. This information will also help people in related fields who need to understand the techniques used in skin permeation studies, and the trends that have been discovered. References accompanying each chapter direct readers to additional sources of information, including mathematical treatments and models not covered in detail in this book.

Three factors appear to be responsible for the enormous increase in publication of skin permeation and sorption data since the publication of Tregear's classic *Physical Functions of Skin* in 1966: (1) the introduction of transdermal patches that can deliver therapeutic amounts of potent drugs to the bloodstream; (2) the search for relationships between local therapeutic response and either tissue concentration or skin flux of an active compound; and (3) the realization that nearly all substances permeate the skin to some degree. Thus, knowledge of ingredient sorption to skin tissues and transport rates for applied substances is vital to the development of effective, well-tolerated skin products regardless of their function.

One result of our recently-acquired knowledge of skin permeation has been the abandonment of the archaic notion that components of cosmetics and other nondrug products used on the skin stay on the skin surface and work their magic from afar. We now know that many effective moisturizers, for example, do penetrate beyond the statum corneum. So do preservatives, insect repellents and ultraviolet radiation absorbers.

Although it is still legally solid, the line between beauty product and dermatological treatment is becoming philosophically blurred as "active" cosmetics and "cosmeceuticals" are introduced. This is a two-way street. Cosmetic companies are beginning to experiment with OTC drugs while pharmaceutical manufacturers seem to have a renewed appreciation for the importance of the esthetic qualities and biocompatability of their products.

Every attempt has been made to keep the notation and terminology uniform. In general, "penetration," "permeation," and "percutaneous absorption" are synonymous in this book. "Sorption" refers to the tendency of a compound to be retained on the surface or within the bulk of a particular skin tissue. "Retention," which has been defined to indicate accumulation within the skin, is not yet in general use.

Many people contributed to the successful completion of this book. I am especially grateful to the other chapter authors for their willingness to share their insights and for putting up with the editors' nagging to meet publishing deadlines. It was a pleasure to work with the staff at Allured Publishing: Stanley Allured, who conceived the project; Nancy Allured, who oversaw it; Kenneth Boltz for designing the book; Sharon Beaver for designing the look of the articles; Janet Ludwig for help coordinating production; Mary Ann Christianson, for typesetting; and Sharon Giammanco for attention to myriad small but necessary chores. Special thanks go to Susan Price for reviewing and editing the manuscripts and lubricating the occasionally squeaky wheels of progress.

Joel L. Zatz

This book is an expansion of a series of articles which dealt with methodology, aspects of product formulation, philosophic and technical questions on permeation research which appeared in 12 consecutive issues of Cosmetics & Toiletries *magazine during 1990 and 1991. The book contains expanded and updated versions of these articles to include as much recent information as possible: several articles published in 1991 have been cited. An additional chapter, reviewing applications of noninvasive instrumental measurements, has been included.*

Contents

Biographies

Joel L. Zatz, PhD, is professor and chairman of the department of pharmaceutics at Rutgers University. He is a Fellow of the Society of Cosmetic Chemists and a member of the editorial boards of the Journal of Pharmaceutical Science and the Journal of the Society of Cosmetic Chemists. His research interests include delivery of drugs to the skin and the design of novel topical delivery products.

Martin M. Rieger, PhD, President of M&A Rieger Associates, has had more than 40 years experience in skin care and OTC drug development. He was president of the Society of Cosmetic Chemists, edited its journal, and received its Medal Award. He has continued to publish technical papers and to edit and contribute to books pertaining to cosmetics and pharmaceuticals.

Dr. Thomas Franz, MD, is associate professor of Dermatology, University of Arkansas for Medical Sciences, Little Rock, AR. He has worked in the field of dermatology for more than 20 years and has devoted most of his efforts to the study of percutaneous absorption.

Dr. Robert L. Bronaugh, PhD, is a supervisory pharmacologist at the Food and Drug Administration in Washington, D.C. His research has involved many different aspects related to the percutaneous absorption and metabolism of topically applied chemicals. He has authored more than 100 articles in the fields of toxicology, pharmacology, and cosmetic science.

Steven W. Collier is a research chemist with the Food and Drug Administration in Washington, D.C. He is interested in understanding the unique metabolic environment of skin, its relationship to the phenomena of percutaneous absorption, and the pharmacological implications of xenobiotics in skin.

Jim Edmond Riviere is a professor of Pharmacology and Toxicology and director of the Cutaneous Pharmacology and Toxicology Center at North Carolina State University. Dr. Riviere has published 200 research articles and three books. His research is focused on quantitating transdermal drug delivery and biologically relevant in-vitro models.

Joel Sequeira is currently an associate director in Pharmaceutical Research & Development at Schering-Plough. He leads a group of scientists in the development of topical, transdermal, oral liquid and inhalation drug delivery systems. His research interests include percutaneous absorption and drug delivery improvements of a variety of dosage forms.

Edward M. Jackson, PhD, founder of Jackson Research Associates, was most recently director of the Research Services and Quality Assurance Department at The Andrew Jergens Company, a subsidiary of the Kao Corporation of America. His current interests are the cellular and molecular events of the inflammatory process. Dr. Jackson is founder and editor of the toxicology quarterly, *Cutaneous and Ocular Toxicology*. He is on the editorial boards of four other toxicology and dermatology periodicals, has published more than 35 articles and has authored chapters in seven books. He has edited two other books, *The Photobiology of the Skin and the Eye* (1986) and *Irritant Contact Dermatitis* (1990).

Kamel Egbaria, PhD, is currently with Procter & Gamble Inc. at the Sharon Woods Technical Center in Cincinnati, Ohio. **Norman Weiner** is a professor at the University of Michigan, College of Pharmacy. They have collaborated for about 3 years in the area of topical application of liposomal formulations and they have published about 25 papers in this area in that period of time.

Gary W. Cleary, PhD, is the founder , chairman and chief technical officer of Cygnus Therapeutic Systems. He has served as an investigator with the U.S. Food and Drug Administration and has held research and management positions at Cutter Labs, Alza Corporation, Key Pharmaceuticals and Genentech. Dr. Cleary's research and technology interests are in the development of controlled drug delivery systems.

Pramod Sarpotdar, PhD, is a senior research investigator in the Sterling Winthrop Pharmaceuticals Research Division where he is engaged in the discovery and development of novel drug delivery systems. Dr. Sarpotdar has spent nine years working in the area of drug delivery.

Jeffrey K. Mills is a research assistant at Rutgers University, Piscataway, New Jersey. Mr. Mills' interests currently center in engineering. His work at Rutgers was to identify noninvasive instrumental approaches for measuring physiological end points following topical application. Mr. Mills has also done research at the Universtiy of Pennsylvania School of Medicine and he is a member of the American Association for the Advancement of Science and the New York Academy of Sciences.

Richard S. Berger, MD, is a clinical professor in the Division of Dermatology at the University of Medicine and Dentistry of New Jersey. In addition to his academic activities, Dr. Berger maintains a private dermatology practice and he has worked in the area of evaluation of safety and efficacy of products intended for the skin. His memberships include the American Academy of Dermatology (Fellow) and the Society for Investigative Dermatology.

Scratching the Surface:
Rationale and Approaches to Skin Permeation

By Joel L. Zatz, PhD

Although early investigators thought that the skin was totally impermeable, we now realize that a few substances overcome the resistance of the epidermis rather easily and most make steady, slow progress through the skin. The literature of skin transport has been growing rapidly (one might say this subject area is in a state of flux) because of its many applications, and because it is also now possible to get better, more precise information on the uptake and transcutaneous movement of molecules than in the past. With the introduction of sensitive analytical techniques and improvement in study methods, we can often quantitate the sometimes infinitesimal amounts of various substances that manage to get into and through the skin.

The skin barrier is constantly put to the test. Whether swimming in the ocean or walking through an ocean of air, whether because of spills or sprays, the skin is bombarded by minute amounts of many chemical agents. Then we have products deliberately put on the skin: dermatologicals to modify skin function, cosmetics to beautify, transdermals to treat some distant organ. Finally, individuals may repeatedly come into contact at their workplace with potentially toxic materials at concentrations thousands of times those encountered by the general population.

Reasons for studying skin permeation

The efficacy of skin treatment products is measured by clinical testing, an expensive, time-consuming process. It is usually possible to replace some clinical testing during product development with laboratory tests that relate to the clinical outcome. To be effective, sufficient quantities of the active ingredient(s) must reach the intended site of action within the skin. Thus, skin uptake and permeation studies are useful for screening ingredients and comparing formulations. In many cases, only comparative results are required.

For cleansers, protectants and other products that are intended to act on the skin surface, passage through, or accumulation within the skin are undesirable. Such products as insect repellents and sunscreens will generally perform for a longer period of time when absorption into the deeper tissues is minimized. Extensive permeation may remove significant quantities from the skin surface, perhaps eventually depleting the protective layer. There is also the possibility of interaction with viable skin tissues, another undesirable result. Here, the function of permeation studies is to identify the extent to which penetration is blocked. On the other hand, sorption to the stratum corneum, the skin's outer layer, may help to prevent loss by physical contact (rub-off).

The prototypic transdermal nitroglycerin product is the ointment, which has been on the market for many years. But with the recent introduction of transdermal patches containing all types of drugs, the possibilities of systemic therapy using the skin as a conduit have been spotlighted. For such products, and for treatments that focus on subcutaneous tissues, skin concentrations are largely irrelevant; it is the amount of material passing through the skin that is important. Here again, skin penetration studies are very useful during product development. Pharmacokinetic models can be used to estimate blood levels in human subjects if the absorption characteristics through human skin are known.

The percutaneous absorption of potentially toxic chemicals, whether product ingredients or environmental contaminants, is a source of concern. The rate and extent of absorption into and through the skin determine the effective dose of toxins that operate on the skin tissues or in systemic circulation. It is not pleasant to think about, but certain agents used in chemical warfare penetrate the skin very rapidly.

Overview of the skin barrier

Although the skin excretes wastes, receives sensory stimuli and helps regulate body temperature, its principal function is to separate and protect the sensitive protoplasmic jelly of the body's interior from an environment that can be very harsh. The skin prevents intrusion of microbes, chemicals and various forms of radiation, and keeps body fluids and tissues from spilling out. Figure 1 in Chapter 5 shows the various skin layers and structure.

It is remarkable that the principal resistance to permeation of most, though not all, substances resides in the paper-thin outer layer of skin called the stratum corneum, or horny layer. This stratum, generated by the underlying cells of the epidermis, is most conveniently thought of as a separate layer when skin permeation is under discussion.

The horny layer is a compact amalgam of dried, dead, elongated cells (corneocytes), the end product of differentiation of the cells produced in the viable epidermis. Keratin, deposited within the corneocytes, provides strength and chemical resistance. Most of the lipoidal material present is found between the compressed cells in the form of neutral lipids.[1] The horny layer is a rather dry tissue, although the actual moisture content depends on the ambient relative humidity. At low humidity, most of the water associated with keratin and other proteins is tightly bound and therefore oriented, so that the tissue has a low effective dielectric constant. Within the cells are low molecular weight hydrophilic substances (such as amino acids and sugars) that are sometimes collectively referred to as natural moisturizing factor (NMF).

Resistance to transport through the horny layer depends on the properties and arrangement of its alternating hydrophilic and hydrophobic layers, as well as their thickness, all of which vary from species to species and even from place to place on the same individual. Additional variables are the local concentration of hair follicles and sweat glands; these provide possible alternate pathways for diffusion.

Experimentally, large permeation differences have been demonstrated depending on skin location.[2] Although relative rates are to some extent a function of the permeant, we can generalize and rank permeability of body sites as follows: genitals > head areas > trunk > limbs.

The horny layer is manufactured by the next skin layer down, the viable epidermis. Highly enzymatically active, the epidermis is crammed with cells in various stages of biochemical alteration. There is constant movement of newly-generated cells upward, from the basal layer toward the skin surface. The rate of cell production matches the rate at which the glue binding the outermost horny layer cells together fails in normal skin. Thus, the thickness of the horny layer in a particular skin region remains essentially constant, although horny layer thickness does vary from place to place.

One consequence of this process is that the horny layer is not totally uniform from top to bottom. The cells at the skin surface are held less securely than those below. Although this would be expected to produce differences in the degree of resistance to diffusion as a function of depth within the horny layer, such differences are generally ignored in theoretical treatments because of the added complexity they would introduce.

Hair follicles and associated sebaceous glands are structurally part of the epidermis. The follicles are lined with epidermal tissue. The sebaceous glands are holocrine glands which produce a lipid mixture (sebum) that is deposited onto the skin surface.[3] The glands themselves, as well as the upper sections of the follicles, which are filled with sebum, are potential locations for the uptake of lipoidal substances. The hair follicles extend down into the dermal region, sometimes reaching into the fatty layer beneath the dermis.

The epidermis has no blood vessels. Nutrients must diffuse into this tissue from the dermis, a much thicker layer that contains many fibers and is responsible for most of the skin's mechanical strength and "feel." Blood vessels and nerve endings are also found here.[3] The junction between epidermis and dermis is highly indented, something like an egg carton. Capillaries extend to just beneath the epidermal-dermal junction.

The dermis is supported by a layer of fatty tissue, referred to as the hypodermis or subcutis, which provides insulation and mechanical cushioning. The thickness of this layer varies greatly from one body site to another. The hypodermis may act as a storage depot for lipophilic molecules that manage to evade the blood vessels as they diffuse through the skin.

Target areas

When a treatment or product is applied to the skin surface, some specific end result is desired. Depending on the goal and the mechanism of action, it will be necessary for active substances to reach target sites within the skin. In some cases, the benefit is due to the product as a whole rather than any single ingredient. Some targets and examples of appropriate materials or product types are listed in Table I.

Products designed to function on the skin surface work best if absorption is minimal. These include cleansing treatments, protective agents (such as insect repellents and sunscreens) and vehicles, like petrolatum, that use occlusion to enhance the retention of moisture by the horny layer.

Table I. Target sites for preparations applied to the skin	
Target	Examples
Skin surface	Soaps, sunscreens, insect repellents, petrolatum
Horny layer	Moisturizers, keratolytics
Sweat ducts	Antiperspirant aluminum salts
Living skin cells	Steroids, local anesthetics, retinoids
Epidermal basal cells	Cytostatic agents (e.g. methotrexate)
Blood	Transdermal patches (e.g. nitroglycerin)
Local muscle tissues	Nonsteroidal anti-inflammatory drugs

Dry skin conditions are often the result of excessive moisture loss from the horny layer because of low humidity conditions or because of exposure to solvents, detergents or other harsh chemicals that leach components of the stratum corneum. Certain moisturizers, such as pyrrolidone-5-carboxylic acid (PCA), function by augmenting or replacing natural hydrophilic substances within the horny layer. Other compounds whose action focuses on the horny layer are keratolytic agents like salicylic acid, used in high concentrations to soften and remove corns and callouses.

A variety of drugs can function only if they are able to reach the viable tissues. Included are: corticosteroids such as hydrocortisone, used to treat a variety of skin conditions; local anesthetics such as benzocaine, for relief of itch or local pain; and vitamin A acid, used in the treatment of acne. The result of treatment using a drug in one of these classes depends on both the drug's inherent potency and also the fraction of the applied dose that reaches the target tissue. Some drugs that are very active when given orally or by injection have failed to work when applied to the skin, apparently due to an inability to reach the target site.

The objective of local therapy is to produce adequate tissue levels of a drug while simultaneously producing very low blood concentrations, thus limiting pharmacologic effects or toxicity in other parts of the body. For topically-administered dermatologics, extensive drug uptake by the blood is usually undesirable, not only because of the possibility of untoward systemic effects, but also because rapid removal by the blood may limit the tissue concentrations that can be obtained. Thus, for substances designed to work in the skin tissues themselves, the optimum situation is to have good skin uptake and minimal penetration into the capillaries.

On the other hand, the blood itself is the target of permeation for transdermal products, whose site of action is a different tissue entirely. For these products, extensive skin uptake may slow permeation, at least at early times immediately following application. Therefore, minimal sorption accompanied by rapid penetration through the skin are the optimum properties for this therapeutic class.

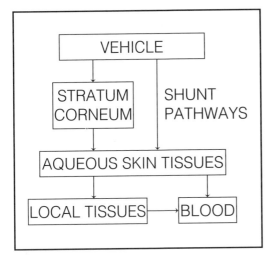

Figure 1. Schematic diagram showing principal permeation routes.

Certain compounds used in the treatment of musculoskeletal pain, notably the salicylates, may be administered by application to the skin. Success with this approach depends on the active compound's permeation through the skin followed by its distribution into the target organ. Here, as with targeting to local skin tissues, extensive loss to the general circulation is counterproductive.

Permeation pathways

Figure 1 is a schematic diagram outlining the pathways leading from the skin surface to the underlying layers and finally the circulation. Two major thoroughfares exist, one through the stratum corneum and the other utilizing the so-called shunts—the hair follicles and sweat gland ducts. Permeation along the shunts avoids contact with the horny layer which, as we said earlier, is the skin's principal barrier. However, it has been estimated that shunts occupy less than 1% of the total surface area of human skin. Therefore, even if permeation via the follicles and glands is faster than the route across the horny layer, the latter is expected to be the major pathway for most substances.[4]

However, recent data suggest that the influence of shunts on permeation has been undervalued. Older publications were reviewed and new results presented in a paper by Illel et al.[5] The authors developed an experimental model using the hairless rat. The skin of this animal, although free of hair, contains hair follicles. These were eliminated by immersion in hot water followed by healing of the treated area. The healed skin was free of follicles. After excision of skin from the animals, in-vitro diffusion studies were performed on both normal and regrown (follicle-free) membranes. Tritiated drugs were applied in acetone solution (100 μl); the cells were left open to the atmosphere, allowing evaporation of the solvent. Some data from the paper are summarized in Table II. For three drugs, removal of hair follicles reduces skin penetration to one-third to one-half their normal values.

Within the horny layer itself, two penetration pathways can be envisioned.[6] One crosses the cells and intercellular spaces (the transcellular route) while the

Table II. Comparison of diffusion through untreated and regrown (follicle-free) hairless rat skin. Data from Reference 5.

Drug	Total Quantity Permeated in 48 Hours[a] (nmol cm^{-2})	
	Intact Skin	Regrown Skin
Caffeine	200 ± 20	1 ± 4
Niflumic acid	176 ± 25	65 ± 6.5
p-Aminobenzoic acid	342 ± 20	172 ± 18

[a]Values are mean ± standard deviation (n=3)

second involves passage only through the intercellular lipid domain. An analysis of available data with intact skin concludes that neither pathway can be ruled out.[6] The relative surface area of the intercellular route is perhaps 1% of the total stratum corneum; furthermore the cellular arrangement would require that diffusing substances taking this route follow a highly tortuous path through the membrane. This could help to account for the very low values of apparent diffusion coefficient exhibited by most substances. Guy and Hadgraft reviewed the evidence favoring the intercellular lipid pathway as the major conduit through the stratum corneum.[7] These authors point out that most of the variability in permeability measurements can be explained in terms of differences in lipid/water partition coefficient.

A two-pathway model for the horny layer has been proposed to explain the ability of molecules with a wide disparity in physicochemical properties to permeate the skin.[8] The "polar" pathway accommodates primarily water, ions and uncharged hydrophilic molecules while the "lipid" pathway handles everything else. The polar pathway has a smaller capacity and so contributes less to the total penetration. The polar route has not been identified with any physiologic component of the stratum corneum. A recent study of simultaneous penetration of lidocaine base (a lipophilic molecule) and water does not support the existence of a separate polar route.[9] Fluxes of the two penetrants through human skin from different donors were proportional. In addition, cationic surfactants produced proportional effects on the flux of both compounds (see also Chapter 7).

Another two-pathway model visualizes the membrane as parallel regions of lipid material and pores.[10] Diffusing molecules take both paths and the total amount penetrating is the sum of the two contributions. In contrast to the "polar" pathway, the pores are nondiscriminating and admit all substances, as long as molecular size is not a limiting factor. According to this model, compounds with moderate-to-high partition coefficients (>1) will be transported through the lipid pathway. The pore pathway would be most important for ions and polar molecules. However, solvents that disrupt the stratum corneum could create additional pores within the horny layer, changing the balance between the pathways. This would explain the loss of permeant discrimination that occurs in the presence of damaging solvents. Although the nature of the pores and their location in native skin is unknown, the model can be used to reconcile much of the known permeation data.

Skin distribution

The time course of concentration in the horny layer following topical administration has been followed by repeated stripping of the skin with fresh pieces of adhesive tape.[11] The compound of interest is labeled with a radioactive atom. Cells adhering to each piece of tape can be monitored for permeant content by liquid scintillation counting. A profile of concentration vs the number of strips then can be constructed. Semilogarithmic plots of such profiles are often linear, suggesting that the horny layer is functionally uniform. However, the number of strips does not correlate linearly with depth within the stratum corneum. The first few corneocyte layers (those nearest the skin surface) are loosely attached, so that relatively large quantities of horny tissue patches are removed by the first pieces of tape. Each successive strip removes smaller quantities.[11]

The stripping technique can be performed both in vitro (on excised skin) and in vivo. The epidermal/dermal concentration profile can be estimated by taking a punch biopsy, slicing the tissue into uniformly thick sections with a freeze microtome, then analyzing each section.

Distribution to other tissues has been estimated in animals by homogenization and analysis following sacrifice. In most cases, distribution is based on measurements of radioactivity of a tagged compound. Autoradiography provides a visual record of accumulation of the label in the skin. Although the high sensitivity offered by quantitation of a labeled compound is invaluable, these procedures may introduce errors because it is impossible to correct for metabolism, chemical degradation and other processes that result in loss of label from the initially-applied compound.

Following application to intact skin, components of a topical formulation partition between the vehicle and the surface of the horny layer. From this point, migration begins. Progress through the horny layer, perhaps the major thoroughfare for most compounds, depends on the size of the diffusing molecules and their tendency to interact with this stratum.

If transport of a compound through the horny layer is rate-limiting, the permeant will develop a substantial concentration gradient in this layer. As a corollary, the horny layer should be able to supply the underlying tissues for some time after application. The horny layer thus can function in a dual capacity, acting both as a barrier and reservoir, storing drugs and other chemicals for a period of time. It is possible to obtain biological effects hours or perhaps days after the topical formulation is first applied to the skin.

Perhaps the most dramatic example of the reservoir effect has been observed with the corticosteroids. Using dermal vasoconstriction as a bioanalytical end point, Vickers[12] showed that corticosteroids remained in the skin for about two weeks after a single application under occlusion. This was demonstrated by removing the occlusive covering, at which time the blanching caused by the steroid disappeared. When the occlusive film was once again applied to the skin, vasoconstriction became apparent once more. As a follow-up to Vickers' work, Carr and Wieland[13] applied an alcoholic solution of labeled triamcinolone acetonide to the forearm of a human volunteer, with and without occlusion, and analyzed these sites by tape stripping after various times. They found that most of the label, shown to represent unchanged drug, was confined to the outermost section of the horny layer and that the same distribution pattern resulted regardless of whether stripping took place just after application or two days later.

The stripping technique has been extended as a means of predicting systemic absorption following topical application.[14] Subjects were divided into two groups and an application of radiolabeled drug was allowed to remain in contact with the skin for 30 minutes. The dose was washed off from both groups; then the stripping procedure was performed on group 1 while urine was collected for 96 hours from the members of grouup 2. The total amount collected in the urine was proportional to the amount recovered in the stratum corneum. This was true even when different drugs (all having about the same molecular weight) and different vehicles were studied.

Bioavailability

The term "bioavailability" may be defined as the extent and rate of absorption of an active compound from a particular preparation. Bioavailability is generally measured in a comparative sense; the absorption from a test product or formulation is compared to that from a reference system containing the same drug. With systemic administration, blood concentration is usually the most appropriate measure of absorption. There is frequently a relation between blood concentration and therapeutic activity. Furthermore, once they reach the bloodstream, drug molecules have no memory of the delivery system that was used. The blood level patterns of test and reference are compared to see whether they are equivalent. Thus, although bioavailability measurements have nothing to do with drug activity directly, it is usually possible to assume that two products containing the same drug with the same bioavailability will be equipotent.

As mentioned above, the bioavailability of drugs administered for systemic action can be measured by analysis of blood concentration over time. This approach can be applied to transdermal products, since the skin merely provides a pathway to the circulation. However, it might be misleading to use blood levels as an indication of the availability of dermatologicals; after all, the "best" formulation in a dermatological series should target the skin tissues and allow minimal systemic absorption.

A reasonable alternative for products that are applied to the skin with local treatment as the goal is to assess the drug level within the target tissue and compare that to some reference application. As with systemic administration, the reference must contain the same active compound. Some indication of drug concentration within the various skin layers may be obtained using the stripping and slicing technique described above. However, the requirement that test permeants be radiolabeled is a limitation when comparison of finished products is the objective.

Another possibility is to make use of a pharmacological end point that correlates with drug concentration in the target area. Vasoconstriction is the most well-known and widely used of several bioassays; it responds to minute amounts of corticosteroids within the skin. When testing a particular steroid preparation, another preparation containing the same steroid is applied at the same time in a double blind study. A judgment that test and reference products are bioequivalent requires that they have the same score (within experimental error) on the assay.

There are various ways of setting up the test protocol when using the vasoconstriction assay. The most versatile involves grading the response (usually from 0 for no response to 4 for maximal blanching) and taking readings over a period of several hours. Visual examination is the most popular means of evaluating the degree of vasoconstriction, although instrumental methods have also been tried.

In the absence of a suitable bioassay, some workers tacitly assume that tissue concentration is proportional to the rate of skin transport and apply in-vitro diffusion methods to compare experimental dermatologic formulations. However, this approach requires validation before it can be applied to a particular case.

Experimental considerations

The experimental approach chosen to measure skin permeation depends primarily on the type of information needed, although external factors, such as cost, time required, and facilities available may also have to be considered. In the following paragraphs, some of the factors that enter into the various approaches are mentioned.

In vivo vs in vitro: In-vivo studies in humans provide us with the most direct, relevant and therefore conclusive information on skin permeation. Bioassays are very useful measures of target area concentration, although they are limited to drug classes that produce a measurable local effect. If the goal of the study is to measure systemic bioavailability or toxic potential, then assays of blood, urine or other appropriate body fluids are suitable. However, the amounts penetrating the skin are frequently quite small, requiring very sensitive assays for quantitation. If a radiolabeled compound is employed, simply following the label is sometimes misleading, as it may be carried by a metabolite rather than the applied compound.

In studying the skin absorption of toxic compounds, ethical considerations make it advisable to perform in-vitro experiments rather than put human beings at risk. Furthermore, there may be occasions when the effect of a caustic chemical or harsh environmental change must be determined. An example would be evaluation of a thermal or electrical burn on skin permeability. In such cases, in-vitro experiments likely to correlate with in-vivo data are very useful.

Other advantages of in-vitro work are lower cost, and the ability to test large numbers of formulations in a relatively short time. Using carefully selected models and experimental conditions, it is possible to screen candidate formulations as well as test the effect of various ingredients on skin penetration. In-vitro data can also be used to identify the rate-limiting skin layer for a given compound.

Table III. Comparison of percent of the applied radioactivity in vivo and in vitro (1 mm split-thickness) in pig skin. Data from Reference 15.

Compound	Time (h)	In vivo[a] Epidermis	In vivo[a] Dermis	In vitro[a] Epidermis	In vitro[a] Dermis
Benzoic acid	1	47 ± 2	10 ± 2	46 ± 11	1.9 ± 0.2
	24	42 ± 2	0.3 ± 0.1	37 ± 5	1.9 ± 0.8
Parathion	1	61 ± 13	5 ± 3	64 ± 8	1.3 ± 0.3
	24	5.9 ± 0.9	0.05 ± 0.02	43 ± 23	26 ± 14
DDT	1	67 ± 11	8 ± 5	74 ± 3	3 ± 2
	24	55 ± 13	0.5 ± 0.2	49 ± 6	6 ± 1

[a]Data given as mean ± standard deviation

Riefenrath et al. reported data for skin penetration and retention of pesticides and other compounds using pig skin as a model.[15] Various parameters, including air flow rate and dose were evaluated. There were significant evaporative losses, particularly at high flow rate of even relatively nonvolatile compounds such as DDT. A direct comparison was also made between permeant levels measured in vitro and in vivo. Data for three compounds at two time points, 1 and 24 hours, are collected in Table III.

With the exception of parathion at 24 hours, the epidermal amounts in vitro and in vivo are remarkably close to each other. Dermal levels were somewhat lower in vitro than in vivo at one hour, but the opposite was true at 24 hours. The latter undoubtedly reflects the lack of an intact circulation in vitro; the average path length through the dermis in vitro is greater than the distance to the capillaries in vivo. Combined totals for the amount of each compound reaching the receptor plus that remaining in the dermis at 24 hours are reasonably close to corresponding amounts showing up during the same time period in urine and fat in the animals.

The suppression of metabolism is a limitation of much in-vitro work. Information on conversion and metabolite transport is necessary for risk assessment, as is determination of the extent to which prodrugs are converted to active compounds during passage through the skin. This is sometimes labeled a "first pass" effect, analogous to the metabolism of compounds by the liver before they reach the general circulation following oral absorption. In some cases, particularly involving compounds with poor water solubility, chemical or biological transformation enhances the rate of penetration through skin by reducing the buildup of permeant in tissues downstream from the horny layer. Further information is found in Chapter 4.

Whole animal studies: In the event that it is not possible or advisable to conduct an in-vivo study using human volunteers, one must resort to either in-vitro work or selection of another species. Let us first consider whole animal studies. The advantages of small laboratory animals, such as mice, rats and rabbits, are their relatively low cost, ready availability and good animal-to-animal uniformity. However, their small blood volume sometimes limits the number of samples that can be taken. Furthermore, because of species differences in the thickness and construction of the stratum corneum, the skin of ordinary laboratory animals tends to be many times more permeable than human skin. In general then, the amount absorbed by the animal represents a maximum; for toxic compounds, this is a worst-case situation.

With large animals, it is possible to perform a series of experiments on each individual. This facilitates comparison of different formulations or types of application of the same compound, since each animal serves as its own control. However, adequate housing is a limitation at many research facilities, and some species such as monkeys are difficult to maintain. One problem with any animal substitute for humans is that there may be significant differences in metabolic pathway for a given compound. This complicates the extrapolation of results from the animal to the human situation.

Animal studies may be used to evaluate skin absorption from different formulations as part of the product development process. Many of the considerations discussed below under "Choice of Membrane" would apply here.

In-vivo skin-flap models: Skin-flap models combine good features of in-vivo and in-vitro experiments. They permit the investigator to work with living systems including gaining access to the vasculature leading to and away from the skin. With this type of model, it is possible to investigate skin metabolism under conditions analogous to those in a living animal and to quantitate permeation of a parent substance and metabolites without interference from processes that may occur in other parts of the organism. These models often provide more information than can be obtained from in-vivo studies. However, the preparation of flap models requires a good deal of surgical skill and is expensive.

One of the questions that skin flaps can readily answer is the influence of blood circulation on drug transport through skin. A porcine skin flap has been used to show that vasodilators and vasoconstrictors influence the rate of permeation of iontophoretically-administered lidocaine.[16] Additional information on this model appears in Chapter 5.

Another flap model utilizes split-thickness human skin grafted onto the athymic (nude) rat.[17] The model can be used for up to six months. There are no major histological changes in the grafted skin. The transport of radiolabeled caffeine across grafted human, pig and nude rat skin followed the same rank order as in previously published in-vivo studies. This model has been used to investigate solvent effects in skin permeation as well as the role of changes in blood flow.

In-vitro studies: The major assumption made when conducting in-vitro experiments is that the horny layer (stratum corneum) is the rate-limiting barrier to permeation. It is further assumed that, since stratum corneum is a dead layer, the skin's barrier properties are not compromised by the removal of skin from the living organism. The possibility of metabolism within the skin is frequently ignored, although progress has been made in designing in-vitro experiments in which the membrane's viability is maintained for a reasonable time.[18]

The assumptions described above are generally valid for polar compounds. However, permeants with high oil/water partition coefficients often present difficulties, particularly if skin metabolism is extensive. The viable tissues (epidermis and dermis), which are essentially aqueous in nature, may represent a significant barrier to diffusion of nonpolar molecules. In a live subject however, much of the permeating material would be picked up by the capillaries just beneath the epidermal/dermal junction. Thus, the path length through full-thickness skin in vitro is significantly longer than that encountered in vivo.

Well-designed in-vitro experiments have been extremely valuable in the development of mathematical models of skin transport. In-vitro studies have been widely used to assess the effect of vehicle and environmental factors influencing percutaneous absorption, and to investigate the mechanisms involved. The type of data obtained in these experiments—direct measurement of compounds coming through the skin—can usually only be inferred by in-vivo studies.

A common experimental setup utilizes two half-cells arranged horizontally, with a membrane clamped between them. Both sides of the membrane are exposed to large volumes of liquid (infinite dose) and have provision for stirring. During the course of an experiment, the composition of the donor (containing the permeant) remains essentially unchanged. This technique has the advantage of yielding relatively reproducible data. Interpretation is straightforward, since the amount penetrated is usually linear with time after a lag period. The slope of this linear portion (amount per unit time) divided by the application area yields the steady-state flux, J_{ss}. From this value, a permeability coefficient, P, which is a function of the permeant, the membrane and the vehicle, can be calculated:

$$P = \frac{J_{ss}}{C_v} = \frac{D_m K_m}{l_m} \qquad \text{(Equation 1)}$$

C_v represents the concentration of dissolved permeant in the vehicle. D_m, K_m and l_m are diffusion coefficient in the membrane, membrane/vehicle partition coefficient and membrane thickness, respectively. With certain assumptions, it is sometimes possible to estimate the partition and diffusion coefficients. Infinite dose studies mimic the conditions found following application of occlusive coverings, such as transdermal devices. However, the occluded membrane frequently behaves differently than when in its more usual "dry" state.

The need to simulate clinical application without occlusion has given rise to the development of in-vivo-mimic cell designs and procedures.[19] These utilize vertical cell arrangements in which only the receptor (which collects substances that diffuse through the membrane) is stirred. Although no universal procedure has been established, small quantities are applied to the membrane surface and left open to the atmosphere, so that changes in variables such as applied volume, drug concentration and vehicle composition, can take place. These "finite dose" conditions are typical of most dermatological and cosmetic applications. An advantage of the vertical cells is their ability to accommodate the application of ointments, creams and other semisolids, while the horizontal arrangement described in previous paragraphs is limited to work with liquids.

The permeation profiles following finite dose application may be complex for several reasons. Among these are changes in composition of the applied film due to evaporation of volatile components, and permeation into the skin. Computer simulation using a multicompartmented membrane model resulted in patterns similar to those often seen experimentally.[20] Depletion of permeant from the skin surface can decrease the rate of penetration by lowering the concentration gradient across the membrane. Depletion was especially important for compounds with a high partition coefficient.

Choice of membrane: Excised human skin is the preferred membrane for in-vitro studies. There are almost always differences in penetration rate between human skin and the skin of other animals. These have been ascribed to variations in the thickness and integrity of the stratum corneum as well as in the density of hair follicles. The thickness of the dermal tissue may be reduced by dermatoming full-thickness skin, or by separating the dermis and using only the upper layers for diffusion experiments.

Human skin is usually obtained from autopsy of cadavers or as excess skin from surgery. A disadvantage of human skin is the large variation in permeability between individuals. If, as so often happens, the skin from several subjects must be used, the inherent variability in skin properties may mask small but significant formulation differences.

If human skin is not available, it is possible to work with animal skin if the data required is comparative. Because of species differences, the actual amount of a compound penetrating through human skin cannot be calculated from animal skin experiments. However, if we are comparing different formulations containing the same permeant, and our interest is in identifying the formulation with the greatest (or least) penetration, in-vitro experiments using animal skin may be useful.

Large animals provide many skin samples, minimizing inter-individual variations in skin structure. However, there are site differences in skin properties, so skin sections from different places on the same individual would be expected to have different permeabilities.

The advantages of small laboratory animals are ease of handling, relatively low cost and ready availability. Skins from these animals tend to exhibit minimal intra-individual differences because of standardized breeding and feeding.

The furry species should be avoided because their fur must be clipped or shaved, which may introduce large errors into the data. Human skin is relatively free of hair, even in those areas that we think of as "hairy." The hairless animal species are easier to work with as they require no clipping or other surface preparation. In addition, the low density of hair follicles brings these membranes closer in that one respect to human skin.

Much of the time, the relative penetration rate of a series of related compounds through hairless mouse or rat skin parallels that through human skin. Although we would not normally expect the value of the permeability coefficient for an animal model and that for human skin to be the same, we can anticipate that changes in permeability due to alterations in vehicle makeup would occur in the same direction in both species, as long as the rate-limiting step resides in the stratum corneum. Thus, if addition of a particular cosolvent were to increase the flux of a drug through hairless mouse skin, we would expect that the same change in vehicle would increase flux through human skin. However, the extent of this effect might be quite different. The larger permeability often found when animal skin is used in place of human skin also serves to reduce the time required for each experiment.

However, caution must always be exercised in extrapolating results from in-vitro studies using animal skin. The skins of most common laboratory animals are more sensitive to the effects of damaging or highly interactive agents than is human skin. Certain compounds which cause a significant increase in the skin penetration of other substances (penetration enhancers) generally have a more pronounced effect when tested on animal models (such as hairless mouse) than on human skin.

Another potential problem in studies involving a comparison of vehicles is most likely to be encountered with hydrophobic compounds, most of which tend to diffuse through the horny layer comparatively well. In such cases, data from animal experiments may indicate little difference between vehicles while effects on human skin could be quite different. If the flux of the compound through the horny layer of the animal skin is near-maximal, a significant portion of the total resistance to permeation can reside in the underlying skin layers. Vehicles and vehicle components do not interact with these layers, so that major differences between vehicles will not be evident. On the other hand, human stratum corneum is generally more resistant to permeation, and the effect of an active vehicle could be much more pronounced.

A simple way of evaluating whether this problem exists is to compare penetration through whole skin and through skin whose horny layer is completely removed by stripping with tape. These flux values allow calculation of a potential enhancement factor (PEF) according to Equation 2.[21]

Data for lidocaine flux through excised human and hairless mouse skin appear in Table IV. The variability found with human skin from different donors is obvious. A low PEF value indicates that the resistance of the viable tissues is important. A high value emphasizes that the stratum corneum is the principal barrier. With a PEF value of only 1.7, the researcher's ability to detect penetration enhancement of lidocaine using a hairless mouse model is minimal. No formulation, no matter how effective (or disruptive to the horny layer), could increase lidocaine permeation by more than 70%. Human skin, despite its higher variability, is the better choice for comparing formulations and evaluat-

$$PEF = \frac{\text{Stripped Skin Flux}}{\text{Intact Skin Flux}} \qquad \text{(Equation 2)}$$

ing penetration enhancers for lidocaine.

An example of a hydrophobic compound that is readily absorbed through the skin is 2,3,7,8-tetrachlorodibenzo-p-dioxin (TCDD). Table V contains in-vitro data comparing skin penetration into a receptor containing 5% polysorbate 80. Stripping produced a very small increase in flux in the mouse skin while a much larger difference was found with human skin, showing, as with lidocaine, that the contribution of the stratum corneum to the total skin resistance is more important in the latter. These data with lidocaine and TCDD

Table IV. Potential enhancement factors for penetration of lidocaine through human and hairless mouse skin. Data from Reference 18.

Skin sample	Potential Enhancement Factor ± SD
Hairless mouse	1.7 ± 0.6
Human, donor G	17 ± 5
Human, donor H	1.2 ± 0.3
Human, donor I	5.6 ± 3.3
Mean human value	8

Table V. TCDD penetration in vitro from mineral oil solution at equivalent concentrations, infinite dose

Species	Steady-State Flux (pg/cm²/h), ±SD		PEF
	Normal skin	Stripped skin	
Hairless mouse	240 ± 27	330 ± 35	1.4
Human (subject 1)	23 ± 3.5	137 ± 21	6.0
Human (subject 2)	50 ± 5.6	160 ± 25	3.2

indicate that hairless mouse is not likely to be a good model to investigate the effect of formulation on the permeation of hydrophobic molecules. Before selecting any model, it is a good idea to determine the PEF.

Sato et al. determined the absorption of nicorandil through several excised skin membranes under infinite dose conditions.[22] They measured skin thickness, conductance and the amount of lipids extracted by either acetone or chloroform:methanol, 1:1. The permeability coefficient of pig skin was closest to that of human skin while hairless mouse, hairless rat and guinea pig had higher values. There was an inverse correlation of permeability coefficient with stratum corneum thickness; stratum corneum/water partition coefficient was proportional to extracted lipids suggesting that differences in the lipid content of the horny layer explained much of the permeation behavior. The addition of isopropyl myristate or Azone® to donor vehicles increased nicorandil flux through human and pig skin to about the same degree while the other animal membranes responded differently.

Molecular determinants of absorption

In this section we identify the major molecular factors that influence skin uptake and transport. Most of the relevant information comes from in-vitro studies under infinite dose conditions.

Partition coefficient: The single most important permeant characteristic influencing skin penetration is distribution into the horny layer. The horny layer has for many years been identified as a nonpolar membrane. Its "solvent" properties have therefore been mimicked by various nonpolar liquids including ether, octanol and isopropyl myristate, usually expressed through an organic solvent (or "oil")/aqueous solution partition coefficient. It is important to remember that the partition coefficient is also dependent on the solvent properties of the vehicle. When water is the vehicle, as is the case in many model studies, an oil/water partition coefficient is relevant to transfer of a permeant from a vehicle to the horny layer. This is not the case when other vehicles are used, although the oil/water partition coefficient may still provide useful information about distribution between the stratum corneum and other skin tissues which are predominantly aqueous in nature.

A recent paper on percutaneous absorption of a series of nicotinic acid esters shows the expected pattern (Figure 2).[23] With water as vehicle, the logarithm of permeability coefficient (P) was proportional to the logarithm of isopropyl myristate/water partition coefficient ($K_{I/W}$) but leveled off at higher $K_{I/W}$ values. Visualizing the horny layer as a lipid membrane, this type of pattern is consistent with the notion that an increase in $K_{I/W}$ puts more permeant into the membrane. This continues as the partition coefficient increases; however, at high values of $K_{I/W}$, transfer from the horny layer to the underlying aqueous tissues becomes less favorable and transport through these tissues controls the rate of the overall process.

With pure liquids, a different pattern emerged.[23] P rose with $K_{I/W}$, reached a peak at $K_{I/W} \approx 1$ and then declined. This was attributed to competition for permeant between the vehicle (the pure liquid is obviously a good solvent for itself) and the horny layer. With hydrophobic liquids, both the donor and the membrane have similar solvent properties; thus, the partition coefficient is low and, in accord with Equation 1, so is permeation rate.

Since the partitioning between vehicle and horny layer is involved in the absorption process, it makes sense to measure this directly rather than relying on surrogate solvents. Unfortunately, there are difficulties in obtaining and interpreting the experimental data. Typically, a piece or pieces of stratum corneum are

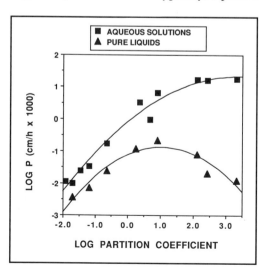

Figure 2. Permeability coefficient of nicotinic acid derivatives as a function of isopropyl myristate/water partition coefficient. Data from Reference 23.

immersed in a liquid containing a known concentration of a drug. After equilibration, which may take several hours or perhaps a day, the concentration of drug is measured and the amount transferred to the membrane calculated by difference or else the latter is measured directly, particularly when radiolabeled compounds are utilized. The horny layer is, therefore, saturated with liquid and does not retain its normal, dry structure during the course of the measurement. It is thus not possible to obtain partition coefficients approximating those for unoccluded skin. Nor is it possible to work with more complex semisolid vehicles which are frequently used in topical therapy. Furthermore, there is the possibility of sorption to structural components of the horny layer; this would influence the partition coefficient but not necessarily diffusion of the molecule. In such cases, permeability is not necessarily proportional to partitioning into the horny layer.

An example of this type of behavior was reported by Anderson and Raykar.[24] They evaluated the effect of several substituents on both partitioning and diffusion through human stratum corneum of p-cresol derivatives and compared their results to data previously obtained with a series of hydrocortisone derivatives. Uptake by the horny layer from aqueous solution was unaffected by delipidization using chloroform:methanol (2:1), suggesting that binding to protein domains within the tissue is most significant. Two solvents, octanol and heptane, were used to mimic the lipids of the horny layer; the behavior of octanol was judged to be closer to that of the tissue, which seemed to have the characteristics of a polar lipid.

Functional group contributions to the permeability coefficient (relative to hydrogen) are collected in Table VI.[24] Positive values indicate a decrease in permeation while negative values mean just the opposite. Values for the two series of compounds are reasonably close. If these results are general, the effect of chemical substitution on skin permeation can be anticipated. Beyond that, there is the possibility that permeation could be calculated *a priori* from chemical structure. Even if it is not possible to calculate the absolute permeability, group contributions provide guidelines for structural modification of molecules to increase or reduce permeation. For example, from Table VI, addition of a methylene group to a molecule would result in about a twofold increase in permeation; addition of –OH would be expected to have a larger negative effect on permeability than –COOCH$_3$.

Table VI. Thermodynamic group contributions to the free energy of transfer from water to stratum corneum at 37°C. Data from Reference 24.

Functional Group	Free Energy Contribution (cal/mol)	
	Hydrocortisone Esters	p-Cresols
—CH$_2$—	-440	
—CONH$_2$	2700	3400
—COOCH$_3$	1400	1100
—COOH	1500	2400
—OH	2400	2500

Molecular size: Considering that the horny layer is a compact membrane and that diffusing molecules follow a tortuous path through it, it might seem obvious that the diffusion coefficient would be inversely related to molecular weight or some other measure of molecular size. Although this is usually taken for granted there doesn't seem to be a definitive study in which size is the only variable. Anderson and Raykar incorporated molecular weight dependence into their analysis of the hydrocortisone and *p*-cresol series of compounds.[24] While permeability correlated well with octanol-water partition coefficient within both series, two distinct correlation lines widely differing in slope were obtained. This was attributed to an effect of molecular size on diffusion coefficient within the membrane. To obtain a single relationship that included all of the data, it was assumed that the diffusion coefficient for each compound, D_m, could be described by the following relationship

$$D_m = D_m^0 \, MW^{-n} \qquad \text{(Equation 3)}$$

in which MW is molecular weight and both D_m^0 and n are constants that depend on the nature of the membrane. From regression analysis, n was calculated to be 4.6, a rather high number reflecting a significant molecular weight effect. The value of n for bulk diffusion is typically between 2 and 3.

On the other hand, Guy and Hadgraft have argued that at our present state of knowledge, all or most of the permeation data in the literature can be explained in terms of oil/water partition coefficients and that, in view of the magnitude of the errors in permeation studies, it may not be necessary to take relatively small differences in molecular size into account.[7] As more data are generated, the precise influence of molecular weight should become clearer.

Charged compounds: The nonpolar nature of the horny layer suggests that charged compounds should encounter high resistance to permeation. This proposition is most easily studied by use of ionigenic compounds, for which the ratio of charged to uncharged species can be manipulated by changing pH of the vehicle. The two species are about the same size, so their diffusion coefficients should have the same value. In such experiments, the possibility of barrier

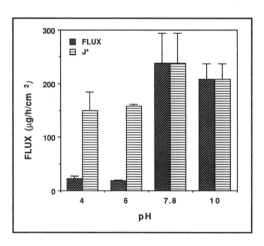

Figure 3. Lidocaine permeation through excised human skin as a function of pH. Shown are the actual flux for 5% systems and J*, the maximal flux for a saturated solution.

alteration at extreme pH values and the membrane's buffering capacity must be kept in mind. In every case studied, the permeability coefficient of the unionized form exceeds that of the charged species, in some cases by two or three orders of magnitude. One reason is the greater solubility of the unionized compound in the horny layer; the second is its poorer solubility in the aqueous donor solvent.

Figure 3 shows lidocaine permeation as a function of pH. Experimental flux values for 5% systems (solutions at pH 4 and 6; dispersions at pH 7.8 and 10) dramatize the significantly higher permeability of the unionized form. Permeability coefficients calculated from the data are 17.7 x 10^{-3} cm/h for the unionized form and 0.336 x 10^{-3} cm/h for the ionized form, a ratio of about 50.[25] Figure 3 also contains calculated flux values labeled J*, flux normalized to saturation. The rationale and calculation method are described in Chapter 6. Significant amounts of ionized lidocaine can permeate the skin. Studies with other ionizable compounds have yielded similar results although the ratio of permeability coefficients (unionized:ionized) vary with the compound. While the introduction of charge always lowers the permeability coefficient, it should not be assumed that charged compounds are locked out of the skin.

Skin binding: The role of binding per se is difficult to study experimentally since, like partition coefficient, it depends on the chemical groups found on the surface of a permeating molecule. Computer simulation can provide an indication of the importance of stratum corneum binding and the patterns to anticipate.[26] Figure 4 shows the model that was used. The stratum corneum (SC) was broken into ten equal segments, five of which comprised the diffusional pathway; the B compartments held "bound" permeant, which was not able to diffuse through the membrane. The distribution between B compartments and the other SC compartments was assumed to be instantaneous and depended simply on the fraction-bound (F SC), which was the variable in these computer experiments. This is analogous to binding at concentrations well below saturation. K was a first-order rate constant for SC transfer. The ratio of K_I to K_{-I} is the SC/DONOR partition coefficient. Other compartments were AQ to represent the viable tissues and SINK which represented the blood in vivo or the receptor in an in-vitro experiment.

Figures 5 and 6 show the effect of binding for a hypothetical drug. The curves in Figure 5 for cumulative penetration as a function of time are of greatest interest

Figure 4. Multicompartmented Membrane Model for permeation of a compound that may bind to elements of the horny layer. Transfer is described by K, the intercompartmental transfer constant. Stratum corneum compartments labeled B contain bound permeant. The AQ compartment represents the viable skin tissues. See text for further description.

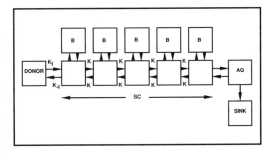

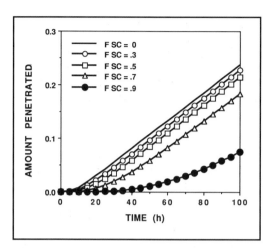

Figure 5. Amount reaching the skin with various degrees of stratum corneum binding, infinite dose conditions. F values shown in figure represent fraction bound. $K = 0.4\,h^{-1}$; $K_I/K_{-I} = 15$; donor conc. = 10 mg/mL; donor volume = 1 mL. Transfer coefficients between stratum corneum and aqueous compartment were 2 hours^{-1}. Transfer coefficient from aqueous compartment to the sink was 5 hours^{-1}. Cross sectional area was 1 cm^2 in all cases and stratum corneum thickness was assumed to be 10 μm.

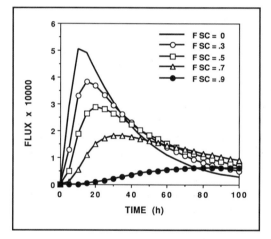

Figure 6. Penetration flux as a function of extent of stratum corneum binding under finite dose conditions. Donor concentration = 10 mg/mL; donor volume = 2 mL. All other parameters were as in Figure 5.

in considering transdermal delivery from a patch or semisolid containing a drug reservoir. The linear sections of the curves are parallel indicating that steady-state flux is unaffected by binding. The major effect was an increase in the lag time, most noticeable at high values of F SC. With 90% bound (filled circles in Figure 5), the lag period was so long that steady-state would not be reached in most experiments. For transdermal delivery then, the effect of binding is to increase the time required to reach constant blood levels, but not the magnitude of those levels.

Figure 6 illustrates the effect of stratum corneum binding on skin penetration following finite dose administration. As the fraction bound is increased, the value of peak flux is reduced, the peak occurs later and it is less sharp. The total amount reaching the SINK is proportional to the area under the curve from time zero to any given time. Clearly, the amount permeating the skin is reduced considerably by binding within the SC. The patterns observed are partially a result of depletion of active compound from the DONOR compartment. At high values of fraction bound, the SC acts as a sponge, soaking up drug molecules from the DONOR and delaying their transit to compartments downstream.

Binding to structural components of skin (which may include proteins and other cell components) represents a consideration separate from oil/water partition coefficient and molecular size. It may help to account for differences in permeation dependence on partition coefficient between chemical families whose binding characteristics are likely to be quite distinct.

Conclusions

Skin permeation and uptake measurements are useful in product development and toxicologic evaluation. The target site of action and intended use of a product determine the type of absorption behavior that is most desirable.

For most compounds, the horny layer, the outermost skin section consisting of a compressed amalgam of dead cells separated by oriented layers of neutral lipids, represents the principal barrier to transport. This makes possible the use of excised skin in in-vitro diffusion experiments. Shunt diffusion via follicles and glands may contribute significantly to the absorption of many drugs.

A variety of techniques may be applied to measure skin permeation. In-vivo data in humans are, of course, most relevant to treatment of humans. When using substitutes, such as in-vivo animal experiments or in-vitro studies, it is a good idea to examine the implicit assumptions, to see whether they are likely to be valid in the particular case. The use of in-vitro and flap models helps to determine mechanisms and highlight the significant factors in skin permeation.

Partition coefficient is perhaps the most signficiant parameter affecting drug sorption and permeation. Although other factors, such as molecular size, undoubtedly play a role, reliable quantitative data are sparse.

Factors Affecting Sorption of Topically Applied Substances

By Martin M. Rieger

Information on retention or sorption of chemical species by skin is unexpectedly scarce. By contrast, extensive data on the interactions between skin and chemicals are available from toxicological or topical therapeutic studies. These types of experimentation are primarily concerned with transdermal permeation, with only limited emphasis on sorptive phenomena.

In order to gain some insight into the retention of chemicals by skin and the mechanism thereof, one must depend in part on studies conducted for entirely different purposes. As a result, systematic generalizations are not available, and validation of concepts is generally not possible until additional data are generated.

The following review is divided into two major parts. Part One deals descriptively with general concepts and accepted principles of sorption, diffusion and permeation. Part Two is a summary and examination of some published experimental data.

Sorption is a loosely used and sometimes poorly defined general term. It may, for example, describe the process that occurs when a dry sponge sorbs a liquid (which may or may not contain a dissolved solute) or a suspension. For scientific reasons, one might wish to differentiate this (sponge-like) sorption of a bulk liquid from the sorption of individual molecules, atoms, or ions by a substance as exemplified by the sorption of water vapor by sulfuric acid, anhydrous calcium chloride or glycerin. As a rule, this latter type of sorption is referred to as absorption, which simply implies the imbibition (or engulfment) of one substance by another. In the case of skin, this phenomenon is illustrated, for example, by soaking a piece of skin in an aqueous solution of sucrose. The skin can absorb the solution (and may swell during this imbibition). At equilibrium, the concentration of sucrose in the bulk solution is essentially identical to that of the solution absorbed by the skin; one may reason, then, that skin does not exclude sucrose, nor has it any specific affinity for this sugar. Under these conditions, a measurement of the sugar retained in the skin (even after drying) can be used to determine the skin's ability to sorb water after soaking in the sugar solution.[1]

The term sorption might also describe the process by which a thin layer of a substance is sorbed by weak interaction (via van der Waals forces) or chemically (via chemisorption) onto a substrate's surface. This type of sorption plays a role in chromatography and catalysis and is the basis of theories of sorption (isotherms). This process is appropriately called adsorption. In the case of skin, one speaks of adsorption whenever a substance (usually in solution) adheres such that its concentration at the (hypothetical) skin/solvent interface is higher than that in the bulk solution. If the substance is not readily or completely removed from the skin by re-exposure to pure solvent, one generally refers to this phenomenon as substantivity. For the purpose of this review, Wester and Maibach's definition of substantivity as "nonpenetrating surface adsorption" will be used.[2]

Exposure of skin to a topically applied substance can result in bulk absorption or in surface adsorption. The latter is of particular interest whenever the interaction between skin and solute results in measurable substantivity. Another phenomenon which plays a role in both sorptive processes is diffusion. The need for diffusion is clearly a prerequisite for absorption by skin. In the case of adsorption, diffusion is required for access to the skin's interior. In the absence of diffusion into the skin, adsorption remains a surface phenomenon. Only if diffusion takes place can absorptive processes occur throughout the bulk of the skin.

In order to gain insight into retentive, i.e., sorptive, processes on or in the skin, three—generally concurrent—processes must be examined:

I.   Diffusion, which describes access of a substance for adsorption or absorption.
II. Absorption, which describes the bulk invasion of the various layers of the skin.
III. Adsorption, which describes some highly specific interaction effecting retention of the invading chemical on certain sites within the skin.

Definitions

The diffusion of a substance into and through the skin represents a typical membrane transport problem. Membrane transport is vital to living organisms (e.g., intestinal absorption) and controls many inanimate systems (e.g., dialysis). Transport is simply movement of a substance through a medium. Membrane transport occurs whenever a substance passes into or across a membrane from one side to the other. Neither the medium nor the substance need be identified; transport may occur through liquid, solid or gaseous media, and the transported substances may include liquids, solids or gases.

Diffusion through skin is transport from one medium to another through restricting partially permeable membranes. In order to facilitate an understanding of such a complex system, investigators have created models to describe the passage of a permeant (or solute) from one compartment (the donor) through the stratum corneum to a second compartment (the receptor).

The simpler models routinely employed in membrane transport are confounded and complicated by the unusual nature of the skin as a multilamellar membrane (Figure 1). One of these layers, the stratum corneum, has been identified as the major barrier to the entry of substances into the body.[3] For most practical purposes, removal of the stratum corneum by stripping or other mechanical means eliminates the barrier properties of the skin and allows entrance of (foreign) substances into living tissue.

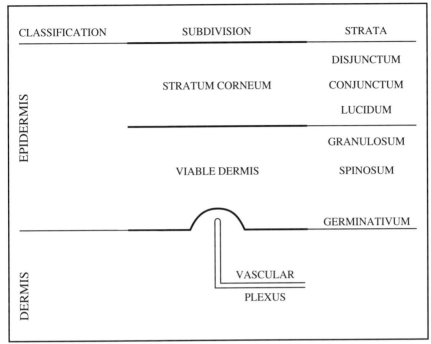

Figure 1. Schematic of skin structure

Diffusion of topically applied substances into skin results in their accumulation within various strata and components of the skin. The ability to diffuse depends critically on the capability of the substance to enter a particular skin layer or reach a specific site. This process is called *penetration* and differs from the process of *permeation*. The latter describes a substance's penetration into a skin layer and its subsequent transfer to other skin layers and ultimately to the vascular system. In order to comprehend the sorptive processes within various skin layers, it is sometimes helpful to view penetration and permeation as complementary forces: Penetration deals with a substance's entry, while permeation is additionally concerned with the substance's exit to some other compartment.

Skin Structure

The morphological features of mammalian and especially human skin involved in skin penetration and permeation are shown diagrammatically in Figure 1. Proceeding from the outside towards the inside layers, one first encounters the stratum corneum (SC). The SC is recognized today as the principal barrier to the entry of topically applied substances into the body. It is composed of layers of dead, essentially hexagonal, flat cells, each about 0.5 µm thick and about 30 to 40 µm long, with SC thickness ranging from about 6 to 15 µm. The uppermost layers tend to flake off, or desquamate, because the biochemical and histological components attaching these cells to each other have deteriorated. The lower layers of the SC, which are those in close proximity to the viable epidermis (VE), are more tightly packed and held together by desmosomal structures. The intercellular space in the SC is filled primarily with lamellar layers of skin lipids. SC can, therefore, be described as a composite structure of dead cells (corneocytes) in a lipid medium.[4-6] The components of this intercellular lipid have been identified, and it has been shown that they differ materially from those of sebum.[7]

It is normal for the thickness of SC to vary from site to site on man. In addition, the lipid content of the SC shows wide variation, averaging about 16% (range 3 to 46%).[1] These features of SC play a vital role in sorptive processes in the skin.

The continuity of the SC (as a smooth continuous layer) is interrupted by the ducts of eccrine and apocrine glands and by hair follicles with their sebaceous glands. The cells in the walls of these cuts and invaginations might not exhibit the same desquamating features as normal SC cells. They also might not contain the lamellar lipid entities believed necessary for the formation of an effective skin barrier. These sites, which probably account for no more than about 1% of skin surface area, nevertheless serve as entry ports for externally applied substances. These so-called shunts possess a cylindrical structure, and the wall of the cylinder represents a sizable area of epithelially derived tissue that may be extensively hydrated or unprotected by terminally differentiated SC.[8] Shunt-diffusion bypasses the SC, is rapid, and may allow passage of molecules normally excluded or slowed down by intact SC.[9]

Autoradiography has been used dramatically by Suzuki et al. to demonstrate how radiolabelled lipids—commonly used in cosmetics or as pharmaceutical vehicles—tend to accumulate in the follicular invaginations of guinea pigs and Angora rabbits.[10] Particularly noteworthy is the presence of labelled lipids in the sebaceous glands, suggesting that these appendageal structures may sorb externally applied substances.

Before leaving the discussion of the SC, it is important to note that, at equilibrium, the water content of the exterior portion of the SC is a function of the ambient relative humidity (RH). By contrast, the water content in the lower SC approaches that of the VE and probably equals that of SC at 100% RH. As will be discussed later, hydration of SC plays a major role in the transcorneal movement of substances, and the presence of large amounts of water in the lower layers of the SC modifies its sorptive and diffusional properties from those in the upper layers.

The VE—which consists primarily of keratinocytes and dendritic cells—is at least ten times as thick as the SC and ranges from about 40 to 50 μm up to 400 μm in the thickest portion of the skin. The thickness of the VE also varies on a microscopic scale since dermal tissue tends to project into the VE in normal (adult) skin. The resulting rete pegs contain the capillary vessels of the micro-circulation, which normally lie about 150 to 200 μm below the skin surface. Despite its thickness, VE is generally believed to possess no barrier properties to the passage of most substances. The VE may, nevertheless, tend to sorb permeating substances before they reach the blood vessels of the vascular plexus or the dermis.

The dermis or the corium is the lowest skin layer which may play a role in skin sorption. Whereas VE is a highly cellular portion of the living skin, the dermis includes a variety of (fibrous) proteins and the components of the connective tissue in addition to cells. The dermis is believed to offer no barrier to the passage of molecules that reach it, except for molecules that may be substantive to specific dermal components.

Permeation: A Requirement for Efficacy

The morphological features of the skin describe the environment with which a topically applied substance may interact. In order to make contact with dermal strata, the substance must penetrate a number of skin layers; in other words, it must diffuse. The processes of diffusion and permeation are, in part, described by Fick's Laws. Current understanding of the diffusion of substances in skin is to a large extent based on information developed by scientists interested in topical drug delivery or topical toxicity. Two types of drug delivery must be clearly differentiated: one is required for therapy of dermatological diseases, and the other concerns systemic drug administration.

In the case of topical dermatological drugs, the formulator's task is to provide an effective drug concentration at the site for a length of period sufficient to produce the desired pharmacological effect. In the case of a steroid, for instance, it might be desirable to have the drug permeate the SC to reach the site of inflammation in the VE or dermis. Since drug diffusion can be both forward and backward, sorption into the lower adipose tissue might still deliver effective dosing over a prolonged period. What must be clearly avoided in this instance is excessive sorption by the SC or rapid passage into the vasculature.

The demands for a topically applied systemic drug are entirely different. For example, nitroglycerin is topically delivered to permeate the SC and the VE rapidly for delivery to the vascular plexus. Storage or sorption in any part of the skin is clearly undesirable in this case since the amount of drug for systemic delivery might be reduced or the release from the sorbing tissue might be insufficient for the desired systemic effect.

The toxic manifestations of topically applied substances may include immediate phenomena (such as corrosion or primary irritation), delayed phenomena (such as sensitization), phenomena which require an additional vector (such as phototoxicity), and systemic phenomena (such as paraquat toxicity). Such reactions cannot occur unless the toxic agent reaches a viable part of the skin. If the toxicant can be stored in or sorbed by a skin layer, it might not reach the viable tissues at all or might be released relatively slowly, thus effectively prolonging the symptoms (as is the case with rhus dermatitis). This type of binding reduces the ability of a toxin to reach living tissue. The sorbed toxicant is ultimately lost from the skin surface by desquamation, and this process may be a means for detoxification.

The case of topically applied cosmetics is complicated by promotional demands and regulatory rulings. In principle, the formulator will try to avoid systemic absorption by the vasculature. Cosmetic effects, as evidenced by visual appearance, are preferably restricted to the surface of the SC. Thus, for most cosmetics, sorption (or retention) on or sometimes in the SC is desirable.

Marketers, formulators and regulators apply differing criteria to cosmetic ingredients intended to exert beautifying effects by reaching skin strata below the SC. However, there is little disagreement concerning the fact that some cosmetic ingredients applied from finished products can be sorbed by and reach all strata of the skin.

In the light of these comments, it is apparent that the compounder's objectives for permeation, penetration or sorption vary from product to product and depend on the desired pharmacological or cosmetic effect. It is also apparent that standard mathematical models based on drug or toxicant permeation studies might have to be modified to fit the specific penetrant or mixtures of penetrants delivered topically. Regardless of these refinements, sorption into skin strata always precedes permeation. Conversely, no substance can penetrate through intact integument unless it is sorbed (or resides even briefly) within the layers of skin.

Diffusion: Physical Concepts

Diffusion in the pharmaceutical and cosmetic literature is frequently equated with transdermal permeation. It is preferable to define diffusion more precisely as the transport of matter resulting from movement of a substance within a substrate.

Diffusion within the confines of SC has been modeled with the aid of three simplying modeling processes:

1. The particle (or molecule or ion) must pass through the vehicle (donor compartment) to the surface of the SC. The step controlling this process is diffusion, which obeys the Einstein $\sqrt{t}$ relationship.

2. The second step, passage into the SC, is controlled by the distribution coefficient K, which will be described in detail below.

3. In the third step, the permeant diffuses through the SC. This is generally the rate-determining step as shown by extensive experimentation in the study of skin permeation.

Fick's Laws are routinely applied to skin permeation data to ascertain the amounts of permenant passing through one or more strata making up the skin. Fick's Laws include a diffusion coefficient which is assumed to create a linear concentration gradient of the permeant within the SC. Gradients of permeants in the SC are, in fact, not linear, and one may infer that the diffusion coefficient for SC in vivo is not constant from top to bottom.[11] Data on the rate at which a permeant reaches its equilibrium concentration in the SC are not readily available. There is no clear cut evidence that the $\sqrt{t}$ relationship of diffusion holds for SC, although the existence of such a relationship is very likely.

Fick's Laws

Fick's Laws are generally viewed as the mathematical description of diffusion processes through membranes. Fick's Laws are applicable whenever the chemical or physical nature of the membrane controls the rate of diffusion. As will be shown in the next few paragraphs, the laws of diffusion cannot be separated from the rules that govern sorption. An excellent introduction to membrane-controlled mass transport was provided about 15 years ago by Flynn et al., and the following discussion is based on their logical development and explanation.[12]

In order to pass from the solvent (or vehicle) to the skin, the diffusing solute molecule must have some affinity for the SC. Once the molecule is within that membrane it can, of course, diffuse in any direction. Progress is, however, not random because the permeant tends to move steadily from the higher population density to the lower concentration. From heat flow concepts developed almost 200 years ago by Count Bertholett, Fick postulated that diffusive flow, which is the flux (J), through a membrane should be proportional to the concentration differences ΔC between the two sides of the membrane and inversely proportional to the thickness *l* of the membrane. The proportionality constant is defined as the permeability coefficient P. It includes the differential diffusion coefficient D and the partition coefficient K; this relationship is known as Fick's First Law:

$$J \approx dC/dl \text{ or } J = P\Delta C = \frac{KD\Delta C}{l} \qquad \text{Equation 1}$$

The units of J are mole/cm^{2}sec, which clarifies the physical meaning: J is the quantity of solute passing through a unit area of the membrane in unit time. In order for any measurable flux to occur, the solute molecules must first enter the SC (controlled by K). Next, the entering solute must concentrate within the SC and begin its time-dependent diffusion process (controlled by D) until the solute molecules reach the border between the SC and the VE. The rate of passage of solute molecules into and through the VE is generally believed to be much larger than its rate of diffusion through the SC. Thus the solute concentration can be expected to be highest at or near the donor site (at which the permeant reaches the SC) and lowest at the receiving site (at which the permeant enters the VE). As long as the solute concentration at the donor site is constant (infinite dosing), flux into the receiver normally continues at a steady-state rate. Under these conditions, the solute concentration near the membrane's (SC) outside will be that in the applied vehicle (C_v) and will decrease steadily to zero on the underside of the SC. If the supply of solute from the vehicle is decreasing (finite dosing) or is stopped, the solute concentration gradient in the SC will disappear, and the tendency of the solute to travel into the VE can be expected to approach zero as ΔC in Equation 1 approaches zero. The time required to reach this point (which is theoretically infinite) can be expected to vary from solute to solute in practice. However, some solute will remain in the SC membrane until this point is reached. The process just described is "passive" diffusion; the only driving force for its occurrence is the concentration gradient across the membrane.

It is another cardinal principle of skin diffusion and ultimately permeation that the diffusing species passes from one layer in the skin to the next. To follow this process investigators routinely assess rates and diffusional resistances from the *concentration* of the permeant. This might not always be correct since the characteristic that determines these rates is not concentration but the (thermodynamically definable) *chemical potential*. In order to conform to common usage, "concentration" will be used in this review, although "activity" would be the preferred term. It is noteworthy that partition coefficients (distribution coefficients) are determined at equilibrium, which is when the chemical potentials in the two phases are the same; this does not mean that the concentrations in the two phases are identical.[13]

Fick's First Law (Equation 1) is applicable only to membranes which are homogeneous from one side to the other, which is equivalent to the statement that P (or KD) is invariate throughout the membrane's thickness. P must also be unaffected by the variable concentrations of sorbed substances which may include constituents of the vehicle as well as the permeating (active or drug) species. This is probably not true in the case of living skin. Attempts to create quantitative skin models that take into account changes effected by topically applied substances have not been entirely successful. Instead, in the pragmatic approach, the subtlety of effects on the membrane are generally ignored. The SC is simply viewed as a barrier that offers some finite—although not invariate—resistance to transport. By analogy, sorption within the SC, and especially in lower skin layers, has received little attention by investigators. Although quantitative data are lacking, one can nevertheless learn much about the process of sorption through use of generally accepted principles. A critical examination of the fundamental assumptions of Fick's First Law reveals much about the features of transport through the SC and by inference about sorption within the SC.

Questions concerning variable membrane thickness and the presence of shunts have already been mentioned. They are generally ignored as a first approximation. (See, however, Reference 14.)

The integrated form of Fick's First Law describes a straight line relationship. The existence of a linear correlation between flux J and time at steady-state permeation has been established in vitro and in vivo for the passage of drugs through isolated SC, full-thickness epidermis, and whole skin. In this type of experimentation, the receptor, which may be either an artificially constituted liquid or the body fluid, must be an infinite sink for the penetrant. The need for infinite dosing from the donor has already been noted.

The initial curvature of the flux vs. time curve, shown in Figure 2, is typical of experimentally observed data.[15,16] The straight line portion begins at point X and can be extrapolated to the time axis, where Q equals zero. The intercept on the time axis is called the lag time, t_L, which can be used to compute the diffusion coefficient from $D = l^2/6t_L$. D (permeant dependent) and l (membrane dependent) play major roles in the shape of the flux vs. time curve. During the time elapsed from the origin to t_L, sorptive and diffusional equilibria must be established before the diffusing molecules pass through the rate-controlling (restricting) membrane. Some or all of the components of the vehicle and of the diffusing species of interest may be retained by or react with functional groupings in the membrane. When point X is reached, these sorptive processes have also reached steady-state or equilibrium levels, and flux per se provides only limited information on factors contributing to sorptive processes.

A slight modification of Equation 1 (by replacing ΔC with C_v) is possible on the assumption that the concentration of the permeant is nil (sink condition) at the receptor interface and that the donor concentration is invariate (infinite dosing):

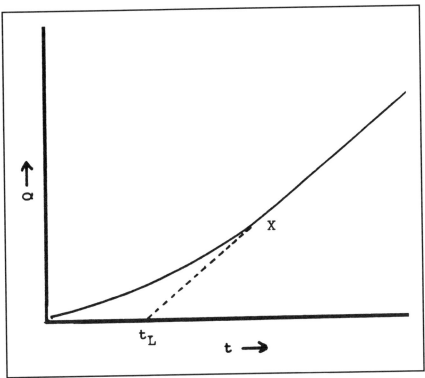

Figure 2. Time vs. permeation curve showing the approach to steady-state flux and the lag time t_L

$$J = \frac{K D C_v}{l} \qquad \text{Equation 2}$$

This equation and related expressions describe the steady-state diffusion of a substance through a (homogeneous) barrier membrane. Since skin is a multi-lamellar structure, the overall flux might be advantageously expressed as a sum of fluxes through multiple layers, with each layer exhibiting its own K, D and l. The diffusive process in the SC, the body's barrier membrane, is slow and rate determining. The diffusive process through the VE, by contrast, is relatively fast, and the rate-limiting step for penetrant diffusion is generally located in the SC. Similar considerations apply to diffusive processes in the dermis and into the vascular bed.[3] As a result, it is common practice to base flux, steady-state measurements, and quantification of the permeability coefficient P on data obtained with the SC barrier membrane (or skin preparations which include SC).

Derivations of Fick's Second Law are based on the consideration of a volume element formed by two planes perpendicular to the diffusive flow.[12] Diffusant enters the volume element from the side of high concentration and exits on the side of low concentration. The masses of diffusant entering and leaving per unit time can then be calculated from the First Law. The equation quantifying the difference between these two masses is Fick's Second Law for unidimensional flow. In real systems a molecule entering the SC can move in three directions. In simplified solutions of Fick's Second Law, the diffusion coefficients in these three directions are assumed to be equal. As a result, Fick's Second Law is commonly presented as:

$$\frac{dC}{dt} = D\left[\frac{d^2C}{dx^2} + \frac{d^2C}{dy^2} + \frac{d^2C}{dz^2}\right]$$ Equation 3

Fick's Second Law teaches that the rate of change of the concentration of a diffusing species in a given volume element of the barrier membrane is proportional to the rate of change in concentration gradient at that point.

Solutions to Equation 3 require a set of boundary conditions, and these are, of course, selected on the basis of utility for the specific experimental condition. For example, the steady state (zero-order) flux situation described above applies to a unidirectional flow during which the concentration in the donor compartment remains constant and in which the receptor compartment is maintained at zero concentration, or sink conditions. The general solution of Fick's Second Law teaches that the permeant's concentration at a penetration depth X is a function of $X/\sqrt{Dt}$. Complex mathematical expressions for the cumulative amount of penetrant (Q) per unit area during any time (t) can be obtained. Equations based on Fick's Second Law can be used to understand the diffusional processes during the lag time and to compute the concentration profile of a diffusant within a given

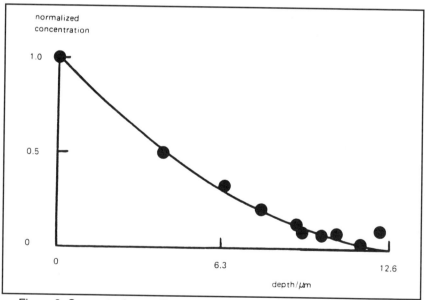

Figure 3. Concentration profile of glycerin vs. depth of penetration into nude mouse stratum corneum, normalized to concentration in outermost layer. Reproduced by permission of the copyright owner, Marcel Dekker, Inc., from Reference 16. [For a similar profile of hydrocortisone in man, see D. Caron et al., *J. Am. Acad. Dermatol.*, **23**, 458-462 (1990).]

restricting membrane.[15,16] An example (Figure 3) taken from Reference 16 shows that the linearity demanded by the First Law is not completely obeyed in real life and that the exponential expressions derived from the Second Law come closer to experimental data.

Control of Sorptive Processes in the Skin

The permeability coefficient P in Fick's First Law (Equation 1) includes not only the partition coefficient K but the diffusion coefficient D. D represents a permeant's mobility within a medium in accordance with the basic postulates of the Einstein equation:

$$D = \frac{\Delta \bar{x}^2}{2t} = \frac{RT}{Nf}$$

where X^2 is the mean square displacement, t is the time, R/N is the Boltzmann constant, T is the temperature, and f is a form factor which depends on shape and volume but is essentially mass-independent. The shape dependence of the diffusion of a solute through a solvent presents a complicated mathematical problem unless sphericity is assumed. The volume dependence, on the other hand, has been simplified to a useful proportionality:[12]

$$D \approx \left(\frac{1}{v}\right)^{1/3}$$

where v is the partial molal volume. This approximation provides some information on factors controlling the rate of diffusion.

Partition coefficients are the gate-keepers controlling access of permeant to SC. A permeant's passage through the SC cannot begin until the permeant has been transferred from the vehicle to one of the SC components. It is the partition coefficient (K) which controls this process. K is routinely determined by analyzing a substance's concentrations in two immiscible solvents, in a solvent and a tissue, or in two tissues at equilibrium.[17] In the case of SC, the partition coefficient K_1 is defined as:

$$K_1 = C_{SC}/C_V \qquad \text{Equation 4}$$

where C_V is the permeant concentration in the vehicle and C_{SC} that in SC.

As a rule, partition coefficients are determined by equilibrating the tissue (SC) with an excess of the permeant in a suitable solvent (frequently water). Under these experimental conditions, the SC can be fully hydrated, and the equilibrium would be established with SC which is not in its normal in vivo condition. It is also apparent that these conditions expose SC to permeant diffusion from directions not encountered during normal practice. The preparation of SC in its normal lipid-rich state is cumbersome, and most investigators substitute various organic solvents for SC. Use of the octanol/water partition coefficient is common,[3] and isopropylmyristate, heptane and hexadecane are additional examples. (See References 16 and 17). The selection of such solvents is based on the assumption that the $K_{solvent/water}$ is a realistic parallel to the value of $K_{SC/water}$. It has also been ascertained that, within a homologous series, skin permeation as determined by flux is proportional to the partition coefficient. Even if unrelated chemical species are arranged in the order of their partition coefficients, flux measurements follow the same pattern. The use of partition coefficients to assess a permeant's ability to partition into SC is a special case of the Mayer-Overton theory of drug absorption with its emphasis on the permeant's lipid solubility.

Several processes can account for the entry of a permeant into SC. The permeant may be more soluble in one or more of the constituents of SC than in the vehicle. The vehicle may volatilize, leaving behind a residue of the permeant, which then slowly "dissolves" in a component of the SC. The vehicle or one of its constituents (e.g., a so-called penetration enhancer) may also enter the SC and travel coupled with or separately from the permeant towards the VE. It is not likely that the permeant diffuses in its (vehicle) solvent through some sort of channel in the SC. Instead, the diffusion coefficient D probably describes the permeant's stepwise progress from site to site. The temporary bonding on a site in the SC must be at least partially reversible if significant transport is to occur at low concentrations of the permeating species. If the binding (sorption) is not reversible, the permeating species probably is subject to covalent binding (chemisorption). The term substantivity is sometimes used to describe this process as well as instances in which binding is favored but not permanent. SC can be expected to contain a variety of sites which may bind a passing molecule or ion more or less effectively. If binding within the SC has some level of permanence, the permeant must first saturate these sites of permanent binding before it can diffuse to lower layers of the SC. Binding of permeant—regardless of permanence—may reduce externally determined concentration levels and may contribute to delays in diffusion as measured via the lag time.

It is apparent that the partition coefficient plays a key role in the initial phases (vehicle in contact with top of SC) of permeation. The partition coefficient of SC probably is not constant throughout the thickness of the SC, varying as a function of lipid and water contents.[18,19] This may create unexpected phenomena since hydration of SC has been shown to increase the penetration of drugs, while K (as defined in Equation 4) might decrease if the SC is fully hydrated. These considerations make it reasonable to assume that SC in vivo exhibits a range of K's. These variables throughout the thickness of the SC mandate that the sorption of permeant will also be variable, as already noted in the opening remarks on Fick's Laws.

K_1 may be defined as an equilibrium distribution coefficient which—if favorable—allows penetration of the permeant into the SC. Once the permeant reaches the VE, it encounters a "new" environment, and passage into the VE is controlled by another distribution coefficient:[20]

$$K_2 = C_{SC}/C_{VE} \qquad\qquad \text{Equation 5}$$

K_2, as defined by Equation 5, is generally assumed to favor transfer of the permeant to VE. A similar distribution coefficient may exist between the VE and the dermis. Ready passage from SC into VE may not always be the case. In vivo one might achieve penetration of a very hydrophobic substance to the SC. Its solubility may preclude passage into VE, and the permeant becomes literally trapped in the SC. The importance of these distribution phenomena to skin permeation of substances in vitro and in vivo has been studied by

Hawkins and Reifenrath.[21] Their studies included compounds whose log K (octanol/water) ranges from 0.01 to 5.0.

If a substance should be retained in the SC, its ultimate removal from the skin must await the shedding of the SC. Analogous cases were reported by Bronaugh and Stewart and others, who observed that absorption of some lipophilic and easily solubilized substances into the receivers of diffusion cells was improved when normal saline was replaced by 6% aqueous oleth-20.[22,23]

The important contribution of partition coefficients to sorption and permeation may be modified appreciably by metabolism within the various layers of the skin.[24]

At the molecular level the diffusant is sorbed and desorbed repeatedly until it reaches the dermis or some other sink. The progress depends on the permeant's shape and the mean square displacement. In addition, this motion is dependent on the rigidity of the substrate's lattice. The presence of small voids and defects is essential, and their availability is temperature dependent. The heterogeneity of the SC, which includes protein platelets in a matrix of lamellar lipids, accounts for defects which may provide sites for the (temporary) sorption or bonding of the permeant. The proteinaceous platelets are surrounded by a hard shell, but the cellular material is generally believed to be at least partially hydrated. In addition, some lipid is covalently bonded to the corneal cell. To date, voids, channels and similar structures have not been identified in SC, but their presence—at least at the molecular level—seems to be a theoretical prerequisite for diffusion.

The polar heads of the (multiple) bilayer lipid palisade in SC may become attachment sites for water molecules. The continuity and directional order of the lipids is interrupted by desmosomal structure as well as void-appearing islands called lacunae. Somehow, diffusing molecules must find their way through this maze to reach lower strata. It is not surprising, therefore, that diffusion coefficients for SC are low (at least one order of magnitude lower than those in water). On the basis of current pictures of the lipid arrangement in SC, a diffusing molecule with some affinity for the lipid should find it easier to move laterally within the SC rather than vertically. The tacit assumption in Fick's Laws that a substance traverses skin perpendicular to its surface and that the area covered by the product on the surface equals the area at the underside is probably unrealistic. This and other complex questions about the mode of diffusion through SC must remain unanswered at this time. Diffusion and site preference of the permeant probably play additional roles in sorption, but lack of information makes any analysis impossible.

Inapplicability of Fick's Laws

Cases exist in which the usual assumptions of Fick's Laws may not be routinely applied. Instances in which permeation is not controlled by SC and other skin layers are probably more common than generally recognized and are of considerable practical importance. One of these is the case in which the penetrant is dissolved in a medium from which passage into the SC is relatively slow or negligible. An example would be that of a substance exhibiting a distribution coefficient favoring the vehicle. For illustrative purposes, one might conceive of a vehicle which, upon application to the skin surface after exposure to poison ivy, might deplete the SC of the toxin and speed recovery from the allergic response. A second example is the use of skin patches for transdermal delivery of a drug. An adhesive vehicle (which releases the drug slowly) then determines the drug's release rate. Diffusion through the SC thus can be relatively fast by comparison to diffusion through the vehicle or to transfer from the vehicle to the SC. For these conditions, Higuchi developed approximate equations in which the amount of penetrant delivered through the skin is proportional to $\sqrt{t}$:[25]

$$Q = 2\,C_v \left(\frac{Dvt}{\pi} \right)^{1/2}$$

where D_v is the diffusion coefficient of the permeant in the vehicle.

A related equation covers the case in which the penetrant is in the form of a suspension.[15] Under these conditions, sorption into the SC and ultimate diffusion through the membrane depend on the availability of dissolved penetrant. The equation describing this case is:

$$Q = [(2C_v - S_v)\, S_v D_v t]^{1/2}$$

where S_v is the penetrant's solubility in the vehicle and C_v is the total concentration of penetrant (suspended plus dissolved).

A most complicated but rather common case involves a penetrant which is dissolved in the dispersed phase of a two-phase emulsion. This case requires an assessment of mobility of the permeant within the emulsion. If movement should be rapid, Fick's equations are applicable as long as the distribution coefficient favors the SC. If movement is slow (very stable or viscous emulsions), diffusion will most likely obey the $\sqrt{t}$ laws.

All previously described models assumed infinite dosing at the SC surface. This makes it possible to assign an invariate concentration of diffusant to the top layer of the SC. In practice, this is frequently unrealistic since a thin layer of vehicle with permeant is applied at t = 0, but the permeant concentration in the

Table I. Effect of applied dose on flux of cortisone*	
Moles of cortisone in donor/cm^2	Total flux in moles/cm^2/hr
4.05×10^{-10}	1.67×10^{-13}
2.40×10^{-9}	1.61×10^{-13}
4.41×10^{-9}	2.80×10^{-12}
1.29×10^{-8}	3.80×10^{-12}
2.04×10^{-8}	5.95×10^{-12}
2.01×10^{-7}	2.80×10^{-11}
4.01×10^{-7}	3.90×10^{-11}

*^{3}H-Cortisone in acetone solution was applied to 2.54 cm^2 of human epidermis in a diffusion cell and allowed to dry. The receptor was charged with water. The exposed SC in the donor compartment was kept dry with Drierite.
(After Reference 26)

vehicle is reduced as diffusion into the SC occurs. Depending on the nature of the vehicle (especially its viscosity), depletion of permeant might be limited to the vehicle/skin interface. Even if equilibration within the vehicle occurs rapidly, diffusant depletion can still alter the flux. Under these conditions, in vitro flux into a receiver, the standard measurement of permeation, includes flux due to permeant sorbed into the SC, as noted by Scheuplein and Ross.[26] Some of their data are included in Table I.

It is likely that intact emulsified droplets (whether o/w or w/o), micellar aggregates, and liposomes cannot enter stratum conjunctum to an appreciable extent as a result of size exclusion. In practice, inunction and shear may drive droplets between those layers of the SC (the stratum disjunctum) which are loosened for desquamation. Exposure of an emulsion to the skin (lipids, proteins, etc.) and to the ambient atmosphere (water evaporation) tends to break the emulsion. The components of the vehicle and the permeant can now be absorbed by the exposed SC in accordance with their (individual) distribution coefficients. This separation of the emulsion's components may hasten demulsification. The permeant might now distribute itself between the water phase, the oil phase, and the constituents of the SC. This process is rapid but not quite instantaneous; however, drying of an o/w emulsion rarely requires more than about two to three minutes. Depending on the condition of the SC, the emulsion's water may either evaporate or hydrate the SC, with accompanying changes in the distribution and diffusion coefficients of the permeant. It is apparent that systems of this type include so many variables that no meaningful analysis of sorption is possible without resort to complex models.

A most interesting observation was made by Wolter et al. almost 20 years ago.[27] These authors reported on the penetration of solid drug substances from two anhydrous vehicles into the SC. They report finding solid crystalline tolnaftate and other permeants by polarizing microscopy in the SC after as many as 30 adhesive tape strippings. Another drug, benzocaine, did not reach as low as eight strippings, but sodium carbonate could be detected after 35 strippings. As expected, the particle sizes found in the first strippings were much higher than those in the lower layers of the SC. Surprisingly, inunction had little effect on depth of permeation. Evidently these experiments, conducted on the forearm of one subject, were not further replicated. If the experiment was valid, the assumption about size exclusion made above may have to be drastically modified, and the importance of inunction, or lack thereof, to permeation will have to be reexamined. In any case, the data suggest that solids can enter the SC and that they would behave as sorbed substances.

Mechanism of Sorption into Skin

As noted in the introductory comments, sorption of a permeant or of any substance by layers of the skin can be of several types. Regardless of classification, the common feature is the presence of the material found at varying concentrations throughout the skin. In light of what has been said before, it seems futile to explain sorption of a substance within the skin by applying the exacting laws governing gas-on-solid or dissolved substance-on-solid sorption. The location (on lipid or on protein) of the permeant is unknown. The number of available sites varies not only as a result of the different phases making up the

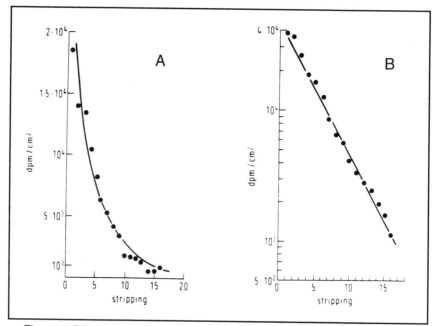

Figure 4. Distribution of radioactivity in stratum corneum after application of clostebol acetate; (A) linear plot, (B) semilogarithmic plot. Reproduced by permission of the copyright owner, Marcel Dekker, Inc., from Reference 28.

skin but also as a result of the tissue's water content.

On the other hand, it is possible to ascertain the "concentration" of the permeant within a given portion of the skin at the instance of sampling.[28] Not unexpectedly, the amount of a topically applied permeant found within the skin drops (probably exponentially) with the distance from the skin surface (Figures 3, 4A and 4B). In SC, such a drop is detected readily, for example by tape stripping after treatment with a tagged substance.

Unfortunately, the normally reported units of concentration are wt/unit area, and no estimate of the thickness of the stripped SC is normally provided, and the stripped layers may not be uniform. A second problem arises from the fact that the stripping properties of skin are affected by the vehicle (and the stripping adhesive) applied to the skin. Stripping is also affected by the contact time of the vehicle with the skin. Tsai and associates suggest that the classical stripping method may not be suitable for comparing drug concentration profiles in skin as a function of depth of penetration or contact time.[29]

Conditions for collecting specimens below the SC in the viable layers are more favorable, and it is possible to construct concentration (in molarity) curves of applied substances as a function of depth or time. The shapes of these curves are variable, depending on the permeant. Some examples are shown in Figures 5 and 6 to prove that distribution is controlled in part by physiological processes rather than exclusively by physicochemical phenomena.[28,30]

Another way of looking at sorption is more trivial: Sorption—without

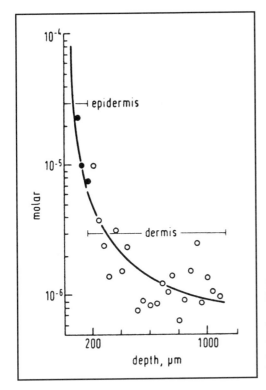

Figure 5. Molar concentration in skin of retinoic acid (0.1% in *i*-propanol) in vivo 100 min. after treatment. Reproduced by permission of the copyright owner, Springer Verlag, Berlin, from Reference 30.

making any assertions about permanence—may be the result of solubility in a dermal constituent. The permeant will be present in solution at the time of analysis. This type of behavior would be expected from treatment with a lipid which might dissolve in SC lipids or with a water-soluble amide which might dissolve in SC proteins. Such a simple process represents absorption: The permeant, by virtue of its solubility, finds suitable albeit temporary sites within the skin and "invades" the tissue. If the permeant remains in solution and if the solvent phase in the SC should be continuous, the permeant can reach the other side of the membrane. Under these highly idealized conditions and at steady-state flux, the concentration of the permeant within the tissue can be expected to show dependence on the partition coefficients on each side of the membrane.

Adsorptive processes are more likely to be encountered by the permeant if it has to pass through phases in the membrane which possesses differing solvencies or affinities for the permeant. For example, a lipophilic compound diffusing through a lipid domain in the SC may reach a hydrophilic barrier, resulting in blockage; the substance cannot reach the underside of the SC but is present (sorbed or trapped) in the SC. Alternately, the permeant may bind through Van der Waals (or hydrophobic) forces to a specific site on the protein hydrophilic barrier and may progress iteratively in short steps from one temporary site to another until it reaches more compatible surroundings. The bonding/ bondbreaking steps described here present an adsorption-desorption process

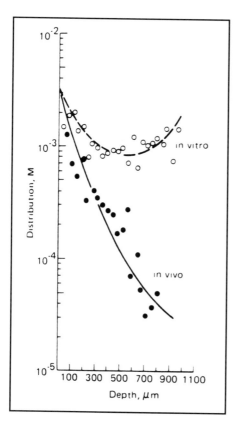

Figure 6. Distribution of hydrocortisone in human skin in vitro (○) and in vivo (●) 100 min. after treatment with 1% glucocorticoid in polyethylene glycol ointment. Reproduced by permission of the copyright owner, Marcel Dekker, Inc., from Reference 28.

which might obey one of the classical adsorption isotherms (BET, Langmuir, Freundlich, etc.). Isothermal studies or the construction of Scatchard plots to determine binding constants for the sorption of materials in SC are complicated. The characteristics of sites vary as a result of hydration. The nature of voids within the SC, especially in the proteinaceous cells, is uncertain. Finally, the permeant may diffuse not as a simple molecule but in combination with a complexing or associated molecule present in SC or in the vehicle (H_2O or propylene glycol).

Anderson and his coworkers have examined permeability of and partitioning into SC in a more formalistic way.[31] On the basis of their results derived from study of a series of 21 esters of hydrocortisone and of p-cresols they suggested recently that SC consists of a polar protein domain and a lipid domain and that the overall permeability coefficient P represents contributions of two barriers in series as defined by the notation:

$$P = \frac{1}{1/P_{lipid} + 1/P_{polar}}$$

and where in accordance with Equation 1:

$$P_{lipid} = \frac{K_{lipid}\, D_{lipid}}{l}$$

K_{lipid} can be related to $K_{o/w}$, the octanol/water partition coefficient of a given compound, which allows for experimental validation of the two-domain concept. The recent data provided by Lambert et al., based on penetration of vidarabine, *n*-butanol, and hydrocortisone, confirm the existence of a parallel polar route for permeation.[32] They define the (total) permeability coefficient P_{total} (t) as the sum of P_{lipid} and P_{polar} (t). The notation "(t)" follows those permeability coefficients that change with time (see discussion about experimental data on "Sorption of Water" later in this chapter).

Adsorption to SC could be limited strictly to the exterior surface. The stratum disjunctum includes voids exposing protein and lipid surfaces, both of which can become adsorptive sites for suitable substances. This phenomenon need not result in transdermal permeation because the adsorbed substance might not be able to enter the compact layers of the SC. For example, a large non-permeating protein molecule may still find an attachment site on the SC.

The magnitude of the binding constant controls the nature of the adsorption, more specifically its reversibility. Reversible adsorption (low binding constant) is required for skin permeation. In simpler terms, the permeant must be able to move through the skin layers. If sorption is irreversible, the penetrating species is found at a site to which it is attached (covalently or coulombically) so tightly that it cannot be dislodged in vivo.

The concept of reversible and irreversible sorption has already been discussed. A reversible sorption mechanism was postulated by Dalvi and Zatz, who observed that in-vitro flux of benzocaine through mouse skin was lower from a saturated solution than from a suspension of benzocaine.[33] If a significant portion of the benzocaine is bound or immobilized in the SC, the drug's concentration in the donor is lowered, thus reducing the flux. When a suspension is used, benzocaine is also sorbed by the SC, but the presence of a suspended solid supplies sufficient drug to maintain a high flux. The type of bonding observed by Dalvi and Zatz was only partially irreversible since most of the sorbed benzocaine could be eluted into the receptor by merely replacing the depleted benzocaine in the donor with water.

It will be apparent that the permeating molecules may encounter bonding sites which show intermediate levels of reversibility and that binding constants depend not only on the permeant but also on the sorbing sites within the skin.

Experimental Data: Generalizations

The general features of the sorption of externally applied substances within the skin has not been studied extensively. Nevertheless, meaningful generalizations become evident from the theoretical concepts described earlier and from the specific and more practical examples reviewed below.

Data on sorption within skin are examined most commonly by determining the concentration of the sorbed substance as a function of depth of penetration, contact time, concentration, vehicle variations, and similar parameters. In another assessment, the site of sorption is of primary interest, and concentration variations play a secondary role. This distinction is sometimes obscured but must be kept in mind in the course of a literature survey.

Skin is a multicomponent tissue, and sorption assessment is made at a given (experimentally convenient) instance. The sorbed substance may be found in one or all of the histologically or morphologically identifiable skin components. Much of the work on receptor sites in skin is performed on systemically administered substances. Sometimes, sorption experiments are conducted by isolating a specific skin component; exposing it to the active, alone or in solution; and then analyzing binding using classical isotherms and plotting techniques. Results from such experiments do not represent in-vivo sorption of topically applied substances (which rarely is an equilibrium process) but involve numerous pharmacokinetically identifiable rate processes.[16,34]

The location of a sorbed substance within skin is complex and depends not only on transfers between layers of the skin but also between domains within each layer. For example, Raykar et al.[1] identified three domains within SC. One of these is the solvent-extractable lipid domain; the second is the protein domain; and the third is an aqueous solvent domain. The last is particularly variable since it can become larger as the result of engorgement of water under conditions of occlusion. In the viable epidermis (VE), several cell types, such as keratinocytes and dendritic cells, display their specific receptors which may account for binding. The lower layers of the skin include cellular portions, ground substance, fibrous components and the skin's appendageal systems. Each of these has specific abilities to bind chemicals, and the ultimate sites for binding and subsequent disposition of topically applied substances are largely unknown.

Feldman and Maibach[35] and Menczel and Maibach[36] provided evidence for the principle that each layer of skin has its own ability to bind or sorb specific permeant molecules. Their data, based on hydrocortisone and differences in the sorption of testosterone and benzyl alcohol within the dermis and the time at which sorption is studied, appear to depend on specific binding sites within skin layers for a specific permeant.

The following discussion emphasizes the description of the fate of substances applied topically to living or excised skin in which penetration occurs from the outside to the interior. In this review, studies in which the sorbate diffuses laterally or from the underside of the dermis are, as a rule, de-emphasized.

Sorption of Water

Sorption of water by SC plays a dominant role in transdermal drug delivery and in the mechanical properties of human skin. Hydration accelerates the passage of drugs through skin and is the basis of cosmetic skin benefit claims derived from moisturizers. Wurster and Yang demonstrated that water vapor sorption by human delipidized callus could not be described by Fick's Second Law because the diffusion coefficient varies with the tissue's water content.[37] The same authors also computed glass transition temperatures at different levels of water sorption by callus. This temperature is lowered from 55°C to as low as 28°C at 67% RH (at which 1 g of callus contains 0.16 g water). Thus, hydration of this tissue at physiological temperatures can change it from a glass (impermeable) polymer to a rubbery (more permeable) polymer.

The dependence of water transmission through SC on water content has been confirmed in vitro on intact SC by Blank et al., using tritiated water.[38] They used a unique diffusion cell which measured the passage of gaseous H_2O/HTO at RH's controlled in the donor and receptor chamber. The authors showed that at increased RH, which means increased water content of SC, the permeability and diffusion coefficients were raised.

Today it is generally accepted that the water content of the bottom layer of SC in vivo is (close to) that of the underlying VE, and that it drops throughout the SC up to the surface, where it is controlled by the ambient RH. The existence of such a profile was confirmed by Warner et al.[18] Examination of data on water content by SC shows that 5% is tightly held and difficult to remove. Another 30 to 40% of water (based on dry SC) is sorbed and desorbed readily, depending on ambient humidity. However, if SC is soaked in water, it may absorb as much as 500% of its own weight[39] and swells to about 400% of its original thickness in 80 hours.[40]

The permanence of water sorption in SC is clearly variable in vivo and must be considered during in-vitro diffusion cell studies. Extensive exposure effects structural changes; Bond and Barry reported that long exposure to aqueous media changes the barrier properties of SC permanently.[41] These investigators report that the barrier properties of mouse skin are destroyed by long exposure (4 to 10 days), whereas human abdominal or scalp skin is much more resistant to water exposure. SC damage probably increases the number of sites accessible for permeant sorption. During a study of ^3H_2O flux through full-thickness hairless mouse skin, Hinz et al. also observed loss of barrier function during prolonged water exposure.[42] They suggest that flux measurements after 24-hour exposure of this type of tissue may yield inconclusive results. The mechanism by which prolonged hydration alters the skin barrier was recently explored by Lambert et al.[32] As a rule, water sorbed by epidermis after 36 and 48 hours of occlusive conditions is quickly lost, as evidenced by high TEWL. In addition, age plays a role in the rate at which TEWL returns to normal under these conditions.[43]

The dependence of the level of water sorption on temperature was reviewed by Potts.[44] He cites the work of Jacques, who concluded on the basis of isotherm analysis that the number of water-binding sites within SC increases with temperature. Although the binding energy of sorbed water should be decreased by an increase of temperature, an increased number of available binding sites seems to dominate the process. The temperature-induced increase in the number of water binding sites may be the result of protein unfolding or of changes in the diffusion coefficient of water through SC or both.

Sorption of water by SC causes both beneficial and adverse effects. Modest hydration, resulting from occlusion, enhances drug transport through the skin. (See Reference 45 for examples.) It may also enhance transport of undesirable substances, such as surfactants brought into skin contact. Prolonged or excessive water sorption causes skin damage (maceration), which is only slowly reversible. Water sorption by SC (in which the donor and the receptor are both aqueous) during in-vitro diffusion chamber experimentation makes it difficult to translate such results to the normal in-vivo situation (in which only the receptor is aqueous in the absence of total occlusion).

In conclusion, water influences the barrier performance of SC more than any other nonirritating substance. The mechanism through which sorbed water affects skin penetration so far has not been investigated in depth. Sorption of water may alter the sorption of other permeants in the SC, but this problem, too, has not been specifically addressed.

The Sorption of Surfactants

Sorption of surfactants by skin membranes is a special case intermediate between sorption of water (just discussed) and sorption of true penetration enhancers (to be discussed later). The interaction between SC and surfactants was reviewed comprehensively by Breuer in 1979.[46] Studies dealing with the penetration of surfactants into SC frequently also deal with the more general topic of surfactant toxicity.[48] Surfactants as a group are generally considered skin permeation enhancers, but there is no agreement on how these compounds function in this fashion.

Anionic Surfactants: Anionic surfactants are sorbed by keratins via attractive hydrophobic binding as well as via coulombic forces. The latter type of binding by positively charged sites in the SC is expected to interfere with a surfactant's permeation through the SC. Soaps and alkyl sulfates are the anionic surfactants of primary interest in drugs and cosmetics. The presence of soap enhances water, glucose, and salicylate transport through skin, but the impact of pH in these systems has not been elucidated. The data on alkyl sulfates are more instructive. Breuer presented data obtained by J. Poret on the sodium dodecylsulfate (SDS) content in vitro and in vivo on stripped SC exposed to ^{14}C-labeled compounds.[46] The data used to prepare Figures 7 and 8 conform entirely to expected distribution patterns. On the other hand, it is remarkable that the nonionic monocapryl glyceride shows the identical pattern to SDS when the quantities are normalized to the second strip. As a rule, data on surfactant sorption are scattered, and attempts to derive generally valid assumptions must be made with caution.

One of the early in-vitro skin penetration studies with radio-tagged surfactants was reported by Blank and Gould in 1959.[48] They applied dilute aqueous preparations (0.005 M) for 20 hours to skin in a diffusion chamber, washed the skin, and then stripped the SC 14 times for autoradiography and other examinations. Under these conditions, most of the radioactivity was found in the initial strips. Very little alkyl sulfate had reached the dermis (Table II), but penetration by soap was much more pronounced.

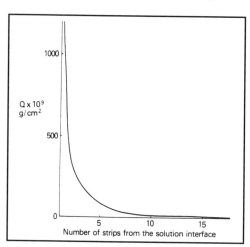

Figure 7. Sodium dodecylsulfate (SDS) in strips of stratum corneum after short exposure to SDS solution. Reproduced by permission of the copyright owner, the *Journal of the Society of Cosm. Chem.*, from Reference 46.

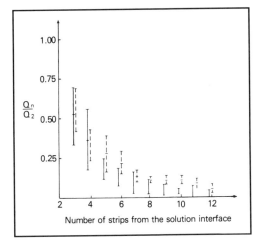

Figure 8. Distribution of sodium dodecylsulfate (SDS) and of monocapryl glyceride (MCG) in stratum corneum normalized to the second strip. Solid line— SDS; broken line—MCG. Reproduced by permission of the copyright owner, *Journal of the Society of Cosm. Chem.*, from Reference 46.

During the study of the permeation of anionic ^{14}C-tagged surfactants, Howes made casual determinations of the amounts of surfactants deposited in rat skin.[49] The data (Table III) permit comparison of SDS retention with that of isethionate; the different experimental conditions make comparison to alkylarylsulfonate sorption impossible.

In the case of alkyl sulfates, sorption reaches a maximum at a chain length of C_{12}. Faucher and Goddard showed that the uptake of sodium lauryl sulfate (SLS) by neonatal rat SC increases with concentration up to 15% SLS.[50] These authors also demonstrated that the uptake of SLS conformed, at least initially, to the $\sqrt{t}$ relationship (Figure 9). By extending their data on bleached hair one may further anticipate that skin sorption of the sodium lauryl ether sulfates (SLES) on SC conforms to the following pattern: SLS >> SLE(2)S* > SLE(3)S* > SLE(12)S*.

*The numbers in parentheses represent the numbers of ethyleneoxide groups.

Table II. Distribution of surfactants in human skin		
	Sodium Laurate* ($mM \times 10^3$)	Sodium Dodecylsulfate ($mM \times 10^3$)
SC Strip 1	77.3	36.5
SC Strip 2	27.4	109.0
SC Strip 3	10.8	8.0
SC Strip 4-9	28.6	24.3
SC Strip 10-14	11.5	14.5
SC Total	156.6	192.3
Epidermis	189.0	21.0
Dermis	221.0	<3.5

*pH at start of experiment was 10.3 and 7.6 after 20 hours. (After Reference 48)

Table III. Surfactant recovery in rat skin
(after 15 min. application and rinsing)

Surfactant	Conditions	Applied Dose Found
Sodium dodecylsulfate	0.5 ml of 25 mM/10cm²	5.5
Sodium dodecylisethionate	0.5 ml of 25 mM/10cm²	1.5
Sodium dodecylbenzenesulfate	0.2 ml of 3mM/7.5 cm²	4.4

(After Reference 49)

In a subsequent paper these authors explored the skin permeation of SLS and concluded that 0.5% SLS (in contrast to myristalkonium chloride and pareth-15-9) enters rat SC with almost no lag time.[51] They also point out that transdermal flux increases with increasing concentration beyond the critical micelle concentration (CMC). On the basis of their results, one should question the notion that only monomeric SLS (or small micelles) takes part in the diffusion and permeation process through SC.

Sorption of SLS as well as that of most anionic surfactants is accompanied by extensive swelling of the SC.[52] All investigators of the sorption of SLS by SC observed changes in the rate of sorption of SLS or in the degree of swelling at the CMC of SLS. The currently accepted explanation of the swelling phenomenon follows: The alkyl sulfates bond to SC hydrophobically and ionically. Evidence

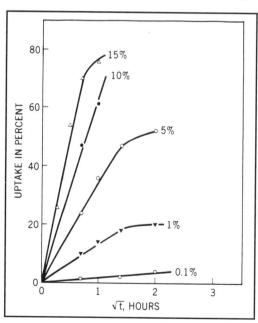

Figure 9. Sorption of sodium laurylsulfate by neonatal rat stratum corneum. Reproduced by permission of the copyright owner, *Journal of the Society of Cosm. Chem.*, from Reference 50.

for ionic bonding is derived from the absence of swelling by nonionic or cationic surfactants. Cationics probably react ionically with negative sites in the SC. This bonding converts hydrophilic sites into hydrophobic sites. By contrast, anionics at neutral pH tend to bind hydrophobically, thus creating additional hydrophilic sites. These interactions are somewhat pH-dependent since anionics are likely to bind to cationic sites in SC created at low phs. These new hydrophobic sites may tend to reduce swelling. This reasoning by Rhein et al. appears sound, in light of the fact that the Mg^{++} and TEA^+ salts of lauryl sulfate effect different degrees of swelling of SC.[52]

The generally recognized interference with SC swelling due to SLS by nonionics seems to be related to interactions between (two or more) surfactants rather than to effects on SC.[53] This assertion is supported by observations of unusual effects due to the association of SDS micelles with polyethylene oxide derivatives.[54] An alternate interpretation could be based on changes in CMC due to the formation of mixed micelles between the nonionic surfactant and SLS. The fact remains that swelling (sorption) is reduced by this combination, and—if Rhein et al. are correct— this phenomenon is directly related to reduced sorption of the anionic surfactant. How any of these concepts can explain the reduction in swelling by the SLESs (up to 6 moles of ethylene oxide) *vis-a-vis* SLS is not clear.[52]

Cationic Surfactants: Cationic surfactants have a different effect on SC from that of the typical anionics. For instance, the alkyltrimethyl bromides, at pH 5 to 9, cause no swelling of human SC, regardless of alkyl chain length.[52,53] Evidence for surface adsorption on keratins of molecules carrying a positively charged nitrogen is overwhelming.[55]

Recent data on the sorption of cationic polymers demonstrate that these cellulose derivatives (MW 250,000 to 600,000) are sorbed very slowly by SC.[56] The diffusion constants, ranging from about $1x10^{-10}$ to $1x10^{-12}$ cm²/sec, show the expected dependency on molecular weight. The observed sorption is too low to be explained by imbibition of polymer-containing water. Instead, SC appears to exclude these polymers to a large extent. Presumably, some of the quaternary polymer chains diffuse slowly by a mechanism of reptation, but no polymer could be detected in the receiving compartment of the diffusion cell. Interestingly, sorption of the low-MW polymer is almost totally inhibited in the presence of a competing quaternary, myristalkonium chloride. One may assume that the negatively charged sites in SC are preferentially occupied by the more mobile myristalkonium chloride.

Permeation studies of quaternary surfactants are somewhat contradictory,[47] but it appears that quaternary surfactants do not appreciably penetrate through SC and do so only after prolonged exposure (6 days) and at high concentration (10%).

In conclusion, quaternaries are probably sorbed by coulombic interaction on and within SC. Initial bonding of the quaternary is so permanent that further quaternary molecules cannot find unoccupied sites in the SC or cannot enter as a result of an adverse partition coefficient.[57] The tenacity of sorption of quaternaries by skin has not been studied specifically, but related studies on hair may be applicable. Scott et al. found that cetyl-trimethyl ammonium bromide (CTAB) sorption by hair and that of dodecyltrimethyl ammonium bromide (DTAB) increases with increasing pH.[57] CTAB was sorbed more efficiently than DTAB, and CTAB was held more tenaciously than DTAB during desorption experiments.

Nonionic Surfactants: Nonionic surfactants of diverse structures can diffuse readily through SC, suggesting that they may also be readily sorbed. For example, the sorption of monocapryl glyceride* has already been noted (Figure 8).[46] Data on the sorption of nonionics by SC are surprisingly sketchy in light of the wide use of these surfactants in topical preparations. Skin sorption of the classic nonionic emulsifiers and stabilizers has not been studied, and conclusions must be drawn from data on the effect of these chemicals on transdermal permeation. This approach is complicated by the fact that nonionics, as a group, have a tendency to lower the chemical activity of permeants, thus also lowering transdermal passage.[58] This effect can be reversed, and permeation can be increased by including 40% or more of propylene glycol. These complex interactions probably are unrelated to sorption of the nonionic by SC. One explanation could involve the permeant's partition coefficient between bulk solvent and micellized nonionics. Alternately, undefined skin damage could result from the combination of propylene glycol and the nonionic.

No truly convincing mechanistic interpretation has been provided for the observation that (low molecular weight) nonionics can effect transmucosal absorption of large molecules such as insulin.[59] Although the mucosa is not a fully keratinized structure, it will not allow such a large molecule to pass in therapeutic levels unless a relatively small nonionic or ionic surfactant is present. Ceteth-10, laureth-9 and laureth-5 allow mucosal permeation of insulin, and this effect is probably related to the interaction of nonionics with some portion of the membrane. Their performance resembles that of the penetration enhancers, and a more detailed discussion follows.

As a general rule—and in the absence of reliable data—it appears reasonable not to ascribe sorptive properties to the nonionics as a group. It is more likely that bulkier nonionics and those possessing long or multiple chains of ethylene oxide groups are not sorbed by SC. On the other hand, smaller molecules with HLBs ranging from about 6 to 12 could be sorbed by the lipid bilayers in the SC via hydrophobic bonding (or solubility) in SC lipids. The resulting disruption, coupled with potential hydration of the hydrophilic side chains, can be expected to facilitate SC permeation.

Penetration Enhancers

Currently, efforts to deliver drugs transdermally frequently depend on the ability to identify suitable enhancers of drug permeability. Penetration enhancers as a group are substances which increase the (rate of) flux of a chemical through SC. The mechanism by which enhancers function is probably unrelated to their effect on the vehicle or on the activity of the chemical in the vehicle. Instead, penetration enhancers presumably disrupt the organization of the barrier. Water, which increases the flux of a chemical through SC, could therefore be viewed as a penetration enhancer.

*This compound is not precisely identified in Reference 46 and may be the glyceryl ester of either capric, caprylic or caproic acid.

One of the first chemicals identified as an enhancer was laurocapram (Azone®). It was soon followed by decylmethylsulfoxide and oleic acid. Substances of this type work in relatively low concentrations and do not act as drug or lipid solvents. They are not very water soluble, and their primary effect is on the lipids within SC, as reviewed by Barry.[60]

The thermal transitions of human SC lipids have been intensively investigated with the aid of Differential Scanning Colorimetry and X-ray diffraction since about 1975. It has been established that penetration enhancers lower transition temperatures and seem to increase the fluidity of the SC lipids.[60,61] Such an effect requires that the enhancer find its way into the lipid phase; that is, it must be sorbed. Once sorbed, the effect of the enhancer is not lost for several days.[62-64] These experimental findings and concepts have recently been broadened by Goodman and Barry to include additional effects on intracellular proteins and on the partitioning of the permeant between the lipid and the protein components of the SC.[65]

Barry utilized schematic models to show how an enhancer intercalates itself into the closely packed hydrocarbon chains of the SC lipids.[60] One of these, for oleic acid, is shown in Figure 10. Barry's models are based on the concept that the enhancer partitions into and disrupts the SC lipid structure, thereby increasing its fluidity. Oleic acid (at neutral pH) and decylmethylsulfoxide can also be viewed as nonionic emulsifiers of low HLB. Nonionics exhibiting similar lipid/water partitioning coefficients could thus be expected to partition into SC lipid and to bind hydrophobically, depending on their bulk and other structural features.

Pretreatment of SC with a penetration-enhancing vehicle reduces the SC's barrier effectiveness. As a result, subsequent drug treatment with no enhancer can provide as much increased transdermal drug permeation as drug treatment in the presence of an enhancer.[11]

Sasaki and collaborators studied the sorption of various N-alkylpyrrolidones by skin and their ability to enhance permeation of drugs of different polarities.[66] Their

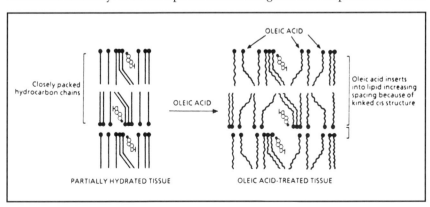

Figure 10. Schematic of mechanism by which oleic acid increases the fluidity of intercellular lipids of the stratum corneum. Reproduced by permission of the copyright owner, Elsevier Science Publishers BV, after Reference 62.

results were explained by them as follows: "All enhancers accumulated to a great extent in the skin...pyrrolidone derivatives enhance the flux of penetrants in skin by increasing the solubility of penetrants in the stratum corneum."

In summary, the effect of enhancers to speed up drug permeation requires their presence (sorption) primarily in the SC lipids. All currently available evidence suggests that effective permeation enhancers are sorbed into SC.

Sorption of Solvents

Sorption of solvents by SC can be expected to depend on the presence of water. The comprehensive permeability data on a number of alcohols, assembled by Scheuplein and Blank,[3] do not allow meaningful interpretation in terms of sorption. Data dealing with the distribution of glycerin within SC were provided by Guy and Hadgraft without details about hydration or the experimental approach (Figure 3, Reference 16).

Despite the fact that information on this subject is extremely limited, the work of Berner et al. on sorption of ethanol, performed on SC and on delipidized (with 2:1 v/v chloroform: methanol) SC, provides some insights into complicated interactions.[67] The amount of ethanol in SC was determined by gas chromatography, and water sorption was assessed with the aid of $^{3}H_2O$. The uptakes were determined gravimetrically (after blotting) on small discs of human SC from the water content (i.e., wet weight minus dry weight minus ethanol content). Some of their results are shown in Figures 11 and 12 in which the volume fraction of ethanol represents the composition of the solution to which the SC was exposed for 24 hours. Up to a volume fraction of about 0.5, the ratio of imbibed water to

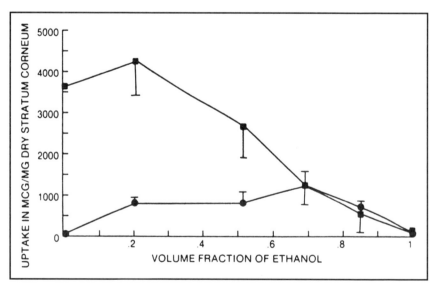

Figure 11. Uptake of ethanol (●) and water (■) by dry stratum corneum from aqueous ethanol at 32°C. Reproduced by permission of the copyright owner, the *Journal of Pharmaceutical Science*, Reference 67.

imbibed ethanol in SC equals that in the solution. At higher alcohol volume fractions, imbibition of both ethanol and water decreases and does not correspond to the composition of the medium. This is attributed to interference with swelling and possible shrinkage of keratin. In delipidized SC, the ratio of water to ethanol is high at low volume fractions but decreases at high volume fractions. The elution of the natural moisturizing factor, which is believed to play a role in the water uptake by SC, may also play a role in water sorption.

These findings—although difficult to interpret—suggest that the two permeants, water and alcohol, are not imbibed in the ratio present in the medium. Even at an alcohol: water ratio of 0.85, water sorption by delipidized SC (on a weight basis) seems to be three times that of ethanol. No comparable data for more hydrophobic alcohols are available. Data from Berner et al. show no significant difference in water sorption of delipidized and normal SC.[67] Delipidization of SC surprisingly enhances the sorption of essentially lipophilic drugs over retention by normal human SC.[17]

Dimethylsulfoxide (DMSO) has been shown by Chandrasekaran et al.[68] and Elfbaum and Laden[69] to be a penetration enhancer at high concentration at which it may exert some lipid solvent effects. The data provided by Elfbaum indicate that the site of action is sorption by protein with attendant protein chain unfolding. The sorption isotherms of scopolamine and of DMSO plus scopolamine on human SC by Chandrasekaran et al. show that, at equilibrium, DMSO does not alter sorption of scopolamine by SC from its sorption from pure water as long as drug activity (rather than weight) is used in the analysis.

Data on skin sorption of most common organic solvents are essentially unavailable. Some information on the sorption of benzene in SC ($9.3\mu l\ ml^{-1}$) can

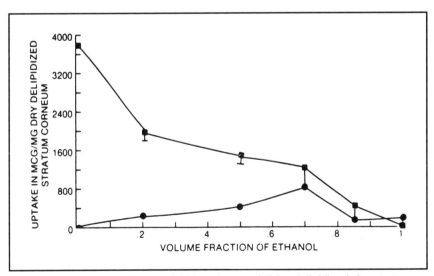

Figure 12. Uptake of ethanol (●) and water (■) by delipidized dry stratum corneum at 32°C. Reproduced by permission of the copyright owner, the *Journal of Pharmaceutical Science*, Reference 67.

be deduced from the data provided by Blank and McAuliffe,[70] but information on other solvents, even such a common excipient as propylene glycol, is essentially lacking. Miselnicky et al. report, for example, that the amount of propylene glycol found in VE after a classical type of in-vitro permeation study was only 5.5% of the applied dose.[71]

In summary, information on the sorption of organic lipophilic and lipophobic solvents by SC is sparse. The limited published data suggest that such solvents are sorbed. The degree of their sorption depends on the presence of water, elution of lipids from the SC, and factors which are highly dependent on experimental conditions.

Reservoir Effect

The ability of SC to act as a reservoir for topically applied agents appears to have been known since about 1954. The early history of this phenomenon was reviewed by Vickers in 1964.[72] The principle of the reservoir effect is best explained via the example cited by Vickers, based on a report by McKenzie and Stoughton.[73] Vasoconstriction from steroids could be demonstrated 7-10 days after topical drug administration (despite normal washing) by reoccluding the site with Saran® wrap. Additional experiments by Vickers and other investigators confirmed that storage of the vasoconstricting steroid took place within the SC.

Since these early studies, the sorption by SC of various drug molecules has been studied extensively.[74] The most comprehensive of these is an in-vitro study in which 17 tagged substances were applied from acetone to 350μm thick sections of rat skin.[71] The underside of the skin was in contact with normal saline as the receptor in a flow-through cell. Twenty-four hours after application, the surface was washed with a detergent solution to remove nonabsorbed substance. Diffusion was allowed to proceed for another two days to permit "unretained material to diffuse from the skin." The results of this extensive study are reproduced in Table IV, in which the compounds are listed in the order of increasing water solubility. The authors conclude that the likelihood of a chemical to form a SC reservoir is predictable from four factors:

1. The substance should not rapidly permeate through the skin.
2. The substance should be poorly soluble in water and oil (octanol).
3. The substance should have an octanol/water partition coefficient larger than 1.
4. The substance should have high affinity for protein (Scatchard plot, see below).

Artuc et al. examined the behavior of five other drug substances on specimens of human VE separated from autopsy skin.[75] The tagged substances were introduced into 2 ml of buffer before varying amounts of dry VE were added.

Equilibration was allowed to proceed for 12 to 36 hours at 40°C, and sorption was determined from the loss of activity in the buffer solution. All five drugs (5- and 8-methoxypsoralen, thiopyronin, α-estradiol, and theophyllin) showed a much higher concentration in the tissue than in the aqueous buffer. The observed drug enrichment in the VE was not due to irreversible binding since the drugs could be removed (or exchanged), and reversible binding was identified as the probable mechanism. An attempt was made to obtain binding constants from Scatchard plots, but the small ratio of tissue sample to surrounding buffer tended

Table IV. Distribution of test compounds following topical administration
(Data expressed as a percentage of the applied dose)

Compound	Amount absorbed*	Skin wash	Epidermis	Dermis	Surrounding tissue	Recovery	K_A** $(\times 10^4 M^{-1})$
AETT	32.50	19.1	13.60	4.89	15.40	87.7	912.90
Testosterone	35.40	55.4	2.63	1.49	4.59	99.8	8.78
Triamcinolone acetonide	14.50	80.9	4.19	0.62	2.92	103.5	8.29
Salicylic acid	11.40	83.4	10.10	1.26	1.70	108.0	4.05
5-MOP	69.90	15.3	1.05	0.65	12.70	99.8	—
8-MOP	66.40	20.1	0.93	0.36	7.36	95.3	4.63
Benzoic acid	30.50	53.0	3.23	0.78	1.94	89.6	2.21
Dihydrotestosterone	29.60	46.5	8.81	2.50	7.09	95.0	21.40
Aspirin	16.70	78.7	6.69	0.88	4.38	107.6	0.45
Hydrocortisone	9.80	71.0	6.92	0.90	3.09	91.9	0.20
Fumaric acid	0.62	98.0	4.81	0.40	0.00	103.8	0
Caffeine	71.80	32.4	0.95	0.16	1.86	107.3	0.40
Propylene glycol	20.30	46.1	1.84	0.27	0.36	68.9	0
Nicotinic acid	9.00	75.5	11.20	1.90	3.27	101.4	0.16
Nicotinamide	15.30	78.2	3.15	0.65	0.88	98.6	0.16
Urea	9.68	85.5	3.03	0.24	0.19	98.7	0
Glycerol	7.34	90.3	5.56	1.07	2.03	106.8	0

*Amount in receptor fluid
**Scatchard Binding Constant
(After Reference 71)

to introduce large errors and unexpected results.

Information on binding activity is highly desirable, and Miselnicky et al. determined the protein binding tendency of the 17 substances studied by them on soluble bovine serum albumen.[71] Their binding constants (from Scatchard plots) are included in Table IV.

Reservoir formation is not limited to SC but can be demonstrated in lower dermal strata.[76]

A somewhat different approach concerning drug sorption within the SC and its subsequent release was taken by Foreman and collaborators.[77] They suggest that occlusion reduces the ability of SC to bind nandrolone irreversibly. These concepts were further supported by in-vitro diffusion cell studies of other steroids in their later publication.[78] On the basis of their studies, the authors postulated that steroid binding sites in normal SC are occupied by water molecules.[78] The latter are displaced by steroid molecules in a reversible fashion, which accounts for release of steroid by water molecules during occlusion. Support for this concept is provided by the more recent data on delipidized SC obtained by Surber et al.[17]

An interesting issue concerning in-vivo studies of skin penetration was pointed out by Watson and Finlay.[79] In order to quantify correctly the amount of drug in skin and that penetrating through skin during long-term studies of a single-dose application, one must take into account the amount of drug sorbed by SC which is lost by desquamation during the course of the study. Their in-vivo data indicate that clobetasol 17-propionate loss due to shedding was about 30% after 48 hours. This so-called "outward loss" was different for the two vehicles tested by these

Table V. Distribution of compounds
(after application of ethanolic solution to rat dorsum)

Compound	Amount found 96 hours after topical application*		Amount in stratum corneum 30 min after application*
	Total permeation	Epidermis plus dermis	
Benzoic acid	26.60	0.50	17.60
Acetylsalicylic acid	6.70	0.85	5.15
Dehydroepiandrosterone	5.28	0.19	1.95
Sodium salicylate	4.98	1.00	3.85
Testosterone	4.32	0.24	2.06
Caffeine	3.73	0.15	2.76
Thiourea	3.23	0.20	2.63
D-Mannitol	2.63	0.30	2.22
Hydrocortisone	0.86	0.04	0.93
Dexamethasone	0.60	0.10	0.41

* in nmol x cm^{-2} application area
(After Reference 82)

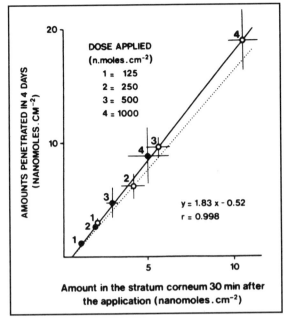

Figure 13. Correlation between the levels of permeation of different doses of benzoic acid after 4 days and their deposition in stratum corneum after 30-40 min. application; ($\bigcirc$–$\bigcirc$) rat; ($\bullet$–$\bullet$) human; and in rat with 10 other radiolabelled molecules (····). Reproduced by permission of the copyright owner, the *Journal of Pharmaceutical Science*, Reference 81.

investigators. As in most cases reported in the literature, a plot of the log of the drug concentration in SC vs. depth in the SC was linear. Deviations from this exponential relationship became more pronounced 48 hours or later after dosing.

The most detailed in-vivo investigation of the SC reservoir for drugs was conducted by Rougier and his collaborators.[80-85] They demonstrated that percutaneous drug delivery, as measured by drug level in the body, was proportional to drug sorption into SC, as measured by the amount of drug present in the SC 30 minutes after dosing. Drug in the SC was quantified by measuring radioactivity in 6 tape strippings after removal of excess from the skin surface by washing.[82] Total drug permeation was determined from the sum of the amount of urinary and fecal excretion and of the drug in the epidermis, dermis and body of the animal. Table V includes experimental results of interest to the topic under discussion. The data show a correlation coefficient of 0.998, even though there are some minor inconsistencies.

The initial animal results were later extended to man in vivo by determining the response to variable topical dosing with labelled benzoic acid (Figure 13).[81,85] The authors concluded that SC sorption of other permeants after 30 minutes could be used to predict their systemic levels in the body after permeation. It is also significant that the level of sorption into rat SC was highly dependent on the vehicle.[83] Despite a 50-fold variation in total body penetration from different vehicles during four days, there still was a correlation coefficient of 0.997 between the amounts sorbed into SC after only 30 minutes and total permeation.

A final check was performed to confirm that a 30-minute SC sorption was predictive of total permeation of four drugs regardless of body site.[84] The rank order of permeability of studied sites was arm < abdomen < post-auricular < forehead. The forehead was approximately two times more permeable than forearm skin to the tested compounds (sodium benzoate, benzoic acid, caffeine and salicylic acid). In light of its predictive aspect, the work of Rougier et al. has attracted much interest among investigators of transdermal drug administration. On the other hand, these data on the sorption in the SC fail to answer questions concerning the mechanism of corneal sorption, of release or of permeation.

Sorption of Miscellaneous Compounds

Tenacious binding of a substance by SC eliminates or at least reduces its systemic absorption. Loose or no binding, on the other hand, only delays the ultimate entry of the substance. A list of about 30 penetrants, together with literature citations, has been compiled by Menczel et al.[86] The list includes hair dyes, pesticides, steroids, metallic ions, and antimicrobial agents. Here we can describe the in-skin distribution of only a few of these penetrants and some other substances.

Typical is the report by Akhter and Barry on aromatic acidic NSAID's.[87] In their diffusion cell experimentation excessive hydration of the human SC was avoided by using full-thickness skin ($\approx$ 430 µm thick) and application of the drugs from a volatile vehicle (acetone). Sorption into SC was readily observed, as was sorption of n-methyl-2-pyrrolidone.

The distribution of indomethacin between epidermis and dermis is affected not only by the choice of vehicle but in addition by the presence of various purported penetration enhancers.[11] Loth cites data on the increase in the amount of indomethacin in skin, epidermis and dermis obtained when excised human skin was treated for 16 hours with the drug in a pasty triglyceride (of caprylic, capric and stearic acids) with 19.8% enhancer.

The data in Table VI represent the increases in the amount of drug found in the presence of enhancers relative to the triglyceride base without enhancer. The polarity of the selected enhancer seems to control permeation through SC,

Table VI. Distribution of indomethacin in excised human skin			
Penetration Enhancer (19.8%)	Increase of Indomethacin in Skin		
	Total	Epidermis	Dermis
None	-	-	-
Glycerylmonooleate	–6	–5	–1
Oleyloleate	10	12	–2
Isopropylmyristate	29	21	8
2-Octyldodecanol	78	47	31
Cetyl/stearyl-2-ethylhexanoate	86	41	45
n-Octanol	90	7	83

(After Reference 11)

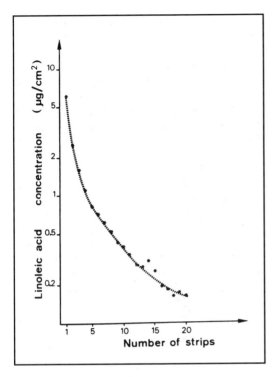

Figure 14. Distribution of ^{14}C-linoleic acid in stratum corneum 24 hours after a single application. Reproduced by permission of the copyright owner, *Journal of the Society of Cosm. Chem.*, from Reference 88.

thus altering the drug levels found in the dermis. Loth provides additional data on the concentration profile of flufenamic acid in human SC, demonstrating that the unctuous triglyceride can provide higher drug levels in the top layers of the SC than vaseline or vaseline/woolwax alcohols ointments. These differences, however, become insignificant in the lower layers of the SC.

In a particularly interesting study, Wepierre and associates explored the deposition of ^{14}C-labelled α-linoleic acid in SC from 100 mg of a 1% emulsion two,

Table VII. Distribution profile of linoleic acid*
in rat stratum corneum

Strips	Time after single application			Time after last multiple application	
	2 hrs	6 hrs	24 hrs	24 hrs	72 hrs
1-5	62±12	27±5	12±3	8±1	8±2
6-20	18±4	6±1	5±1	7±1	6±1

*Sum of [14]C- linoleic acid in mg/cm² found in first five strips and in last 15 strips

(After Reference 88)

six, and 24 hours after a single application.[88] The distribution within the SC, as determined by adhesive tape strippings, was exponential 24 hours after inunction with the emulsion (Figure 14). In addition to the expected decrease with depth within the SC, their data also disclose a decrease at each depth with time elapsed since inunction (Table VII). In the multiple application program 50 mg of emulsion was applied once daily for six days with no rinse or wipe-off until prior to stripping or biopsying. It is remarkable that multiple repeat applications yielded relatively low levels of linoleic acid in the SC. This supports the finding that linoleic acid permeates the SC and accumulates in the VE and dermis (Figure 15). Only small amounts are trapped in the SC. These probably represent distributional levels of linoleic acid between the SC, the VE, and the dermis.

The presence of α-linoleic acid in dermis raises some questions about the existence of sink conditions in vivo. This is a crucial issue in subdermal tissue loading since the polyunsaturated fatty acid evidently was not "captured" by the circulatory system. This type of permeant accumulation or sorption in lower strata may play an important role in topical therapy, a subject critically reviewed by Guy and Maibach in 1983.[89]

Sorption of fatty acids by SC appears to be a general phenomenon, as demonstrated, for example, by Golden et al.[61] The presence of various extrane-

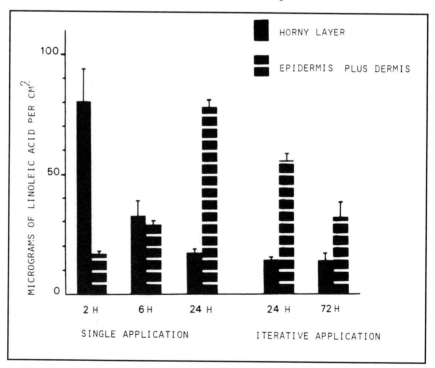

Figure 15. Distribution of ¹⁴C-linoleic acid in stratum corneum and in the viable epidermis plus dermis after a single application or multiple applications. Reproduced by permission of the copyright owner, *Journal of the Society of Cosm. Chem.*, from Reference 88.

ously administrered C-18 fatty acids in pig SC accounts for spectral shifts, for altered transition temperatures, and for changes in the flux of salicylic acid, as shown in Table VIII.

The unusual partitioning of nicotine and of phosphate-buffered nicotine into hydrated human SC is the subject of a paper by Oakley and Swarbrick.[90] Their data shows that the unionized and ionized forms of nicotine partition into different domains of the SC (in accordance with the general precepts of the pH-partition hypothesis). Their work demonstrates that unionized nicotine partitions into the lipid fraction of SC, while the ionized form diffuses into the hydrated—perhaps proteinaceous—fraction of the SC. There is general agreement on the existence of protein and lipid domains in SC. However, agreement on the precise location of a permeant within the SC during its passage through the SC is lacking.[1,91]

Sorption of lipophilic substances by SC and their persistence on the skin despite washing procedures are important for the performance of cosmetic products. Typical are the studies by Iwata et al.[92] and by Klimisch and Chandra.[93] In the former, sorption of ^{14}C-labelled lipid materials into guinea pig foot pad SC was measured by immersing a piece of SC (conditioned at 55% RH) into a sample solution and wiping it before the sorbed lipid was counted. N-Dodecane was relatively poorly sorbed from squalene (S) or castor oil (C) but sorbed more readily from triethylcitrate (T). Lauryl alcohol was sorbed more extensively from S than the hydrocarbon. Lauric acid was extensively sorbed from S; but its sorption from C or T was equal to that of lauryl alcohol. The resistance of silicone oils to removal from skin by washing with soap was demonstrated in the second study.[93] Although the term substantivity could be used for the reported observations, it appears more likely that the residual polydimethylsiloxane found on the skin merely was incompletely removed by the soap wash.

Another study is worthy of note, since it showed a remarkably high degree of retention of tagged isostearoyl lactylate on porcine skin after application from a cream.[94] In this case, repeated rinsings with water failed to remove a large portion of the initially deposited lactylate.

Table VIII. Effect of C-18 fatty acids on pig stratum corneum

Fatty Acid	IR Frequency (cm^{-1})	Transition Temperature (°C; by DSC)	Salicylic Acid Flux (mg cm^{-2} h^{-1})
Octadecenoic	2918.1	62.5	1.21
cis-6-Octadecenoic	2919.0	60.5	0.79
trans-6-Octadecenoic	2919.0	62.0	0.97
cis-9-Octadecenoic	2920.0	59.0	3.81
trans-9-Octadecenoic	2919.4	61.5	2.35
cis-11-Octadecenoic	2920.1	57.0	5.53
trans-11-Octadecenoic	2918.8	61.0	1.11
None	2918.8	62.0	-

(After Reference 61)

The SC sorption of several radiolabelled cosmetic ingredients by human skin grafted on the athymic nude mouse was tested by Petersen et al.[95] In these experiments the SC was stripped four hours after application and subsequent washing, and the amount of radioactivity recovered in 20 strippings was determined. The percentage of recovered radiolabelled substance was about 7% in the case of lactic acid (pH 7.0), 6% in the case of alanine (pH 6.0), 17% in the case of urea (pH 7.2), and 4.5% in the case of p-aminobenzoic acid. These results demonstrate that human SC does have the capacity of sorbing low molecular weight hydrophilic substances.

Stripping with adhesive tape was used to demonstrate that several dyes (Basic Red 76 [CI 12245], Basic Brown 16 [CI 12250], Basic Brown 17 [CI 12251], Basic Yellow 57 [CI 12719], and Solvent Blue [CI 61554]) are retained almost quantitatively within human SC.[96] This experiment was an attempt to confirm absence of systemic human toxicity of cosmetic dyes by demonstrating their retention by SC.

Penetration into and retention by SC of typical UV-absorbing sunscreens is clearly desirable. The recently published data of Hoppe and Sauermann[97] suggest that the distribution of both oil-soluble and water-soluble sunscreens in SC (applied from 1% i-propanol solution to man) follow the exponential pattern typified by Figures 3, 4A and 7. One hour after application, the concentration (weight/unit area) of the water-soluble sunscreen in the first stripping is about 1/4 that of the oil-soluble sunscreens. After about ten strippings, the concentrations are much reduced and more comparable. These findings are not unexpected and conform to currently accepted principles.

It has been known for some years that certain antimicrobial agents can be adsorbed onto human SC during normal washing (soap or surfactant) procedures. The presence of the residual bacteriostat on the skin can be demonstrated quite readily by microbiological techniques[98,99] or radiographic procedures.[100] On the other hand, no scientific investigations of the mechanism of adsorption and of release of the antimicrobial have been performed. The principles underlying this phenomenon affect the performance of surgical scrubs and industrial hygiene products. Some of the major concerns, including that of residual activity, were reviewed a few years ago by Kaul and Jewett.[101]

The presence of ^{14}C-trichlorocarbanilide (TCC) on guinea pig skin was clearly demonstrated by Rutherford and Black.[100] As is the case with other sorbed substances, TCC levels are highest on the skin surface, dropping to low levels at a skin depth of 200 μ. In man, TCC was found in the follicles, sebaceous glands and the sweat glands. In the case of zinc pyrithione, sorption by guinea pig skin seems more pronounced than that of TCC. The more recent tape stripping results (human) and the skin permeation (rats) data of North-Root et al. demonstrate again that the deposition of TCC in lower layers of human SC is minimal and that the amount of TCC permeating rat skin is exceedingly small.[102]

It is likely that high concentrations of topically applied antimicrobial drugs are found only on the skin surface. For example, 90% of the applied dose of econazole does not penetrate deeply into SC.[103] Unless the antimicrobial drugs are substantive, they may therefore be readily removed by washing.

Dansyl chloride is a fluorescent chemical that reportedly binds only to "dead" SC when applied from acetone solution or from 5% dispersion in soft paraffin.[99,104,105] Dansyl chloride is chemically bound to SC from soft petrolatum, reaching the lower layers of SC in man after about 24 hours of application as shown by tape stripping. Dansyl chloride is tightly bound by chemisorption to SC and retained until the SC is sluffed.

By contrast, another highly reactive chemical, 2,4-dinitrochlorobenzene in 0.2% ethanolic solution, can penetrate guinea pig SC rapidly to reach the dermis, as reported by Nakagawa.[106] Dinitrochlorobenzene, which forms the powerful allergenic dinitrophenyl hapten, is rarely encountered by man.

On the other hand, Ni^{2+} is one of the most ubiquitous sensitizers. $^{63}Ni^{2+}$ readily diffuses through the epidermis to the dermis in the presence of surfactants.[107] More recently, the storage site of Ni^{2+} in human skin (in vitro) was again identified as the epidermis.[108] These investigators report in addition that the amount of Ni^{2+} found in the epidermis increased with the time after application and was highly dependent on the vehicle used.

The slow penetration of heparin and its deposition in the dermis have been known for almost 30 years (see Reference 30 for a summary). This phenomenon has played a role in the assessment of the upper range of the molecular weight of compounds that can permeate the skin. A surprising report dealing with the in-vitro deposition of a glycosaminoglycan (GAG) in human dermis appeared much more recently.[109] Elling demonstrated the presence of the GAG polysulfuric acid ester by metachromatic staining of cells in the dermis. In these experiments, no evidence for the presence of the GAG in the "superficial epithelial cells" was obtained. Confirmation of these data appears desirable because the ability of such a large molecule to pass through SC without evidence of sorption is completely unexpected.

Concluding Comments

Examination of theoretical concepts makes it possible to identify some of the factors controlling the sorption of topically applied substances into various layers of skin. Although the published theoretical framework is directed toward explanations of skin permeation, some important factors concerning sorptive processes in skin can be deduced inferentially. For this purpose, factors which generally form the basis of comprehensive reviews of skin permeation can be fruitfully examined to determine how these factors affect skin sorption.[30,110-114]

The information (experimental data discussed in the last half of this chapter) devoted to practical aspects of sorption is essentially limited to casual observation of sorption. The only exceptions to this generalization are data dealing with SC as a drug storage organ. It is apparent that—as a rule—quantification of a compound's sorption within the skin is not the primary goal of the investigator. Thus, data on the site(s) of sorption, chemical or physical characteristics of the sorbate, and permanence of sorption within the skin are essentially lacking. In this chapter both general concepts and experimental data were examined with the goal of deducing some information on skin sorption.

Reviews of the subject of skin permeation identify many contributing factors.[30,109-113] An effort has been made in this review to address most of the factors shown to impact skin sorption (Table IX).

Despite the scarcity of hard data on skin sorption and desorption, these two phenomena can contribute to toxic manifestations and pharmacological effi-

Table IX. Factors affecting skin permeation and sorption		
Biological		
	Thickness	Hydration
	Age	Region
	Blood flow	Species
	Metabolism	
Permeant factors		
	Molecular weight	State of dissociation
	Partition coefficient	Concentration
	Solubility	Molecular size (diffusivity)
	Binding	
Vehicle factors		
	Penetrating properties	Release
	Accelerant	Thermodynamic activity
	Occlusivity	pH
	Surfactant	
Physical factors		
	Temperature	Time
	Climate	
Trauma		
	Mechanical	Chemical
	Disease	

cacy. The retention of a substance in the skin can be reversed by subsequent administration of a second substance. The initially sorbed material is then freed to continue its passage toward the VE. The potential for the displacement of a bound glucocorticosteroid by a second steroid was demonstrated by Baker et al, who showed, for example, that corticosterone could displace cortisol in rat epidermis (see also Reference 78).[114] One can also conceive of chemical interactions between two substances within the skin or of inactivation due to complexation. One may well wonder how many sensitizers have been "identified" by patch test when, in fact, the body responded to a previously sorbed substance which had been innocuously stored in the SC. Sorption by SC or VE also plays a key role in the decontamination problems faced by health professionals in agricultural and industrial hygiene.[116]

The growing awareness of the contribution of epidermal sorption to pharmacological efficacy and systemic and local toxicity is expected to serve as an impetus to more extensive investigations of skin sorption phenomena.

In Vivo Methods for the Assessment of Percutaneous Absorption in Man

By Thomas J. Franz, Paul A. Lehman and E. Lynn McGuire

There has been an explosive growth of interest in the field of percutaneous absorption over the past decade and, as a result of increased investigative efforts, our understanding of the movement of drugs and toxic substances through the skin has greatly matured. In surveying the expanding literature in the field, it can be noted that the majority of studies make use of animal and in vitro models.

The utility of these models has been amply demonstrated over the years, and it is clear that their use will continue to predominate. However, as extrapolation of results to humans is the ultimate goal, it is also clear that some questions can only be addressed or, at the very least are best addressed, through human studies. Yet, unfortunately, studies conducted on living persons represent only a small percentage of those conducted in the field of percutaneous absorption.

Though the latitude of experimental design is often restricted when working with human subjects, these limitations are seldom crucial and are more than balanced by data which are eminently relevant and not subject to extrapolation error. Since human experimentation represents one area in the field where increased activity is sorely needed, this discussion will focus on some of the more common and simple methods used to measure percutaneous absorption in live human subjects.

Historical Perspective

The systematic investigation of the permeability of human skin did not begin until the 1950s. It was largely the result of radioactive tracers becoming available for medical use. The pioneering studies were quite crude by today's standards but, nonetheless, were effective in demonstrating the limited and variable permeability of skin. Early efforts were directed at corticosteroid drugs because they were the new therapeutic drugs of that era and interest in their topical use was great.

The first human study of percutaneous absorption which successfully demonstrated that the skin was permeable to topically applied drugs was conducted by Malkinson and Ferguson.[1] Using radioactive (^{14}C) hydrocortisone (HC) incorporated at 2.5% in an ointment base, they showed that topical application of a finite dose to the forearms of two subjects resulted in the appearance of radioactivity in the urine over the entire collection period of six days. Total urinary excretion of hydrocortisone was estimated to be less than 1% of the applied dose. The peak rate of urinary excretion of radioactivity was seen during the second day, implying that either the rate of HC metabolism or excretion from the body is slow, or that its rate of absorption through the skin is slow. We now know that the latter explanation is the correct one.

In a subsequent study Malkinson et al.[2] measured urinary excretion of radioactivity following topical application of 2.5% ^{14}C-cortisone acetate (CA) in an ointment base. Application of a finite dose was made to the forearms of three subjects; the protocol was similar to that used previously for HC. The results were also similar—radioactivity was detected in the urine over the entire six-day collection period and less than 1% of the applied dose was excreted by this route. The only difference observed was in the peak rate of excretion, which occurred during the first rather than the second day, implying a faster rate of absorption for CA than HC.

Using a different experimental approach, the "disappearance" technique, Malkinson[3] studied the absorption of testosterone as well as both HC and CA following topical application. In this study absorption was assessed by measuring the disappearance of radioactivity from the surface of the skin using a thin end-window, gas-flow beta detector. Each compound was incorporated in an ointment base at 2.5% and applied as a finite dose to 1 cm[2] of the flexor forearm. Testosterone (T) was also applied from a second vehicle consisting of 1% ethanol in petroleum ether. Permeation at sites from which the barrier layer had been removed by tape-stripping was studied as well as on normal skin.

When applied to normal skin, absorption of HC and CA as judged by the disappearance technique was not detectable when the observation period was limited to 4-6 hours (Figure 1). In stripped skin, however, significant absorption was seen with HC but not CA. Surface radioactivity had dropped to 10-22% of the initial activity by six hours. No absorption was noted for T during the first six hours when applied to normal skin from an ointment vehicle, but surface radioactivity dropped to 75-85% of the dose by 6-7 hours when an ether vehicle was used. Absorption of T from the ointment base was only detectable when the observation period was extended (decreasing to 41-58% of initial activity at 48 hours), or following application to stripped skin (decreasing to 9-22% at three hours).

In a subsequent study, Malkinson and Kirschenbaum[4] used both the "disappearance" technique and urinary excretion to measure the percutaneous absorption of another corticosteroid, triamcinolone acetonide. When applied to normal skin, urinary excretion of radioactivity was similar to that seen with HC and ranged from 0.6-2.3% of the dose in two subjects. When applied to stripped skin, only 20% of the activity was detectable on the surface after 20-24 hours.

A number of conclusions can be drawn from these early studies on percutaneous absorption in human subjects. It is evident that the use of radioisotopes made the detection of low levels of absorption possible. However, the technique used was of critical importance. The measurement of compounds having a slow rate of absorption, e.g., corticosteriods such as hydrocortisone and triamcinolone acetonide, is not possible with the disappearance technique. It lacks the necessary sensitivity. Presumably, for compounds displaying a very rapid rate of absorption, or in situations where absorption through damaged skin is being measured, the disappearance technique might prove adequate. It has the

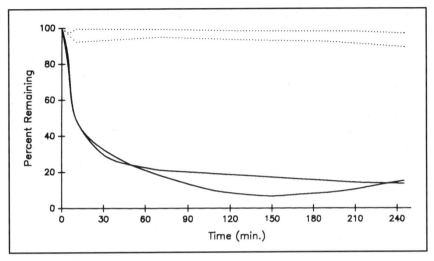

Figure 1. Disappearance of ^{14}C-hydrocortisone from surface of skin following application as 2.5% ointment to normal skin (dotted lines) or stripped skin (solid lines). Data redrawn from Reference 3.

advantage of great simplicity since it does not require the quantitative collection of urine or feces, nor is there need for the processing and analysis of numerous specimens.

However, one major objection to the use of the disappearance technique is that it equates disappearance with absorption. There are numerous situations where this assumption is invalid. Obviously, compounds which exhibit any degree of volatility could never be accurately measured with this technique. Likewise, loss of topically applied materials to the environment can occur through the normal physiological process of exfoliation, whereby the outer cells of the stratum corneum are shed as new cells form at the inner surface. Thus, even if the site of application were protected to prevent wash off or rub off, the continuous microscopic shedding of corneocytes results in loss of surface material which could erroneously be perceived as "absorption." This becomes an even greater problem in diseases with increased epidermal turnover such as psoriasis. Thus, for the disappearance technique to have reliable applicability, some definition of the conditions surrounding its use must be established for a given compound.

The successful use by Malkinson of urinary excretion as a means by which to quantitate the absorption of topically applied drugs set the stage for subsequent investigators. To this day, it remains the standard method for assessment of percutaneous absorption.

Urinary Excretion Method

The most detailed, systematic investigations of percutaneous absorption in living man are those of Feldmann and Maibach.[5-8] Like the earlier studies of

Malkinson, the compounds initially evaluated were the corticosteroids and the technique used to quantify absorption that of urinary excretion of radioactivity. Modifications of this technique have subsequently been made by others to better suit the compound, formulation, or conditions of application (or exposure in the case of toxicants), but the basic elements of the protocol have remained the same and will be examined in detail here.

In the Feldmann and Maibach protocol, the compound of interest was dissolved in acetone and applied to a defined area on the volar forearm at a dose of 4 μgrams/cm². This dose was chosen because it approximates the very small doses of corticosteroids used by patients in a clinical setting. The size of the application site was variable from compound to compound and determined by the interplay of three factors:

1) the specific activity of the compound under study (μCi/mg),
2) the radioactive dose (total amount of μCi to be applied), and
3) the drug dose (4 μgrams/cm²).

Compounds having a low specific activity required larger areas of application in order to achieve the desired radioactive dose, yet not exceed the target drug dose. On the other hand, compounds of very high specific activity required dilution with cold drug if the 4 μgram/cm² dose was to be maintained without exceeding either the desired or safe radioactive dose.

Following application of the compound under study in an acetone vehicle, the acetone was gently blown dry so that it did not remain on the skin for more than 15 seconds. This brief exposure to a lipid solvent such as acetone was not felt to be damaging to the lipid barrier of the skin. The application site was then left unprotected but the subjects were instructed to avoid bathing for 24 hours. All urinary output was collected over the next 5-10 days and analyzed for radioactive content. In order to correct for radioactivity excreted via other routes, an intravenous (IV) dose of the same compound was given. Determination of the fraction of an IV dose excreted in the urine allows for the calculation of total absorption following a topical dose according to the following equation.

$$\frac{\text{Total}}{\text{Absorption}} = \frac{\text{total urinary excretion (topical dose)}}{\text{fractional urinary excretion (IV dose)}}$$

Thus, one assumption upon which this technique is based is that the relationship between the routes of excretion following an intravenous dose are the same as when the drug enters the systemic circulation through the skin. If 75% of drug molecules entering the systemic circulation via an intravenous dose are excreted in the urine, then 75% of drug molecules entering the systemic circulation percutaneously are assumed to be excreted in the urine.

Although the literature contains no critical evaluation of this assumption, one situation of potential concern can be envisioned. When the compound of interest is directly injected into the blood stream, it is the unmetabolized parent compound which is injected. When the same compound is applied to the skin, it cannot be assumed that it is only the unmetabolized species that enter the bloodstream. The skin has significant metabolic activity; there are a number of studies which have demonstrated simultaneous metabolism and absorption of topically applied drugs.[9-11] Thus, one critical assumption underlying the use of the urinary excretion method needs further evaluation.

Specific Considerations

Proper use of the urinary excretion method requires that consideration be given to a number of specific details. Among these are site of application, the size of the dose, application time, collection time and fecal collection. All of these factors can significantly affect the results. Failure to adequately consider the impact of each can lead to results which are either erroneous or not directly applicable to the clinical or use situation.

Site of Application: Since it is now well known that there are regional variations in percutaneous absorption,[6,12,13] the site chosen for application of the radioactive material should reflect its intended site of use or exposure. This is particularly true for products intended for use on the face or scalp where absorption is generally much higher than elsewhere on the body, often 5- to 10-fold higher. Intertriginous areas (axillae, groin) also deserve special consideration since the increased hydration of the skin at those sites also results in significantly increased absorption. One area that has invariably been found to be of unusually high permeability is the scrotum. It appears to be the highest absorbing site in the body.

Generally, differences in absorption observed over the rest of the body (trunk and extremities) are not as great as those observed in the previously mentioned sites, with the exception of palms and soles which tend to show somewhat lower rates of absorption. Guy and Maibach[14] have taken data on regional variation based on the use of two pesticides (parathion and malathion), as well as hydrocortisone, and constructed absorption indices for five anatomical sites (See Table I). Although it is possible that regional differences in absorption may be found to have more compound or vehicle dependence than seen with those three compounds, the indices can serve as a useful first approximation.

The forearm is the most popular site of application because it is the most convenient site for both subject and investigator. It is also a convenient site for the design and construction of relatively simple devices to protect the applied

Table I. Penetration index for five anatomical sites*		
Site	Based on Hydrocortisone	Based on Pesticides
Genitals	40	12
Arms	1	1
Legs	0.5	1
Trunk	2.5	3
Head	5	4

*From Reference 14

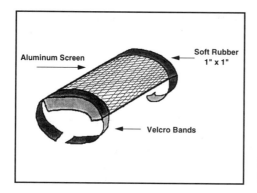

Figure 2. A homemade device
to protect a topical application
to the forearm.

material from ruboff. This is an important consideration from the standpoint of both experimental design and control and, if radioisotopes are being used, from the standpoint of radiation containment and safety. Inexpensive devices can be made from materials obtained at a hardware store. For example, a forearm device can be constructed from heavy aluminum screen (0.25" x 0.5" grid; manufactured to protect entrance screen-doors from pets), dense soft rubber floor mat (1" thick) and Velcro® closure strips. The materials are cut to desired dimension and assembled with cyanoacrylate adhesive (Figure 2).

One drawback to the use of the forearm as the site of application, aside from the relevance issue, is its relatively small available surface area. When much larger areas are required, e.g. because of radiation dosimetry considerations or the need to apply large amounts of drug for the determination of blood levels, the trunk becomes the next logical choice.

Repeated Application: Since the use of most topical preparations involves multiple applications to the same skin (or chronic exposure in the case of toxicants), it may be of importance to determine if repeated applications lead to changes in the absorption profile. This is particularly critical in situations where there is reason to believe that chronic use may lead to barrier damage.

Several human studies have been conducted using labeled drugs in which percutaneous absorption has been measured first through previously untreated skin and, approximately one week later, through skin that has continued to receive daily treatment with an unlabeled version of the same formulation.[15,16] In these studies no evidence of a significant change in absorption was noted after one week of continuous treatment (Table II). Since the limited number of compounds examined to date makes it impossible to generalize to other chemicals or chemical classes, this will continue to be an area which needs further evaluation.

Drug and Formulation Dose: Since percutaneous absorption is known to obey Fick's law, careful consideration is generally given to the concentration of drug in the dosing formulation. For the data to be meaningful, drug concentration should approximate the use condition. In the case of commercial or development formulations, the concentration is usually fixed and not subject to experimental

Table II. Effect of repeat application on percutaneous absorption[a]				
	Minoxidil	Hydrocortisone	Testosterone	Estradiol
Dose 1	3.9 ± 2.9	2.6 ± 0.7	22.1 ± 6.9	9.9 ± 2.3
Dose 2[b]	2.4 ± 1.0	3.4 ± 1.4	20.2 ± 6.8	10.8 ± 4.7

[a]Data from References 15 and 16, expressed as % of Dose ± S.D.
[b]Dose 2 given at Day 7, day 9 for minoxidil.

variation. However, what may be forgotten is the equally important issue of formulation dose. Though the *concentration* of the test drug is fixed (e.g., 1%), total drug *dose* to the skin (μgrams/cm²) is a function of the amount of formulation applied (Figure 3). Relevant data can only be obtained when the formulation dose approximates use conditions. For creams and ointments, it has been observed that subjects generally apply 2-3 mg of product per cm² of skin.[17]

However, the tendency in protocol design is often to apply much larger amounts of formulation since:

1) there is greater ease and accuracy in the application of larger doses, and

2) the analytical task is made easier.

The fallacy in this approach, however, is that both the rate of absorption and total absorption are a function of the size of the applied dose under finite dose conditions.[18] Thus, the use of inappropriately large formulation doses can lead to a significant overestimation of total systemic absorption, as well as of maximum flux rate and peak blood level.

Application Time: It is advisable to apply the test formulation for a specific period of time and then remove it. This may be dictated by radiation dosimetry considerations but, even if not, it is generally relevant to experimental objectives. Most topically applied compounds are poorly absorbed through the skin. The source of the flux, even after many hours, continues to be drug remaining on the surface of the skin, not that inside the skin (Figure 4). Thus, physical removal of the surface source (e.g., by washing) results in a rapid decline of the flux.

When trying to duplicate clinical or use conditions, one should consider the length of time the product would normally remain on the skin. For many

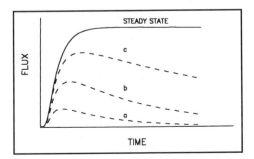

Figure 3. The relationship between amount of applied formulation, where a, b, and c represent increasing amounts, and the rate of drug absorption (flux). Application of an "infinitely" large amount would result in attainment of a steady-state flux.

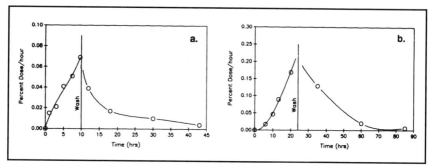

Figure 4. The effect of a skin surface wash on the rate of urinary excretion of topically applied drugs; (a) a soap and water wash of the face 10 hours following a single appplication of 0.05% retinoic acid cream (Reference 19), (b) soap and water wash of the trunk 24 hours following two applications (q 12 hrs) of sulconazole nitrate cream (Reference 20).

products, removal may be linked to the daily bathing routine and 24 hours is a reasonable application time. For others, such as facial products applied at night (e.g., retinoic acid), removal at 8-12 hours seems more appropriate since this would approximate the timing of a morning face wash. Drugs to which the skin is exposed via shampoo or bath would obviously have even shorter contact times.

Collection Time: Urinary collections should be continued until background levels of radioactivity are reached. Although this commonly will be 5-7 days, longer times may be necessary for some compounds (those with long turnover times). Failure to appreciate this factor can result in significant experimental error. Two examples from the literature illustrate this point.

Total absorption of nicotinic acid and thiourea following application from an acetone vehicle were originally determined to be 0.3 and 0.9% of the applied dose, respectively.[8] This data was based on a five-day collection period. Subsequent experiments found that measurable levels of radioactivity could be found in the urine for at least 21 days and that total absorption was, in fact, four-fold greater for thiourea and ten-fold greater for nicotinic acid.[21] (A portion of the error in the original estimate of nicotinic acid absorption was also due to an erroneous intravenous correction factor.)

Compounds for which the rate of excretion continues at low levels for long periods of time must be dosed with sufficiently high levels of radioactivity to make long collection times feasible. This may necessitate use of a large area of application. One can anticipate this type of situation, and plan accordingly, if intravenous administration of the drug is done prior to topical administration. Increasing the size of the area of application will allow application of an increased total radioactive dose while at the same time maintaining any desired drug dose (μgrams/cm^2) or formulation dose (mg/cm^2).

Another issue related to collection time that shouldn't be ignored is the *frequency* of collections, particularly during the early phase of the experiment. Accurate determination of the kinetics of absorption of rapidly absorbed compounds is possible only if frequent urine specimens are collected at early times (Figure 5). One hour collection intervals are recommended for at least the first 4-6 hours. This can be accomplished by having the subjects drink 5-10 fl.oz. of water prior to drug application and every two hours thereafter. By pushing fluids it is generally possibly for volunteers to void by the clock at hourly intervals.

Fecal Collection: Simultaneous collection of feces should be incorporated into the protocol in situations where this represents a significant route of excretion for the compound under study. This will usually be known from animal studies or if a prior intravenous study has been done in humans. Fecal collection is absolutely essential in cases where this route represents the main route of excretion and only limited amounts of drug are excreted in the urine. When the urinary route of excretion is very low, the IV correction factor can become quite large and is subject to high variablilty. This has the potential to introduce significant error into the calculation of total absorption, if one is relying solely on urinary excretion data.

DDT is a compound that illustrates the problem. In the monkey, Bartek and LaBudde[22] found that only 0.4% of an intravenously administered dose was excreted in the urine, giving a correction factor for topical application of 250 (100/0.4). Use of this factor to estimate total absorption of DDT in the rhesus monkey following topical application led to the erroneous value of 375% of the applied dose. Thus, the larger the IV correction factor, the greater the error introduced into the calculation of total absorption when using only urinary excretion data.

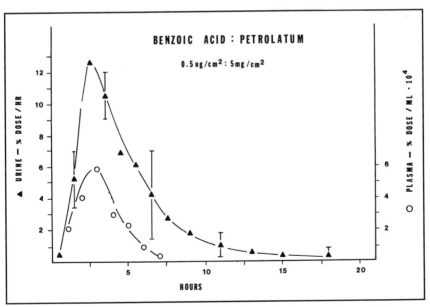

Figure 5. The correlation of drug plasma levels and urinary excretion rate from the topical application of ^{14}C-benzoic acid in a petrolatum vehicle.

Blood Collection

Although the determination of blood levels is an essential component of studies involving other routes of administration, its utility in topical drug studies is problematic because of the combination of 1) low total absorption, and 2) slow rates of absorption. Very sensitive methods of assay are generally needed for the identification of plasma levels of topically applied materials. A case in point is that of topical retinoids currently used in the treatment of acne. Isotretinoin 0.05% gel (13-cis retinoic acid, Isotrex®) was applied twice daily for four weeks at an excessive dose to 1900 cm² of skin in order to determine steady-state blood levels. However, at no time during the study were detectable levels found in any of the volunteers using an HPLC assay sensitive to 20 ng/ml. [23] The same was found to be true for the all-trans isomer of retinoic acid (Tretinoin, Retin-A®) in a similar, but not identical, subchronic dosing study.[24] These results can be contrasted with oral studies of Isotretinoin (Accutane®) absorption in which steady-state blood levels of 160 ng/ml and peak levels over 400 ng/ml were measured (Physicians Desk Reference).

In the future the development of more sensitive assay procedures will facilitate the determination of blood levels of topically applied agents. For example, using the technique of radioimmunoassay (RIA), it was possible to determine plasma levels of the corticosteroid betamethasone 17-benzoate in patients treated for seven days under occulsion.[25] Drug levels were found to vary from 0.3 to 5 ng/ml in these patients, all of whom had some form of eczema or psoriasis.

Stable Isotopes: An alternative to the use of radioactive isotopes are the stable elemental isotopes such as ^2H and ^{13}C. When stable isotopes (nonradioactive) are incorporated into the test compound its molecular weight increases slightly (+1 for each replacement atom) without appreciable alteration of its chemical-physical properties. Measurement of their presence in the collected samples is by mass spectrometry, most often following analytical isolation by chromatography.

There are several advantages to the use of stable isotopes:
1) when a radioactively labeled compound is not available and other assay procedures are too insensitive,
2) when radiation dosimetry considerations exceed safe limits or unduly restrict the conduct of the study,
3) when one wishes to study infants, children or child-bearing/breast-feeding females where radioactivity exposure is contraindicated,
4) when the test compound is also an endogenous chemical and use of a radioisotope is impossible for one or more of the above reasons.

The measurement of stable labeled compounds by mass spectrometry insures high sensitivity for detection as well as the ability to specifically detect the labeled compound separately from an endogenous source by mass weight difference. With the recent introductions of small bench-top mass spectrometers which cost no more than other routine chromatography equipment, mass spectrometry has become affordable to more laboratories.

An excellent example for the study of percutaneous absorption where use of a stable isotope proved to be the critical factor is provided by West et al.[26] The permeability of preterm infant skin was assessed with $^{13}C_6$ benzoic acid. After topical exposure of the infants, their urine was collected and analyzed for benzoic acid and its primary metabolite hippuric acid by GC/MS. Use of the stable isotope permitted the measurement of the absorbed ^{13}C-benzoic acid and its ^{13}C-hippuric acid metabolite separately from the excretion of the infant's endogenous benzoic acid and hippuric acid. There was no risk to the infants from the test compound or its label and, because of this, important data demonstrating the increased permeability of preterm infant skin was obtained.

Mass Balance Method

A recently introduced modification of the urinary excretion method is the mass balance technique,[27] which has the advantage of being able to account for all topically applied material. The basics of the method are patterned after the original Feldmann and Maibach protocol.[5,7] Radioactive compounds at a dose of 4 μgrams/cm^2 are applied to the forearm of human volunteers. Percutaneous absorption is assessed from the excretion of radioactivity in urine corrected for excretion via other routes. However, with the new technique the application site is covered with a semirigid polypropylene chamber* which is taped to the skin. Absorption can be measured under either occluded or nonoccluded conditions by employing the chamber in either closed or vented fashion. To vent the chamber, holes are drilled such that approximately 50% of the surface area is open to the atmosphere. To prevent loss of drug from the surface through desquamation, the holes are covered with 0.2 micron pore-size Gore-Tex® membrane.** This material does not retard transepidermal water loss and therefore does not lead to increased hydration of the stratum corneum.

Twenty-four hours following application, the chamber is removed and analyzed for trapped radioactivity, and the application site is washed using a standardized washing procedure. All wash material is also analyzed for radioactive content. The application site is then covered with a new chamber which remains in place for six days. At the end of this period, the chamber is removed and analyzed for radioactive content and a second wash performed. Following the wash, the application site itself is stripped ten times with adhesive tape† and the tape is analyzed for radioactive content.

With this new method, it is possible to account for what is normally the single biggest source of loss following topical application, that which is lost from the surface of the skin from desquamation, ruboff and washoff. In addition, tape-stripping the stratum corneum at the end of the experiment recovers any test compound remaining (possibly bound) within the barrier. In principle, it should be possible to account for all of the applied radioactivity material and, thus, avoid one of the questions that always accompanies the estimation of total percutaneous absorption: Where is all of the unrecovered material?

That this new method does, indeed, result in better accountability and truly approach total mass balance can be seen from examination of the results obtained on four steroid compounds by Bucks et al.[27] as presented in Table III. For comparison, data obtained in human subjects on the percutaneous absorption of minoxidil,[15] the imidazole antifungal sulconazole nitrate,[20] and retinoic

---

* Hilltop Research Inc., Cincinnati, OH
** W.L. Gore and Associates, Inc., Elkton, MD
† Scotch Brand Tape, 3M, St. Paul, MN

Table III. Comparison of recoveries:
Mass balance versus urinary excretion method

Compound	Total Absorption	Total Recovery
Urinary Excretion Method		
Minoxidil	3.9%	47%
Sulconazole	6.7	43
Retinoic acid	1.1	51
Mass Balance Method		
Hydrocortisone	4.4	89
Estradiol	3.4	100
Progesterone	13	96
Testosterone	18	96

Data taken from References 15, 19, 20, 27

acid[19] as measured by the urinary excretion method are also included.

Total recovery of the four steroid compounds using the mass balance technique with vented (nonoccluded) semirigid polypropylene chambers ranged from 89-100% of the dose. In fact, three of the four compounds showed 96% recovery or better. In contrast, total recovery of minoxidil, sulconazole nitrate and retinoic acid (in which the standard urinary excretion method was used) was only 50% or less. Thus, the applicability of the mass balance method can be easily appreciated.

That material lost from the surface of the skin does indeed represent a significant portion of the total applied dose is shown in Table IV. Of the four steroid compounds shown in Table III, the amount which was trapped in the chamber accounts for 30-55% of the total recoverable radioactivity.

Stratum Corneum Stripping Method

Techniques other than those related to urinary excretion can be used to measure percutaneous absorption in vivo. The disappearance technique, mentioned earlier with its limitations, is one example.

Table IV. Disposition of topically applied steroids

Compound	Chamber	Wash	Strip	Absorbed	Total
Hydrocortisone	30%	54%	2.5%	4.4%	89 %
Estradiol	39	58	0.1	3.4	100
Progesterone	55	27	n.d.	13	96
Testosterone	47	30	n.d.	18	96

Data taken from Reference 27; n.d. = not determined

Another technique, introduced by Rougier's laboratory, utilizes a unique approach to the problem.[12] This technique quantifies total absorption through the measurement of stratum corneum uptake. They have shown that total absorption can be quite accurately estimated by stripping and analyzing the stratum corneum for drug content 30 minutes following application of the test drug. Furthermore, they have shown that the accuracy of the technique is independent of factors known to influence percutaneous absorption. Such complications as variation in dose, vehicle, application time, or anatomical site do not invalidate the method. It has also been shown to be valid in animals as well as humans.

The basis for the technique is quite simple and follows logically from the known properties of the stratum corneum barrier. The stratum corneum is unique among biological barriers in that its dimensions are of the order of microns, not angstroms. The fact that it is a thick barrier, and that diffusivity within it is quite low, results in permeating species being contained within its interstices for a substantial period of time. Thus, following application of a test compound to the skin, there is a period of time during which that fraction which has partitioned into the stratum corneum will be totally contained within. If one quantitatively removes the stratum corneum before significant diffusional loss to the lower layers occurs, one has a measure of total absorption. What this method does not yield is data pertinent to the rate of absorption, such as the time to maximum rate or steady-state, or the magnitude of either of those parameters.

An example of the relationship between stratum corneum content and total absorption is shown in Figure 6. An almost perfect correlation is observed between absorption of the four compounds (benzoic acid, benzoic acid sodium salt, caffeine, acetylsalicylic acid) at various sites in human subjects, measured by the traditional urinary excretion method, and their stratum corneum content 30 minutes after application.

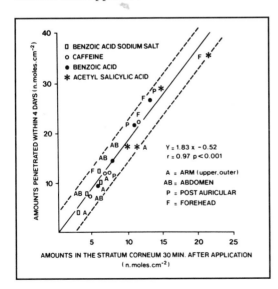

Figure 6. Correlation of total absorption, based on urinary excretion at four days, versus stratum corneum content at 30 minutes. A good linear relationship can be noted independent of compound or anatomical site (from Reference 12 with permission).

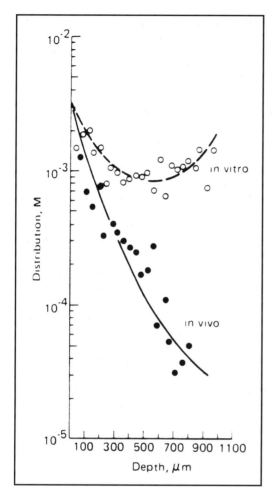

Figure 7. Distribution of hydrocortisone in human skin as determined both in vitro and in vivo by the skin sectioning technique (from Reference 28 with permission).

Skin Sectioning Method

Another specialized technique which adds a new dimension to the in vivo measurement of percutaneous absorption is the skin sectioning technique, largely popularized by Schaefer.[28] Whereas other techniques focus on the quantitation of either total absorption or the rate of absorption, skin sectioning is primarily designed to determine drug content and drug profile within the skin itself (the target organ). The basic elements involve full-thickness skin biopsy and histologic sectioning of the tissue obtained to determine the drug's concentration profile within the skin.

Following topical application of the drug of interest for a defined period of time, the surface is carefully cleansed to remove all unabsorbed material. The horny layer is then removed by multiple tape-stripping and, under local anesthesia, a biopsy is taken from the application site down to and including subcutaneous fat. The biopsy is immediately frozen, placed on a cryomicrotome, and cut into multiple 10-40 micron sections parallel to the skin's surface. Sectioning proceeds from dermis to epidermis, rather than in the reverse direction, so as to avoid carryover of drug from the more highly concentrated upper tissues. Drug concentration in each section can be obtained by any of a number of analytical techniques, but usually radiotracers are used for simplicity.

Since the efficacy of topical therapy is dependent upon the attainment of adequate drug levels within the skin, the above technique is useful for directly assaying the ability of a given formulation to achieve the maximum or desired level. Although in theory, the same approach could be taken in vitro, it has been shown that there are differences between the results obtained in vitro and in vivo (Figure 7). It would appear that the lack of microcirculation in vitro can affect dermal drug content, even though it is without effect on the overall rate of absorption.

Radiation Dosimetry

Because of the considerable complexity of regulations regarding the experimental use of radioactive materials in human subjects, a complete discussion of this issue will not be attempted. Rather, a brief overview of the standards pertaining to radiation dose limits for individuals and guidance for further information is provided below.

Regulatory agencies involved in establishing limits for radiation exposure to individuals from the use of radioactive materials include the Nuclear Regulatory Commission (NRC) and the Food and Drug Administration (FDA). The NRC

Table V. Dose equivalent limits for NRC licensees
(10 CFR 20, 1989; NRC, 1986)

Population	Organ or Tissue	Dose Equivalent Limit, rem Calendar Quarter[1]	Annual[2]
Adult	Whole body[3]	1.25	-
(Occupational)	H_E^4	-	5
	Lens of eyes	-	15
	Skin of whole body[5]	7.5	50
	Hands/forearms/feet/ankle	18.75	-
	Extremities	-	50
Public[6]	H_E	-	0.1

1. Present limits in 10 CFR 20.
2. Limits in 10 CFR 20, to be effective January 1, 1994, limits for minors are one-tenth of the adult limits.
3. Whole body; head and trunk; active blood-forming organs; lens of eyes; or gonads.
4. When internal and external doses are both received, this is actually called in Part 20 the Total Effective Dose Equivalent (TEDE), the sum of the external, deep-dose equivalent and the committed effective dose equivalent (H_E) for internal exposures, excluding the lens of the eyes, the skin and the extremities. See Table VI for details on H_E.
5. The area of the skin to be used for dose calculations is 1 cm^2.
6. The NRC may authorize up to 0.5 rem for an individual member of the public.

establishes limits for both occupational workers and members of the general public,[29] although radiation exposures encountered through diagnostic or therapeutic medical procedures (including research studies) are specifically excluded. The present standards governing occupational exposure are given in Tables V and VI.

A full assessment of potential detriment to an individual must include an evaluation of the radiation dose received by each of the organs listed in Table VI as well as the dose to five other organs or tissues receiving the highest exposure. For radiation sources incorporated into the body, a knowledge of the fate of the materials must be applied to compute the dose. This may be accomplished through the use of metabolic models for different elements (e.g. Reference Man[30]) or, more appropriate to the situation encountered by the dermatopharmacologist, through the use of pre-existing biological data on the compound under investigation. In the present scheme, one would compute the dose to individual organs (H_t), and, using those values, which are limited to 50 rem/yr, compute a parameter termed the Effective Dose Equivalent (H_E). This is found by summing each individual organ weighted dose in accordance with Equation 1:

$$H_E = \Sigma \ (W_t \cdot H_t)$$ (Equation 1)

where W_t is taken from Table VI. H_E is limited to 5 rem/yr.

As stated previously, both routine medical procedures and research uses of radioactive material operate under a different set of dose limits than those that apply to occupational workers and members of the general public. For routine medical procedures, there is no regulatory limit on radiation dose to either a specific organ or H_E.

For experimental procedures, aspects of radiation safety and radiation dose to patients or volunteers are addressed in protocols of studies carried out under one of the following: an Investigational New Drug (IND) issued by the FDA; the local Radiation Safety Committee; or a Radioactive Drug Research Committee (RDRC) authorized by the FDA. The requirements of the IND application and local policies may vary somewhat. However, the requirements of studies carried out under the auspices of an RDRC are clear and are as follows:

Table VI. Organ dose weighting factors used in computation of H_E

Organ or Tissue	W_t
Gonads	0.25
Breast	0.15
Red bone marrow	0.12
Lung	0.12
Thyroid	0.03
Bone surfaces	0.03
Remainder	0.30*

*0.30 results from W_t = 0.06 for each of 5 "remainder organs," the 5 organs in addition to those tabulated that receive the highest doses.

1) The study must be done with an approved drug.
2) The study must be done for the purpose of giving information regarding basic metabolism and kinetics and must not be done as part of a clinical trial.
3) In contrast to other medical studies, doses to individuals are strictly limited as follows:
    a. 3 rem single dose and 5 rem annual or total dose to the whole body (or H_E), active blood forming organs, lens of the eye or gonads, and
    b. 5 rem single dose and 15 rem annual or total dose to any other organ.

These doses must include the dose from other medical procedures carried out during the study, e.g. x-rays.

Special Concerns of the Skin: At present increased attention has been focused on skin dosimetry calculations because of a unique situation which has arisen in the nuclear power industry.[31] Very high radiation doses to localized areas of skin can result from small "hot particles" that lodge on a worker's skin. It has become generally accepted that the radiobiological consequence of this situation (i.e., high doses to small, discrete areas of skin) is not nearly as significant as if larger areas of skin were involved. However, it is also believed to be imprudent to calculate skin exposure by averaging the dose to a localized area over the entire surface area of the skin. Currently, the recommendations from the NRC state that the dose should be calculated by averaging over an area no smaller than 1 cm². Although this applies specifically to occupational exposure, the concept can be applied to volunteer subjects and patients as well. Thus, though most experimental situations will usually involve application to areas of skin larger than 1 cm², and skin dose will be calculated using the size of the actual application area, when the application area is smaller than 1 cm², skin dose should be calculated by averaging over an area of 1 cm².

Another important technical issue that must be considered is the target or site for dose determinations. Since only the basal cell layer is the mitotically active layer of the epidermis, it has generally been taken to be the target of concern for irradiation. Knowledge of its depth from the skin surface is essential to the calculation of dose as most of the applied radioactive compound will not be absorbed into the skin but remain on the surface. For routine radiation protection purposes, the depth at which these cells lie is taken to be 70μm,[32] although this is known to be a function of body location and can vary from 40-150 μm.[33]

Dose calculations: For radioactive materials applied to and transported through the skin, the computation of dose to an individual can be viewed as a consideration of three separate cases:
1) Dose to the basal cells of skin due to the radiation emanating from the distribution of radioactivity fixed on the surface of the skin.
2) Dose to basal cells due to the transport of radioactivity through the skin compartment, i.e., the fraction of applied dose that is taken up or absorbed into the skin.
3) Dose to all other organs of the body due to translocation of radioactivity from the skin compartment into the body via the blood stream.

Case 1 calculations describe the dose due to the radioactive source lying on the surface of the skin whose emissions reach the basal cell layer. Geometrically, the source is usually described as a thin plane or circular source. To perform the calculations for a distributed (non-point) radioactive source, it is customary to resort to the use of a computer program. For photon-emitting sources (gamma or x-rays) the MICROSHIELD computer code may be used.[34]

For the more usual case of electron- or beta-emitting radionuclides, the VARSKIN computer code[35] has been used successfully in common medical applications.[36] The dose is determined by inputting the parameters of nuclide activity, activity area, target area, target depth and length of irradiation time.

The dose to the basal cells from the Case 2 component of total irradiation can be calculated by applying the following principles and assumptions. Assume that the uptake into the skin is immediate and uniform and that the transport out of the skin compartment follows first order kinetics with rate constant k. The dose can then be determined by application of the MIRD schema.[37] In this approach the dose to any target (D_t) can be calculated as:

$$D_t = \tilde{A} \cdot \Delta/m \qquad \text{(Equation 2)}$$

and

$$\tilde{A} = \int_0^{t_i} A_o \exp(-kt)dt \qquad \text{(Equation 3)}$$

where $\tilde{A}$ = cumulated activity (μCi-hr), exp(-kt) = time-activity function, Δ = constant for particular nuclide in g-rad/μCi-hr, m = organ mass in grams, and A_o = fraction of activity applied to skin surface that is absorbed (all of which is assumed to be absorbed instantaneously at t = 0). (Note: 1 rad = 1 rem for most radionuclides used in medicine.)

For Case 3, similar principles as applied in Case 2 are used to compute the dose to other organs. H_E is subsequently calculated or, alternatively, the tables in MIRD 11 may be used. A major problem frequently encountered at this point in the calculations is lack of good information on organ uptake and retention. Whereas the data needed to calculate target dose in Cases 1 and 2 can be easily obtained from in-vitro permeation studies on human cadaver skin or a suitable animal model, the data needed for Case 3 can only be obtained from detailed in-vivo animal studies. Since the type of information needed requires determination of organ radioactivity at multiple points in time, thus the sacrifice of multiple groups of animals, it is not unusual to find those data lacking. When that situation occurs, organ dose can be calculated using the rates of urinary and fecal excretion as estimates of organ clearance and, in addition, employing conservative assumptions.

An Illustrative Example of Dose Calculations

An experiment is planned in which volunteers receive a dose of 10 μCi of ^{14}C applied topically to the skin over an area of 100 cm^2. The substance will be applied in a cream consisting of 1.5 gm. The cream will be removed after a five-hour period. Biological uptake assumptions are as follows:

1) Approximately 5% will be absorbed through the skin into the body.
2) Biological half-time for transport through the skin compartment will be assumed to be equal to that derived from the blood time-activity curve, found to be 50 hours.
3) Data for other organs: Liver-uptake = 1% of initial activity on skin, $T_{1/2,Liv}$ = 100 days; Intestine-uptake = 1% of initial activity on skin, $T_{1/2,GI}$ = 55 hours; Whole body-uptake = 5% of initial activity on skin, $T_{1/2,WB}$ = 100 days.

In these assumptions, a lack of data necessitated a long biological $T_{1/2}$ be estimated conservatively for the liver and whole body.

Case 1 Calculations: Dose due to activity layer on skin irradiating basal cells.
The VARSKIN code requires the assumption of a circular area and we estimate a radius r=5.64 cm for our 100 cm^2 area on the skin (r=$\sqrt{\text{Area}/\pi}$). We assume the basal cell depth to be 40 µm. Since the mass of the substance applied is 1.5 gm and the density is approx. 1 gm/cm^3, the thickness L of the layer on the skin is v/πr^2, where v = volume or mass. Substituting r=5.64 cm and v= 1.5 gm, L=150 µm.

We will assume that the ^{14}C is distributed uniformly through the substance. Since the dose is a function of depth, the total dose will be found by

$$D(T)= \int_{X_{min+b}}^{X_{max+b}} \frac{dD(x)}{dx}\,dx$$

where dD(x)/dx = differential dose at depth x, x_{min+b} and x_{max+b} represent the minimum and maximum distance of the activity from the basal cells, and b represents the basal cell depth. This dose can be approximated by making three separate calculations with VARSKIN.

$$D(T) = D(x_{min+b})+D(x_1)+D(x_{max+b})$$

where 1/3 of the activity (3.33 µCi) is assumed to lie along the planes at distances x_{min+b}, $x_1=[(x_{min}-x_{max})/2]+b$, and x_{max+b}. Inputting these parameters into the VARSKIN code, we have the following results:

D(40µm) = 0.53 rad, D(115µm) = 0.032 rad, D(190µm) = 0 and D(T)=0.56 rad.

Case 2 Calculations: Dose to skin due to activity in skin compartment.
Since the fraction taken into the body was assumed to be 5%, we will assume an initial activity in the skin of 10 • 5%=0.5µCi. From MIRD 4, Δ = 0.105 g-rad/µCi-hr for ^{14}C. The mass of the skin compartment is assumed to be 100 cm^2• x_s cm, where x_s is the full thickness of the skin, assumed to be 0.1 cm.[30] Thus, the mass is 10 gm.

Finding the cumulated activity first, we integrate Eq. 3 from time t=0 to infinity, which reduces to:

$$\tilde{A}=1.44 \bullet A_0 \bullet T_{1/2} = 1.44 \bullet 0.5mCi \bullet 50hr = 37\mu Ci\text{-hr}.$$

Then from Eq. 2:

$$D=0.105 \text{ g-rad}/\mu Ci\text{-hr} \bullet 37\mu Ci\text{-hr}/10 \text{ gm, or } D=0.38 \text{ rad}.$$

Case 3 Calculations: Dose to internal organs.
We may compute the dose to each tissue by using Eqs. 2 and 3 and knowing their masses, or by using the equivalent method of MIRD 11:

$$D_t = \tilde{A} \bullet S$$

where D_t represents the dose to organ t from activity in a source organ s (or t), and S = Δ/m in units of rad/µCi-hr, tabulated in MIRD 11 for each source and target organ pair.

For each of the organs known to have an uptake, we then have their individual doses:

$D_{Whole Body}$ = 1.44•(10µCi•5%)•2400hr•1.5x10^{-6}rad/µCi-hr = 2.6x10^{-3} rad.
D_{Liver} = 1.44•(10µCi•1%)•2400hr•5.8x10^{-5}rad/µCi-hr = 2.0x10^{-2} rad.
D_{GI} = 1.44•(10µCi•1%)•55hr•3.9x10^{-4}rad/µCi-hr = 3.1x10^{-3} rad.

To compute H_E, we assume the dose to the other organs listed in Table VI is represented by the dose to the whole body, and the dose to the "Remainder" is given by the dose to the GI tract and liver. Since the GI tract can be treated as four separate organs—stomach, upper large intestine, lower large intestine and small intestine—we then have:

$$H_E = (W_{WB} \bullet H_{WB}) + (W_{Liver} \bullet H_{Liver}) + (W_{GI} \bullet H_{GI})$$
$$= (0.70 \bullet 2.6 \times 10^{-3}) + (0.06 \bullet 2.0 \times 10^{-2}) + (0.24 \bullet 3.1 \times 10^{-3})$$
$$= 3.8 \times 10^{-3} \text{ rem} = 3.8 \text{ millirem.}$$

The total skin dose from Case 1 and Case 2 is 0.56 + 0.38 = 0.94 rem, well below any applicable dose limit. The maximum dose to any other organ was found to be 20 millirem to the liver. The whole body dose was found to be 2.6 millirem and H_E was found to be 7.8 millirem, also well within guidelines.

In Vitro Methods for Measuring Skin Permeation

By Robert L. Bronaugh and Steven W. Collier

The absorption of chemicals through skin can be measured by in vivo or in vitro techniques. The rate limiting process in percutaneous absorption seems to be the passive diffusion of chemicals through the barrier layer. For most compounds, the rate-controlling membrane is the stratum corneum; but for lipophilic, water-insoluble compounds, diffusion through the viable epidermis is the limiting step.

Absorption has frequently been measured by in vitro techniques because of the simplicity of the experimental conditions. One can accurately sample directly beneath the skin in a diffusion cell, as opposed to the relatively tedious sampling from blood, urine and feces required in an in-vivo experiment to measure the skin permeation rate.

In-vitro studies can minimize or eliminate the use of animals by promoting the use of human tissue and by better utilization of animal tissue. Since human skin is unique in terms of its barrier and metabolic properties, it is the most relevant membrane to use in an absorption study. Potentially toxic compounds often can only be studied in vitro with human tissue. When animal tissue is needed, an animal can be sacrificed before experimentation and will provide the skin for many diffusion cells.

Significant metabolism can occur in the skin during the absorption process. Biotransformations in skin can most readily be studied by in-vitro techniques that maintain the viability of skin. Metabolism observed in biological samples from in-vivo skin permeation experiments cannot be readily separated into the amount that occurred in skin and the amount that occurred in other organs of the body.

For cosmetic scientists, the absorption of cosmetic ingredients into and through the skin can be of major importance. In a general sense, for cosmetic purposes one does not want extensive percutaneous absorption, but rather a sustained local effect at or near the surface of the skin. Enhanced effects of a cosmetic product might be achieved by modifying its formulation to minimize the skin permeation of active ingredients. Safety concerns can arise from the absorption and subsequent systemic distribution of potentially toxic agents or impurities such as nitrosamines that have been found in certain cosmetic products.[1]

In Vitro Methodology

Cell Design: Although many different designs have been utilized for diffusion cell studies, there are really only two basic types: the one-chambered and the two-chambered cell. Each type has its own place in percutaneous absorption studies.

Variations of the two-chambered cell have been used for years to create conditions in which the diffusion of a compound in solution can be measured from one side of the membrane to the other.[2] An infinite dose (one that is large enough to maintain constant concentration during the course of an experiment) is added to one side of the membrane and its rate of diffusion across a concentration gradient into a solution on the opposite side is determined. Usually the solutions on both sides of the membrane are stirred to ensure uniform concentrations. Studies comparing permeation through skin to Fickian diffusion through a membrane are performed in this fashion.

The two-chambered cell is useful for studying mechanisms of diffusion through skin. It also is applicable to the measurement of absorption from drug delivery devices where compounds are applied to skin at an infinite dose and a steady-state rate of delivery is desired.

The exposure of skin to permeating substances usually occurs under conditions that are different from those created in the two-chambered cell. Some substances are intentionally applied to skin in creams or lotions during the use of drug and cosmetic products. Other chemicals, often of toxicological interest, come in contact with skin in a wide variety of vehicles in our environment. Often, the amount of penetrating substance on the surface of the skin is relatively small, and as permeation proceeds, a steady-state rate of absorption is not attained (finite dosage).

For these examples, absorption of the chemicals through skin can only be studied in a one-chambered cell. The surface of the skin in this type of cell is open to the environment, so that thin layers of material can be applied in vehicles relevant to exposure in vivo. The skin is not excessively hydrated by continued exposure to an aqueous solution as in the two-chambered cell.

The chamber beneath the skin serves as a container for the receptor fluid that is continually stirred; samples are taken through a side-arm for subsequent determination of rates of absorption. If desired, infinite doses can also be applied to the skin in the one-chambered cell for determination of steady-state absorption kinetics. Finite dose techniques and the design of a static diffusion cell were described by Franz.[3]

A flow-through cell system[4] was introduced to automate sample collection from a one-chambered cell. It also facilitates the maintenance of viability of skin since the nutrient receptor fluid is continually replaced. The receptor fluid is pumped beneath the skin through a receptor with a volume of only 0.13 to 0.26 ml (depending on skin surface area of diffusion cell). This small volume allows the receptor contents to be completely flushed out with flow rates of 1.5 ml/hr or greater. Similar values (Table 1) have been obtained with the flow-through and static cells in terms of the amount of material absorbed and the time course of absorption.[4]

Special attention may be necessary in measuring the permeability of highly volatile compounds when the skin is not occluded to prevent evaporation. The short walls on the tops of some diffusion cells can protect the skin surface from air currents and it has been suggested that this protection may be responsible

Table I. Comparison of In-Vivo and In-Vitro Absorption (Percent applied dose absorbed)			
		In Vitro	
Compound	In Vivo	Flow Cell	Static Cell
Cortisone	19.6 ± 1.3 (4)	20.1 ± 1.1 (6)	22.8 ± 2.7 (5)
Benzoic acid	37.0 ± 2.8 (8)	28.3 ± 3.0 (6)	35.5 ± 5.2 (5)

Values are the mean ± S.E. of the number of determinations in parrentheses. Compounds were applied in a petrolatum vehicle. The values obtained for each compound by the three methods were not significantly different from each other when compared by the 2-tailed Student's t-test, $p < 0.05$. (From Reference 7).

for differences between in vivo and in vitro results.[5,6] Diffusion cells have been designed to collect evaporating material above the surface of the skin.[7,8] These cells have proven particularly useful in studies of the effectiveness of mosquito repellents.

Some important factors must be considered in an in vitro study that are not a concern with an in vivo experiment. These factors are:

• Preparation of skin,
• Choice of receptor fluid,
• Provision for adequate mixing of receptor contents, and
• Maintenance of physiological temperature.

Preparation of Skin: When human skin or when most animal skin is used in the diffusion cell, a split-thickness preparation of skin should be made. A chemical that permeates human skin in vivo does not travel through the full thickness of the skin but is taken up into the blood in the highly vascular region of the papillary dermis just beneath the epidermis. Most, if not all, of the dermis should be removed so that it does not serve as an artificial barrier to absorption. This is particularly important for hydrophobic compounds because the aqueous viable tissue of the epidermis and dermis offers significant (and sometimes the primary) resistance to permeation. For animals with very thin skin such as the rabbit and mouse, removal of the dermal tissue is not as important; moreover, because of the thin membrane it is somewhat difficult to do.

The application of heat is a relatively simple procedure that can be used for separating the epidermis from the dermis of human and other nonhairy skin.[9] Besides not working with most animal skin, this method would also be unsatisfactory if viable epidermis is required for metabolism studies.

The skin is immersed in water heated to 60°C for approximately one minute and the epidermis can then be peeled away from the dermis. Hair remains in the dermis, and if present, will leave holes in the epidermal sheet.

Soaking skin in 2M solutions of sodium bromide or sodium thiocyanate loosens the epidermal-dermal junction[10] and hair stays in the epidermis as it is peeled away. The epidermis of laboratory rodents is extremely fragile, especially after the hydration that results in the use of this method.

A technique suitable for both human and animal skin is the separation of skin by the use of a dermatome.[11] Any hair shafts are severed and remain in the follicles so no leaks are created at the appendegeal openings. Dermatome slices of 200 to 350 μm from the surface of skin have been used routinely in our studies. A thinner section of skin (200 μm) can be prepared without damage to barrier properties when hairless skin is used (for example: human, hairless guinea pig). Thicker sections (350 μm) should be prepared with hairy skin.

Preparing slices of reproducible thickness requires some practice, as the depth of the cut is not determined solely by the dermatome layer thickness adjustment but partly by the angle with which the dermatome is held and the pressure with which it is moved across the skin. We have found that stretching the skin tightly over a flat surface aids in making a good cut.

The hair on animal skin must first be lightly shaved with an electric clipper before the dermatome is used. Care must be taken to leave some stubble on the skin surface to avoid cutting too closely and damaging the skin. A depilatory should not be used for hair removal, as this procedure is known to damage the barrier properties of skin.[12,13]

Choice of Receptor Fluid: The selection of the receptor fluid has become an increasingly important decision as investigators strive to create in vitro conditions that can adequately duplicate the situation in vivo. For measuring the absorption of water-soluble compounds, the use of normal saline or an isotonic buffer solution may be sufficient.

Recently, it has been demonstrated that some chemicals are metabolized significantly during the percutaneous absorption process.[14] The viability of skin can be maintained for 24 hours in a flow-through diffusion cell using a physiological buffer as the receptor fluid.[15] Metabolism and percutaneous absorption can be measured simultaneously as discussed below in the Metabolism section. The combined information gives a more complete picture of absorption since the actual permeating species are identified.

Many members of important classes of chemicals such as fragrances, pesticides, and petroleum products are highly lipophilic and readily enter and diffuse through the stratum corneum. The measurement of the percutaneous absorption by in-vitro methods of these water-insoluble compounds requires special techniques, and is a frequent source of experimental error.

When applied in vivo, hydrophobic compounds are taken up by blood perfusing the skin directly below the epidermis. When these compounds are applied to the skin in vitro, they are absorbed into the skin but will not partition from it into a saline or aqueous buffer solution. Analysis of the receptor fluid suggests that little or no penetration of skin is taking place.

We examined a number of receptor fluids for their ability to facilitate partitioning from skin and thus give permeation results comparable to the in-vivo absorption of several fragrance ingredients.[11] The absorption of ^{14}C cinnamyl anthranilate and ^{3}H cortisone from a petrolatum vehicle was measured through rat skin (Table II). Cortisone was a control compound with sufficient water solubility that its permeation was not limited by partitioning into the receptor fluids. If a receptor fluid enhanced the absorption of cortisone (in addition to the fragrance ingredient) the increase in absorption was considered to be due to an alteration of the barrier properties of the skin by the receptor fluid.

Table II. Effect of Diffusion Cell Conditions on the Absorption of Cinnamyl Anthranilate (Cortisone Control)

Receptor Fluid	Cinnamyl Anthranilate % Absorbed (5 Days)	Cortisone Permeability Constant x 10^5
Normal saline (4), whole skin	5.0 ± 0.3	3.8 ± 0.7
1.5% Volpo 20 (4), whole skin	5.4 ± 0.9	-
Normal saline (4)	5.8 ± 0.4	7.1 ± 0.5
1.5% Volpo 20 (10)	15.5 ± 1.2	6.1 ± 0.5
6% Volpo 20 (8)	27.9 ± 1.8	7.0 ± 0.9
20% Volpo 20 (8)	18.3 ± 1.8	9.3 ± 0.9
Rabbit serum (4)	8.8 ± 0.6	6.8 ± 0.8
3% Bovine serum albumin (4)	12.1 ± 1.2	5.4 ± 0.2
50:50 Methanol:water (4)	27.1 ± 2.0	17.2 ± 0.2
1.5% Triton-X (4)	17.9 ± 1.1	10.8 ± 0.5
6% Triton-X (4)	38.4 ± 2.9	14.5 ± 1.3
6% Pluronic F68 (4)	7.3 ± 1.3	9.8 ± 0.6

Although rabbit serum or a serum albumin solution would be desirable from a physiological standpoint, they were less effective in enhancing absorption than the nonionic surfactants and organic solvents used. The most effective receptor fluid that could be used without apparent damage to the skin was the nonionic surfactant polyethylene glycol 20 oleyl ether.*

Caution must be exercised in the selection of a suitable receptor fluid to avoid alteration of the barrier properties of the skin. Agents that enhance the partitioning of hydrophobic test compounds may also remove lipid-soluble constituents of the skin. A water solubility of less than approximately 10 mg/l (in combination with good lipid solubility) would indicate a potential problem in a diffusion cell with a standard aqueous receptor fluid.[11]

Recently, we have found it necessary to take a different approach in our studies of the absorption/metabolism of hydrophobic compounds. The use of a lipophilic receptor fluid can destroy metabolic activity of skin. Percutaneous absorption can alternatively be measured if one includes the materials absorbed into skin and remaining there at the end of the experiment as part of the absorbed compound.[16] If an epidermal membrane is used and if the receptor fluid is stirred and contains protein (4% bovine serum albumin), then the artificial dermal reservoir is eliminated and the receptor fluid contents more accurately reflect rates of skin permeation of hydrophobic compounds.[17]

Mixing of Receptor Contents: In most diffusion systems this step can be readily accomplished by some kind of automatic stirring device in the receptor fluid. In a flow-through cell with a small receptor volume (less than 0.5 ml), the agitation from the fluid flowing through the cell can be sufficient to provide adequate mixing.

* Volpo 20, Croda Inc., New York NY

As mentioned above, we have recently observed that, for water-insoluble compounds, an increased partitioning of the test compound into the receptor fluid is observed when the receptor contents are mixed with a small stirring bar. Presumably the same effect could be achieved by increasing the flow rate of the receptor fluid. However, this would dilute the receptor fluid levels of absorbed material and possibly make analytical methods more difficult.

Maintaining Skin Temperature: In-vitro percutaneous absorption studies have been conducted with skin surface temperatures ranging from an ambient temperature of 22°C[18] to as high as 37°C.[19] The diffusion of molecules through the skin is temperature-dependent. A reasonable guideline would be to expect a doubling in absorption with a 10°C increase in temperature. Although average body temperature is 37°C, the skin surface temperature is somewhat lower. The temperature of the skin surface of personnel in our laboratory averaged 32°C, but varied with the temperature of the room at different times of the year.

The method of maintaining a physiological temperature will determine the temperature setting of the water bath that is needed. Cells submerged in a water bath should be heated to exactly the temperature required. For cells that are jacketed or mounted in heated blocks, the circulating water must be heated to higher temperatures to allow for the loss of heat during the process. Water heated to 35°C and circulated through holding blocks for our flow-through diffusion cells produced a skin temperature of 32°C.[4] Temperatures are likely to vary slightly between human and animal skin.

Skin Metabolism and Percutaneous Absorption

The skin of the average human is an organ of approximately 4 kg with a surface area of 1.8 m².[20] The outer layer, the epidermis, is a differentiated tissue of ectodermal origin weighing approximately 225 g which completely regenerates itself on an average of every 45 days.[21] Other than the hemopoietic system, this level of cellular replacement is unique to the skin, requiring metabolic capacities sufficient to meet enormous protein and lipid synthesis and bioenergetic needs. It is not surprising that an organ possessing such great metabolic capabilities for endogenous compounds would also be capable of xenobiotic metabolism.

Traditionally, the study of percutaneous absorption has focused on the physicochemical processes of passive diffusion. Though the diffusional processes through such a structurally complex organ as the skin and its associated adnexal appendages are sufficiently challenging to measure, model, and predict, it is simplistic not to consider cutaneous metabolism if one's goal is to assess the toxic or therapeutic potential of the penetrating compound.

As interest has grown in the variety and extent of xenobiotic biotransformations by skin, investigations have demonstrated the existence of cutaneous phase I and phase II metabolic systems. Teleologically, these activities might be interpreted as the body's second line of defense against dermal exposure to toxic xenobiotics, a first pass metabolism which detoxifies and prepares compounds for rapid elimination shortly after absorption. The types of metabolic processes found in skin have been extensively reviewed.[22,23]

In vivo, the extent of cutaneous metabolism is difficult to differentiate from systemic metabolism. Frequently the rates of cutaneous metabolism are low compared to those of the liver[16] and the detection of metabolites is sometimes precluded by the quantity of blood which must be collected. When venous effluents are collected for analysis, the contribution of skin metabolism is confounded with that of metabolism in the plasma.

The predominant experimental techniques for cutaneous enzyme activity have used epidermal homogenates[24-27] and epidermal cells in culture.[28] Isolated cells or subcellular fractions, while advantageous for some specific studies of cutaneous metabolism in vitro, are farther away from the situation in vivo than intact skin. Indeed the architecture of the epidermis with its water and ionic gradients[29,30] and pH effects[31] appear to affect its metabolism and differentiation. The use of intact skin may be a more useful model for estimating metabolic rates and processes encountered in vivo, and has been used by a few researchers for skin metabolism studies.[13,15,16,32,33]

Skin Organ Culture: Successful culture of human skin was achieved over 70 years ago by Ljunggren[34] although not widely studied until the second half of this century. Blank et al.[35] were successful in maintaining viability of human skin on agar and utilized this in-vitro system for the study of fungal infections. Reaven and Cox[36] described a skin organ culture system for the study of environmental effects on skin growth.

For examining cutaneous metabolic effects during the percutaneous penetration process, it is convenient to maintain the viability of skin sections in the flow-through diffusion cell. The requirements of cells for their growth and replication include proper pH, osmolality, the proper ratio of potassium and sodium, phosphate, calcium, magnesium and chloride.[37] These requirements are met through the use of an appropriate balanced salt solution (BSS). In addition to BSS, the proper temperature must be maintained and dissolved oxygen sufficient to meet the metabolic requirements of the cultured cells must be available. For protein synthesis, the required amino acid precursors must be present. Other growth requirements include vitamins, lipids (essential fatty acids, phospholipids, lecithin and cholesterol), hormones, attachment and spreading factors, and carbohydrate energy sources.[38-40] As required for protein synthesis, the lipid, attachment and spreading factors, and hormonal requirements are typically met by a serum supplement.[41]

Maintaining Viability in Diffusion Cells: Percutaneous absorption/metabolism studies are conducted for finite durations, thus active multiplication of the perfused tissue is not necessary for most investigations. At the same time, the high concentrations of amino acids, vitamins and lipids are occasionally sources of interferences in analytical assays for parent compound and metabolites.

In order to develop a simplified medium to function as a receptor fluid in flow-through diffusion cell studies which would maintain skin viability and not interfere in most analytical procedures, a series of physiological buffer solutions was prepared and perfused under freshly obtained dermatome sections of fuzzy rat skin in flow-through diffusion cells.

The ability of the skin sections to maintain aerobic and anaerobic glucose utilization at initial rates and maintain metabolism of topically applied steroids, and the histological appearance of the skin following 24 hours of perfusion were used to assess viability.[15]

Minimal essential media (MEM) with a 10% fetal bovine serum (FBS) supplement, Dulbecco modified phosphate buffered saline (DMPBS),[42] a balanced salt solution[43] buffered (25 mM) with N-hydroxyethyl-piperazine-N'-2-ethanesulfonic acid (HEPES) to yield a HEPES buffered Hanks balanced salt solution (HHBSS), and a phosphate buffered saline solution with glucose (PBSG) were tested for their ability to maintain skin section viability.

Prior to metabolism study, the receptor fluid reservoir, transfer tubing and diffusion cells are first sterilized by flushing with a 70% ethanol solution. The receptor fluids are sterilized by filtration through a sterile 0.2 μm cellulose nitrite filter. The sterilized receptor fluid is then pumped through the diffusion cell apparatus to flush out any residual ethanol solution before mounting the skin section. As shown in Figure 1, MEM (+FBS), DMPBS, and HHBSS are able to sustain glucose utilization, steroid metabolism and histological appearance for 24 hours. Figure 2 is a transmission electron micrograph of the lower portion of the viable epidermis following perfusion with HHBSS for 24 hours. Visible is a basal cell with normal nucleus, nucleolus, and mitochondria, and an intact basement membrane.

Testosterone and estradiol are extensively metabolized in the skin. Estradiol yields estrone as the primary metabolite. Testosterone metabolites co-chromatograph with standards for 5-androstane-3,17-dione, and 4-androstane-3,17-dione or 5-dihydrotestosterone.

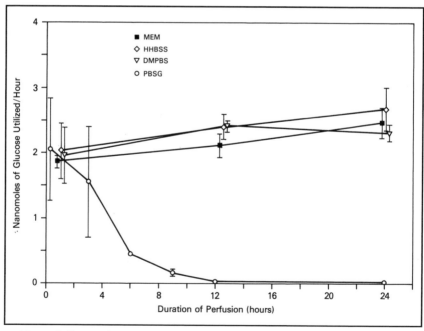

Figure 1. Rates of aerobic glucose utilization by fuzzy rat skin in flow-through diffusion cells. Mean of three determinations + SEM.

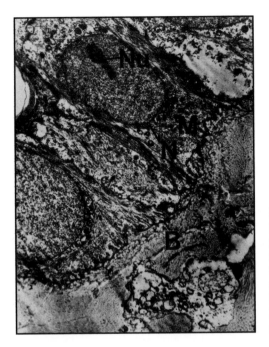

Figure 2. Transmission electron micrograph (x9600) of the stratum germinativum of a dermatome skin section perfused for 24 hr with HHBSS, showing normal mitochondria (M), nuclear membrane (N), and nucleolus (Nu). The basement membrane (B) is also visible.

The amounts of metabolite(s) recovered in the receptor fluid fractions are expressed as a percentage of the total radioactivity penetrating into the fraction (Table III). The percentage of estrone appearing in the receptor fluid remains constant at ca. 20% throughout the 24-hour duration of the experiment for skin sections perfused with MEM or HHBSS. PBS perfused skin shows declining rates of metabolism consistent with its inability to sustain glucose metabolism.

No estrone was recovered from distilled water control perfusions when gentamicin sulfate was added. Exclusion of gentamicin sulfate from the distilled water perfusate shows baseline recovery of ca. 3% estrone from the receptor fluid. The final distilled water fraction (18-24 hr) contained twice the amount of estrone as the preceding fractions. Presumably the estrone formation in the gentamicin deficient distilled water is due to bacterial metabolism rather than mammalian cell metabolism. The supplementation of MEM with 10% FBS results in an apparent reduction of metabolism which is believed to be the result of binding of estrone to the serum protein, thereby masking metabolism.

Testosterone absorption/metabolism experiments were conducted with Osborne-Mendel rat skin. HHBSS, MEM and MEM supplemented with 10% FBS all were able to maintain testosterone metabolism. Distilled water perfusion shows very small quantities of metabolites at levels less than 5% of those found with the other receptor fluids.

These results indicate that the receptor fluids MEM, DMPBS and HHBSS are able to sustain viability of thin dermatome skin sections in flow-through diffusion cells. The use of thick skin preparations is not only undesirable from a percutaneous diffusional perspective but also might limit duration of viability

Table III. Effect of the Receptor Fluid on the Measurement of Steroid Metabolism in Diffusion Cells

Metabolite Formation (% of Sample Radioactivity)

Fraction Compound and Receptor Fluid	0-6 h	6-12 h	12-18 h	18-24 h
ESTRADIOL		**ESTRONE FORMATION**		
MEM+FBS	1.1 ± 0.04	1.4 ± 0.04	2.1 ± 2.1	3.0 ± 2.4
MEM	19.4 ± 2.6	20.3 ± 1.9	22.4 ± 1.8	23.8 ± 2.5
HHBSS	20.8 ± 1.3	20.1 ± 1.4	21.3 ± 1.3	20.6 ± 1.6
PBS	17.2 ± 2.0	16.2 ± 3.3	7.7 ± 1.1	5.3 ± 1.3
Water	2.3 ± 1.0	3.1 ± 0.8	3.2 ± 0.7	6.7 ± 0.8
Water + Gentamicin	0	0	0	0
TESTOSTERONE		**METABOLITE FORMATION**		
MEM+FBS	28.0 ± 3.1	34.2 ± 5.7	27.5 ± 7.7	26.3 ± 11
MEM	36.1 ± 8.0	35.1 ± 4.7	32.9 ± 11	35.5 ± 3.0
HHBSS	34.4 ± 3.0	42.4 ± 2.6	33.0 ± 3.1	26.5 ± 4.2
Water	2.1 ± 0.4	0.5 ± 0.3	1.4 ± 0.7	2.1 ± 0.5

Values are the mean ± S.E. of 4-6 determinations. MEM = minimum essential medium; FBS = fetal bovine serum; HHBSS = Hepes-buffered Hanks' balanced salt solution; PBS = phosphate-buffered saline; estradiol was applied to fuzzy rat skin (5 μg/cm^2) and testosterone was applied to Osborne-Mendel rat skin (50 μg/cm^2).

by limiting diffusion of perfusate and dissolved oxygen to the viable epidermis. Skin utilizes most glucose anaerobically, producing lactate. The maintenance of viability in static cells is complicated by the cumulative depletion of glucose from the receptor fluid and the necessity of a buffer capacity large enough to maintain physiological pH. The use of PBSG or distilled water does not maintain skin viability in flow-through diffusion cells and would not be expected to do so in static cells.

Adequate measures must be taken to insure the microbiological integrity of the diffusion cell system. The apparatus must be sterilized prior to each study. The receptor fluid must also be sterilized and since viable primary skin tissue cannot be sterilized, antibiotics must be used.

Serum use might be justified in the study of lipophilic compound penetration and metabolism as a means of providing a more lipophilic receptor fluid. However, the variability[44] of serum and its intrinsic ability to metabolize some compounds is of concern. The use of bovine serum albumin for this purpose instead of whole serum may represent a less costly and better defined alternative.

The leaching of an esterase and a deaminase from skin into the receptor fluid in static diffusion cells has been reported.[45,46] In such a situation, retention of enzymatic activity in the receptor fluid results an over-estimation of cutaneous metabolism. Hydrolytic enzymes such as esterases occur in the cytosol and the endoplasmic reticulum. They are also present extracellularly in the stratum corneum. While it may seem unnecessary to maintain skin section viability for the study of hydrolytic biotransformations, cell lysis might increase leakage of hydrolytic enzymes into receptor fluid fractions thereby exaggerating cutaneous metabolic effects. When determining the contributions of cutaneous metabolism in an absorption study, suitable blanks must be performed to correct for any non-enzymatic changes in the parent compound.

Intact viable dermatome skin sections from mice, rats, hairless guinea pigs, and humans have been used in flow-through diffusion cells to study the penetration and metabolism of estradiol, testosterone,[15] AETT, BHT,[16] benzo[a]-pyrene, 7-ethoxycoumarin,[47] and azo colors.[48] The extent of metabolism of a percutaneously absorbed compound cannot be assumed to be negligible. By using and maintaining viable skin in vitro, the investigator can readily assess the effects of cutaneous metabolism on topically applied compounds.

In Vivo and In Vitro Comparisons

Human Skin: Only a few comparisons have been made between the results of in-vivo and in-vitro percutaneous absorption studies. Burch and Winsor[49] found excellent agreement in transepidermal water loss between excised human skin and that of human volunteers. Franz[3,50] compared the in-vitro permeation of 12 organic compounds to in-vivo results previously obtained by Feldmann and Maibach.[51] Good agreement was obtained; the few discrepancies could be explained by experimental differences.

The results of in-vivo and in-vitro permeability measurements of 16 compounds in the same laboratory using standardized methods were summarized by Anjo et al.[52] Flux in vivo was determined from urinary excretion data (with correction for incomplete urinary excretion), and rates were measured in vitro with a flow-through system.[53] A direct correlation was obtained between the two methods when a plot of the log transformations was used. Careful examination of each compound shows that, with some, a good correlation of the methods cannot be obtained. In some cases differences can be explained by a lack of solubility of the compound in the dermal perfusate; other differences cannot be explained at present.

Bronaugh and Franz[54] have compared the absorption of benzoic acid, caffeine, and testosterone applied to skin in solution in different vehicles (Table IV). Because benzoic acid ionizes in water and ethylene glycol, benzoic acid data were collected only when the petrolatum vehicle was used. Reasonably good agreement was obtained between in-vivo and in-vitro measurements, with the data expressed in terms of either the rate (% dose/hr) or the total amount absorbed. A significant difference in the percent absorbed in this comparison was obtained only with testosterone (petrolatum and ethylene glycol vehicles). This was consistent with a trend toward lower values in the diffusion cell experiments. In the in-vitro studies, the permeability constants determined for the compounds in each vehicle (petrolatum, water gel and ethylene glycol gel) correlated with either the stratum corneum-vehicle partition coefficient or the

Table IV. In-Vitro and In-Vivo Comparison				
	In Vitro		In Vivo	
Compound	% Dose/Hr (Steady State)	% Absorbed	% Dose/Hr (Maximum)	% Absorbed
Benzoic acid				
Petrolatum		46.5±5.9	13.2±0.7	60.6±10.7
Caffeine				
Petrolatum	1.4±0.1	40.6±2.2	1.0±0.2	40.6±6.1
Ethylene glycol	0.8±0.2	32.2±7.3	1.7±0.3	55.6±11.7
Water	0.1±0.02	5.1±0.5	0.1±0.03	4.0±0.5
Testosterone				
Petrolatum	1.0±0.1	39.4±1.2*	1.7±0.3	49.5±5.8
Ethylene glycol	0.7±0.1	23.7±2.0*	1.2±0.4	36.3±0.4
Water	1.8±0.2	41.1±6.8	2.1±0.3	49.2±4.7

Values are the mean ± S.E. of 5-20 determinations.
*Significant difference from value in vivo by Student's t-test, p <0.05.

percent saturation of the vehicle. Caffeine penetrated most readily from a petrolatum vehicle whereas the greatest testosterone absorption was from a water gel.

In-vitro studies with human skin require that care be taken to ensure that the integrity of the barrier layer has not been damaged at some point prior to assembly of the diffusion cell. Scrubbing of the skin in preparation for surgery or autopsy can damage the stratum corneum. Measurement of the absorption of a standard compound, such as ^{3}H-water, has proven useful as a screening tool.[55]

Animal Skin: A number of in-vivo and in-vitro comparisons have been made with animal skin, with the general conclusion that similar results should be expected if the methodology is sound. As with human skin, compounds that are essentially insoluble in water may not partition freely into the diffusion cell receptor fluid unless it is made more lipophilic.[11]

When comparisons not in agreement have been reported, it is likely that experimental errors such as in the choice of receptor fluid may be responsible. Tsuruta[56] suggested that differences between his in-vivo and in-vitro absorption data for chlorinated solvents might be due to differences in their respective solubility in body fluids (in vivo) and in normal saline (in vitro).

Bronaugh et al.[57] measured the skin permeation of three compounds in the rat, using a petrolatum vehicle, in order to compare in vivo and in vitro absorption results. Benzoic acid, acetylsalicylic acid, and urea were selected because of the expected differences in rate of permeability caused by their solubility properties. The in vivo and in vitro absorption values compared well. (See Table V for acetylsalicylic acid data.)

Bronaugh and Maibach[5] measured the percutaneous absorption of five nitroaromatic compounds through excised human and monkey skin in diffusion cells (Table VI). Absorption through monkey skin was also measured by in-

Table V. Percutaneous Absorption of Acetylsalicylic Acid in Rats		
	Total Absorption (% Applied Dose)	
Days	In Vivo	In Vitro
1	8.5 ± 1.6	8.8 ± 1.2
2	7.9 ± 2.0	8.5 ± 1.2
3	4.0 ± 0.9	4.6 ± 0.5
4	2.8 ± 0.5	4.3 ± 0.4
5	1.9 ± 0.5	2.9 ± 0.1
Total	24.8 ± 4.4	29.0 ± 3.1

Results are expressed as the mean ± S.E. of 4-5 determinations.

vivo techniques. Results were compared with previously reported human in-vivo studies on 2,4-dinitro chlorobenzene and nitrobenzene. No significant differences in absorption were found in values obtained by the different procedures except for nitrobenzene, a compound that is highly volatile and therefore difficult to compare accurately.

The skin permeation of fragrance ingredients was examined by in-vivo (Rhesus monkey) and in-vitro (human) techniques.[6] The compounds (safrole, cinnamyl anthranilate, cinnamic alcohol and cinnamic acid) were applied to skin in an acetone vehicle. Because of the lack of water solubility of safrole and cinnamyl anthranilate, a 6% solution of the nonionic surfactant PEG-20 oleyl ether was used as the receptor fluid to measure the absorption of these compounds. The greatest difference between in vivo and in vitro absorption

Table VI. Percutaneous Absorption of Nitroaromatic Compounds				
	% Applied Dose			
	Human		Monkey	
	In Vivo	In Vitro	In Vivo	In Vitro
p-Nitroaniline		48.0 ± 11.0 (9)	76.2 ± 8.4 (4)	62.2 ± 6.1 (6)
4-Amino-2-nitrophenol		45.1 ± 8.0 (5)	64.0 ± 6.2 (6)	48.2 ± 7.8 (5)
2,4-Dinitrochlorobenzene	53.1 ± 6.2 (4)	32.5 ± 8.7 (8)	52.5 ± 4.3 (4)	48.4 ± 3.9 (11)
2-Nitro-p-phenylenediamine		21.7 ± 2.6 (7)	29.9 ± 6.9 (3)	29.6 ± 4.3 (5)
Nitrobenzene	1.5 ± 0.3 (6)	7.8 ± 1.2 (6)	4.2 ± 0.5 (4)	6.2 ± 1.0 (5)
			41.1 ± 2.0 (3)[a]	

Values are the mean ± S.E. of the number of determinations in parentheses. Only with nitrobenzene were there significant differences (Student's t-test, 2-tailed, $p < 0.05$) between the values determined for the compounds by the four different methods. The value for the human in-vivo study was significantly different from the results by the other three procedures. Also, there was a significant difference between the human in-vitro and the monkey in-vivo values.
[a]Diffusion cell tops covered with parafilm.

values occurred with safrole, which was the least well absorbed and the most volatile compound (Figure 3). Cinnamic acid absorption through human skin (17.8 ± 4.9%) was significantly lower than through monkey skin (38.6 ± 8.3%). The values for absorption through human and monkey skin did not differ significantly for cinnamyl anthranilate or cinnamic alcohol.

Good agreement between in-vivo and in-vitro animal studies has been found by other investigators. Ainsworth[58] studied tributyl phosphate in the rabbit and pig; Sekura and Scala[59] measured alkyl methyl sulfoxides in the rabbit; and Creasey et al.[60] compared the permeation of water and tripropyl phosphate in the rabbit.

Animal Models for Human Skin: Human skin is unique and is therefore preferable for assessing the absorption and metabolism of a chemical in contact with human skin. Its use, however, is limited by the small supply that is available. It is therefore necessary to use the skin of animals, particularly for repetitive studies or mechanistic studies that require large amounts of skin. Many of the published in-vitro comparisons of human and animal skin are summarized in Table VII.

Tregear[61] was one of the first to compare the skin permeability of laboratory animals. His work supports the use of the weanling pig as a model for human skin. The sparse hair density combined with a thick stratum corneum make the

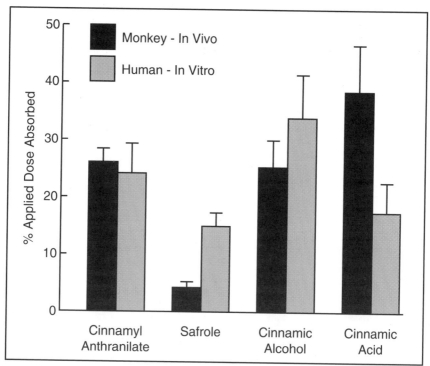

Figure 3. Percutaneous absorption of fragrance ingredients in monkeys and humans.

Table VII. In-vitro comparison of the permeability of animal skin relative to human skin[a]

Reference and Compounds	Pig	Monkey	Rat	Guinea Pig	Hairless Mouse	Mouse	Rabbit
Bronaugh et al. [39]							
Acetylsalicylic acid	1.2		1.0		4.9	8.7	
Benzoic acid	0.2		0.6		2.0	2.0	
Urea	1.5		4.8		0.9	5.8	
Bronaugh and Maibach [8]							
p-Nitroaniline			1.3				
4-Amino-2-nitrophenol			1.1				
2,4-Dinitrochlorobenzene			1.5				
2-Nitro-p-phenylenediamine			1.4				
Nitrobenzene			0.8				
Tregear [35]							
Ethylene bromide	0.8		2.3	1.5			
Paraoxon	1.4		3.3	3.0			
Thioglycolic acid	3.3		3.0	2.3			
Water	1.4			1.0			3.3
Chowan and Pritchard [55]							
Naproxin				2.3			3.5
Durrheim et al. [15]							
Butanol					1.8		
Ethanol					1.5		
Octanol					0.6		
Stoughton [38]							
Betamethasone					1.8		
5-Fluorouracil					1.1		
Hydrocortisone					1.5		
Walker et al. [40]							
Water			1.1	4.8	3.8	1.5	2.7
Paraquat			37	268	1461	51	109
Foreman et al. [42]							
Nandrolone			0.4				
Allyl estrenol			1.1				
Van Hooidonk et al. [43]							
VX				3.1			
Soman				2.0			

[a]Human skin in all studies was assigned a value of 1.0

use of pig skin attractive. It should be pointed out that donor pigs must be young pigs (either mini-pigs or standard size), since the skin appears to become less permeable with age, particularly in animals older than six months.

Reifenrath et al.[62] have demonstrated a high correlation between the permeability values for weanling pig skin (in vitro) and values for human skin (in vivo) for nine organic compounds.

Monkey skin has been shown to compare favorably in permeability with human skin both by in-vivo[63] and in-vitro[5,6] procedures. The comparisons of monkey data with the human absorption in vitro of nitroaromatic and fragrance compounds have already been discussed. Although the monkey is a hairy animal, the hair density is sparse in the abdominal area which seems best suited for permeability studies.

The pig and the monkey are probably the animal models of choice but their use presents major disadvantages; they are expensive to purchase and, because of their size, difficult and expensive to handle and care for. Since no animal skin has permeability characteristics identical to those of human skin, it may not be worth the extra effort to use pig or monkey skin, but may be more desirable to use one of the common laboratory animals such as the hairless mouse, the rat, or the guinea pig. The rabbit is generally considered to have skin that is more permeable than human skin, but this could be considered advantageous from the standpoint of providing a margin of safety in toxicity evaluations.

Hairless mouse skin was reported to give permeability values similar to those obtained with human skin for the series of C_1-C_8 alcohols.[19] Good agreement in permeability between human and hairless mouse skin was also reported by Stoughton[64] for several anti-inflammatory steroids. But better agreement between human skin and other animal skin has sometimes been reported.[65,66] Behl et al.[67] have recently found that human skin is an order of magnitude less permeable to hydrocortisone than is hairless mouse skin.

Bronaugh and coworkers[65] compared the absorption of benzoic acid, acetylsalicylic acid, and urea in the skin of humans, mini-pigs, rats, mice and hairless mice (Figure 4). Pig skin was found to have a barrier most like that of human skin, but rat skin was superior to the skin of the mouse and hairless mouse for the two faster penetrating compounds. When urea was the test compound, the hairless mouse skin was superior to that of the other animal species possibly because of reduced appendageal absorption of the slow-penetrating compound. Studies in addition to ours have indicated that rat skin can give absorption values similar to those from human skin.[64,66]

A sex-related difference in the absorption of chemicals was found in the back skin of the Osborne-Mendel rat.[70] Permeability constants were approximately twice as high when female skin was used. Because this difference was not seen when castrated male rats were compared to female rats, a hormonal influence on skin permeability was demonstrated. Knaak et al.[71] have also observed reduced absorption in male rat back skin; their studies were performed with the Sprague-Dawley strain.

Regional differences in permeation were seen in the male rat; the abdominal skin was consistently more permeable than that of the back.[70] Wester et al.[72] have also observed regional differences in the monkey. As in humans,[73] the ventral

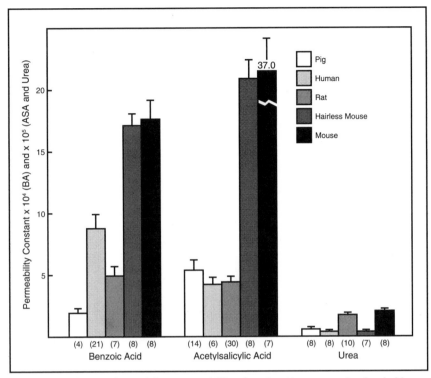

Figure 4. Comparison of the permeability of excised human and animal skin. Values are the mean ± S.E. of the number of determinations in parentheses.

forearm had low permeability and the scalp was 2-3 times more permeable than the forearm. The back and the abdomen were not examined. With male hairless mouse skin, Behl et al.[74] found similar absorption in the back and abdominal regions.[73-75]

We have recently used the hairless guinea pig for most of our animal studies. The lack of hair eliminates the need for clipping prior to a permeability study. More importantly, thin dermatome sections (200 mm) can only be prepared with hairless skin.

Absorption through Damaged Skin: It is not unusual for chemicals to come in contact with skin that has a damaged barrier. It is therefore important to be able to create or simulate a damaged skin barrier for evaluating the absorption of substances applied to nonintact skin.

In a few studies, the stratum corneum has been removed by repeated stripping with cellophane tape and observing the effect on absorption. Blank[76] reported that with excised human skin, tape stripping of the membrane resulted in an increased permeation of water approaching two orders of magnitude. In the most comprehensive "tape-stripping" study, Flynn and coworkers[77] have shown that the magnitude of the absorption of a series of alkanols through tape-stripped hairless mouse skin was determined by the lipophilicity of the molecules.

Table VIII. Water Permeation Through Damaged Human Skin (In Vitro)

Treatment of Skin	% Dose Absorbed (24 Hr)	% Dose/Hr (Maximum)
None (7)	2.7 ± 0.1	0.12 ± 0.01
Abrasion		
1 time (10)	10.7 ± 1.6	0.52 ± 0.09
3 times (7)	30.2 ± 9.4	2.4 ± 1.0
4 times (8)	33.8 ± 7.1	2.4 ± 0.9
Tape stripping		
12 times (7)	56.9 ± 7.2	3.6 ± 0.7
Depilatory (3)	3.2 ± 0.3	0.16 ± 0.02
Depilatory + abrasion		
4 times (7)	32.9 ± 7.1	2.0 ± 0.6

Values are the mean ± S. E. of the number of determinations in parentheses.
Treatment with depilatory was for ten minutes followed by a water rinse. Abrasion lines across the surface of the skin were made the indicated number of times with a 19-gauge hypodermic needle.

Table IX. Nicotinic Acid Absorption

Condition of Skin	% of Applied Dose Absorbed	
	In Vivo	In Vitro
Normal	6.8 ± 0.8 (5)	5.3 ± 1.1 (4)
Abraded	47.4 ± 5.3 (5)	50.9 ± 6.4 (4)
Tape stripped		57.5 ± 2.9 (6)
UV irradiated		
1.5 minutes	21.8 ± 3.6 (5)	6.5 ± 0.8 (12)
		13.0 ± 1.3[a] (11)
60 minutes	51.1 ± 5.1 (5)	

Values are the mean ± S. E. of the number of determinations in parentheses.
Nicotinic acid was applied in Vaseline Intensive Care Lotion at 5 mg/cm^2. No significant difference was obtained between the in-vivo and in-vitro results with the normal and abraded skin (Student's t-test, $p < .05$). Compound applied to skin 3 days after UV irradiation except as indicated.
[a]Compound applied 4 days after irradiation

In clinical studies, Felsher and Rothman[78] found a 3- to 10-fold increase in transepidermal water loss in patients with psoriasis and exfoliative dermatitis. Skin was abraded with a hypodermic needle to measure the increased absorption of lead through damaged skin in human volunteers.[79] When a single line was made at the site of application, a slightly more than two-fold increase in total body lead was obtained.

Bronaugh and Stewart[80] compared in-vitro methods for damaging the skin. They found that abrasion (one mark across skin) with a hypodermic needle would produce a mild damage; but after four marks across the skin, the increase in absorption of water was only slightly less than with tape-stripped human skin (Table VIII). Similar permeation values were obtained by in-vivo and in-vitro abrasion (Table IX). It was difficult to simulate damage caused by mild (1.5 min) UV irradiation. Mild damage to skin in vitro must be achieved by physical methods. The absorption of seven compounds was measured through normal and abraded skin (four marks).[80] The penetration of compounds that are poorly absorbed through skin may be increased by several orders of magnitude by abrasion.

Conclusions

If done with care and by proper techniques that overcome inherent problem areas, permeation can be reliably measured by in-vivo or in-vitro techniques. If the study cannot be performed with human skin, an animal model must be selected. Hairless animals allow for best preparation of the barrier layer for in-vitro studies. Ideally, some studies should be done with human skin to "calibrate" the animal skin for the test compound. The measurement of skin metabolism provides additional data that can aid in the evaluation of efficacy or toxicity of the absorbed material.

Biological Factors in Absorption and Permeation

By Jim Edmond Riviere

The quantitative prediction of the rate and extent of percutaneous penetration and absorption of topically-applied drugs and chemicals is complicated by the biological variability inherent to skin. In order to gain a perspective on this phenomenon, one should appreciate that mammalian skin is a dynamic organ with a myriad of biological functions. The most obvious is its barrier property which is of primary relevance to percutaneous absorption. Another major function of mammalian skin is thermoregulation since maintenance of body temperature is one of the defining characteristics which distinguishes mammals from lower vertebrates. Three cutaneous mechanisms are primarily responsible: thermal insulation provided by pelage and hair, sweating, and regulation of cutaneous blood flow.

Other functions of skin include mechanical support, neurosensory reception, endocrinology, immunological affector and effector axes, glandular secretions, and keratin, collagen, melanin, lipid and carbohydrate metabolism. These varied functions result in an organ which has a complex microanatomy composed of many different structures and cell types, as can be appreciated from examining Figure 1.[1] This complex microanatomical structure should be acknowledged when considering biological factors which may alter permeation of topically-applied chemicals.

In order to ascertain how these functions could interact with compound penetration through skin, it is important to define the basic phases in permeation where altered structure or function could have an effect. Figure 2 illustrates simple stages in percutaneous absorption viewed as the fate of a topically-applied drug once it is dosed on the surface of the skin.

A large percentage of the dose of any topically-applied chemical never penetrates the rate-limiting stratum corneum barrier. This may be due to pharmaceutical factors such as vehicle-retention or binding to the application device. If the compound is volatile, dose may be lost by evaporation. Chemical binding to surface stratum corneum (substantivity) may be lost by exfoliation. This fraction of the applied dose has not penetrated the skin.

Compound which has entered the stratum corneum is available for further disposition within or through the skin. It is generally accepted that the stratum corneum functions as a lipid barrier to compound penetration. Note that, for certain compounds, route of entry into the skin may be via appendages such as

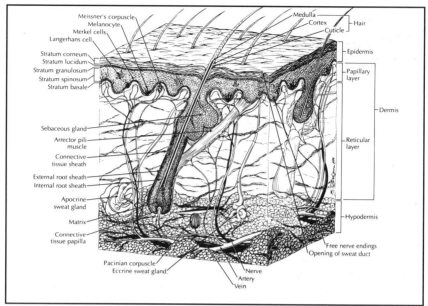

Figure 1. Schematic diagram of cutaneous microanatomy (From Reference 1)

hair follicles or sweat ducts.

Compound entering the skin after topical application has three possible fates:
- complete absorption into the cutaneous microcirculation,
- formation of a so-called reservoir by binding to stratum corneum or subcutaneous fat where it subsequently may be very slowly released into the capillaries, or
- metabolism by cutaneous enzymes.

Compound which enters the cutaneous capillaries is considered systemically absorbed. For consistency in this chapter, compound which is in the skin but has not been absorbed into the capillaries will be considered to have only penetrated the skin while that fraction which has entered the capillaries will be considered to have been absorbed. Permeation will be considered as describing drug which has either penetrated or has been absorbed.

It is important to consider these stages when trying to interpret how altered biology affects the rate and extent of cutaneous permeation. This scheme also needs to be considered when interpreting experimental studies conducted using in-vitro and in-vivo systems. Depending on the time course of an experiment, much of the compound which has penetrated into the skin may ultimately be systemically absorbed.

In shorter studies, this fraction of dose would not be detected in the reservoir of an in-vitro system, or in blood or excreta (e.g. urine, feces) in vivo. It could be detected using mass-balance techniques which determine the amount of drug which remained on the surface of the skin. Studies which do not differentiate the amount on the surface (by washing or tape stripping) from that actually penetrated into the skin are difficult to interpret. The optimal design would differentiate the penetrated drug (amount actually in the skin at the end of an experiment) from that easily removed from the surface by washing or wiping. Similarly, if radiolabelled compounds are used, the contribution of metabolism to total absorption is difficult to ascertain. Figure 3 illustrates how various biological (organismic) or extrinsic (ecologic) factors could alter the intrinsic properties of skin, and thus may modulate percutaneous permeation. The intrinsic properties are those which may have a direct effect on determining the fraction of an applied dose which either penetrates into or is absorbed through the skin. Various biological and extrinsic variables could affect these processes and result in changes in the amount of chemical which penetrates or is absorbed. For instance, various dermatologic diseases may alter the cutaneous permeation of a topically-applied compound.

It is the purpose of this overview to briefly consider some of the biological factors which have been demonstrated to modulate the rate and/or extent of topical drug permeation. A knowledge of these processes gives a framework upon which a classification of inter-individual differences in skin permeation

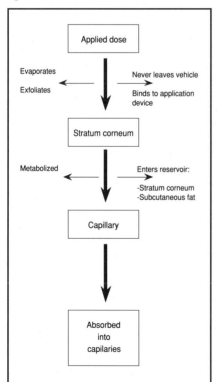

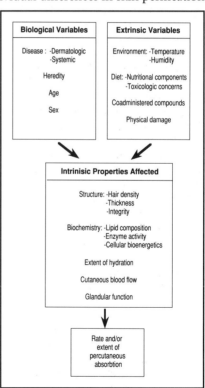

Figure 2. Fate of a topically applied compound.

Figure 3. Factors which could modulate the rate and/or extent of percutaneous permeation.

could be based, since these differences would be a direct consequence of the individual's cutaneous biology.

This review will not deal with pharmaceutical differences in formulation nor the physiochemical or biophysical properties of compound diffusion through the stratum corneum, two topics which have been adequately addressed by other authors in this book. Where appropriate, this chapter will use data generated in the author's laboratory to illustrate principles. The perspective is that of the skin as an intact organ, with its unique anatomic structure and physiologic functions defining its possible interactions with chemicals and the environment.

Integrity of the Stratum Corneum

A primary focus of much of the research on disease effects is on the integrity of skin's barrier properties. The importance of intact stratum corneum to the skin's barrier function has been amply demonstrated in vitro and in vivo.

Penetration through the stratum corneum is generally directly correlated to the compound's lipid partition coefficient.[2-6] Removal of stratum corneum by adhesive tape stripping, keratolytic agents, abrasion, or by blistering using suction or cantharidine results in enhanced compound penetration with a return to normal flux when stratum corneum is regenerated. Additionally, altering the structure of the epidermis without complete removal of the stratum corneum may also enhance permeation, as evidenced in studies using skin with proliferative dermatologic disorders. The importance of the intercellular lipids to these barrier functions can be appreciated when they are removed by solvent treatment (e.g. ether, chloroform/methanol). In such delipidized skin, penetration of hydrophilic compounds (such as hydrocortisone or benzoic acid) was reported to be greatly enhanced in in-vivo guinea pig studies.[7]

Conditions such as eczema, which result in thickened skin with maintenance of an intact structure and lack of parakeratosis, may retard absorption because of the increase in absorptive path length. Similarly, regional and species differences in the thickness of skin or in epidermal structure would also affect compound permeation.

In contrast, absorption through psoriatic skin is enhanced.[8] This may be secondary to altered epidermal structure as well as to changes in vascular perfusion.[9] Similarly, absorption is enhanced in congenital ichthyosis, a condition clinically marked by dry, scaly skin.[10] In a condition similar to that of diseased skin, the barrier function of the skin of preterm infants is not fully developed, as evidenced by enhanced phenylephrine and theophylline absorption.[11-12]

Systemic disease states could also potentially alter the rate of topical drug absorption. For example, diabetes is known to alter the structure of epidermal basement membranes and capillary function such that compound diffusion out of cutaneous capillaries is enhanced in chronic diabetics.[13-15] Such alterations associated with development of systemic disease would be expected to alter absorption of compounds where capillary function is an important process. The potential effect of such microvascular diseases on the transdermal delivery of peptides merits further investigation.

Although the stratum corneum is the primary barrier to percutaneous absorption for most compounds, some small polar compounds may preferentially pass through the so-called "aqueous pore pathway." This is composed of either adnexial structures such as hair follicles and sweat glands or a nonlipid pathway through protein-rich structures such as keratinocytes.[3-5] For these compounds, differences in the density of hair follicles and sweat ducts in different species or between different body sites may also account for altered rates of compound permeation. A similar scenario may also occur when drugs are administered by iontophoresis.

These factors should be considered when comparing absorption of compounds in different animal species. In the commonly-utilized laboratory rodents, the skin is much thinner and has a greater hair density than that of humans. Thus for the majority of compounds studied, penetration is much greater and more rapid in mice, rats and rabbits than in humans. The absorption through skin from hairless rodent species is less, but still is often greater than that seen using human skin. Of all the animals studied, primate and porcine skins most closely resemble human skin in respect to compound penetration.[16-18] In addition to differences in skin structure between species, cutaneous blood flow also varies greatly.[19] The selection of an animal model finally rests on the purposes of the study. If safety is the primary concern, then rodents are often used since they overestimate absorption in man and provide a direct tie-in to the other animal toxicology tests conducted. However, in the pharmaceutical arena, other species are often used since the goal is to predict, as closely as possible, the flux seen in man.

Skin Hydration

Hydration of skin is a major factor affecting the rate and extent of percutaneous absorption. A primary method of increasing skin penetration is by the use of occlusive dressings, as was demonstrated by Wurster and Kramer[20] for methyl, ethyl and glycol salicylates, and by Feldman and Maibach[2] with hydrocortisone absorption in humans. This effect is usually more important for nonpolar than polar molecules,[21] and is most likely secondary to an increase in diffusivity of the penetrating molecule.

However, hydration may also affect the partitioning and concentration gradient of the penetrating molecule in the stratum corneum as well as the overall thickness of the effective barrier. Changes in these parameters could alter the size of the stratum corneum reservoir for different penetrants, an event which would change the shape of the permeation profile.

Occlusion prevents surface evaporation of endogenous water which results in stratum corneum hydration. Environments with high relative humidity (greater than 80%) may also result in significant skin hydration.[22] An assessment of the degree of hydration can be made by monitoring the permeability of the stratum corneum to water through measurement of transepidermal water loss (TEWL). Recent in-vitro studies in our laboratory with the organophosphate pesticide parathion demonstrated much greater fluxes when relative humidity was 90% compared to 60% or 20%.[23] The effect of hydration has also been demonstrated using in-vitro model systems in which the epidermal surface (donor reservoir) is immersed in water; in this case the relative humidity is effectively 100%. In in-vitro diffusion cell studies where the donor chamber is fully immersed in fluid (e.g. infinite-dose static cell studies), one is actually studying the absorption across fully-hydrated skin, a situation rarely encountered in vivo in humans. This limitation should be recognized when extrapolating data from such studies.

Cutaneous Blood Flow

The dermis of the skin is richly perfused by a large network of capillaries which functions to modulate cutaneous blood flow in response to thermoregulatory needs. When the environmental temperature exceeds body temperature, cutaneous blood flow increases so that heat is lost through the skin. In contrast, blood flow is decreased or even totally shunted in cold temperatures to prevent surface heat loss. In extreme cases, frostbite is the result. The average blood flow to the skin has been reported to vary from 0.5-100 ml/min/100 g. Normal resting blood flow in human skin ranges from 3-10 ml/min/100 g. When ambient temperature exceeds 43°C it can increase ten-fold.[13]

From a pharmacokinetic viewpoint, cutaneous blood flow should not affect the rate or extent of compound absorption unless the rate of presentation to capillaries is so rapid that capillary uptake rather than stratum corneum penetration becomes the rate-limiting process. However, blood flow may theoretically modulate the size of cutaneous depots by shifting the fraction of penetrated drug which is absorbed into capillaries to be deposited into a depot. This could be either a result of rate of capillary perfusion or a function of the number of capillaries being perfused since shunting is a major mechanism for thermoregulation. Capillary permeability to large molecules may also be a function of perfusion. In the design of dermatological compounds where high skin concentrations are desired, cutaneous vasoconstriction should increase skin concentrations at the expense of vascular uptake into the systemic circulation. Although this phenomenon may be beneficial for dermatologics, it would reduce the bioavailability of transdermal preparations. Formation of cutaneous depots may not alter total systemic bioavailability, but rather may simply prolong the absorption phase, since most penetrated drug may ultimately be absorbed by the cutaneous microcirculation.

Danon and coworkers[24] demonstrated that the in-vivo topical absorption of methyl salicylate was increased threefold in humans when they were exposed to high ambient temperatures or underwent strenuous exercise. Increased blood flow was presumed to be the major factor, although increased skin hydration or sweating also should have contributed. The cutaneous clearance of hydrophilic methotrexate was increased by dermal perfusion, an event which decreased the attainment of effective antipsoriatic concentrations in the viable epidermis.[25]

Even in in-vitro systems, increasing temperature may increase the rate of chemical absorption, as was demonstrated in our laboratory with parathion.[23] Thus high environmental temperature may alter the rate of absorption by both thermodynamic and physiological factors. As was previously discussed, humidity also alters penetration. These two factors, temperature and humidity, are primary variables in assessing the effect of environment on percutaneous permeation. Table I lists results from in-vitro flow-through diffusion cell studies using porcine skin conducted with three different concentrations of parathion, and demonstrates the significant effect that changes in humidity and temperature may have on the transdermal flux of a topically applied compound.[23] One also appreciates from this data the dependency of fractional absorption (% dose absorbed) on dose, with decreasing fractional absorption occurring with increased dose. In spite of this dose-related decrease in absorption efficiency, the actual amounts absorbed (% absorbed x dose) still increase with dose.

Progress in this area has been hampered by the avascular nature of in-vitro diffusion cell and cell culture models. Although temperature and humidity effects may alter flux in in-vitro diffusion cell studies, the further interaction of changes in blood flow cannot be assessed. The use of vascular skin flap preparations is ideally suited to investigate this phenomenon. Benzoic acid absorption across the rat-human skin flap (RHSF) was reduced when vasoconstriction was induced by either phenylephrine iontophoresis or decreased body temperature.[26,27] These preliminary studies demonstrated a rebound effect when normal blood flow was resumed, supporting the concept of a perfusion-mediated cutaneous reservoir.

Table I. Effect of temperature and humidity on the percutaneous absorption of parathion in vitro in porcine skin

Applied Dose of Parathion (μg/cm^2)	Temperature Skin (°C)	Air (°C)	Relative Humidity (%)	Relative Absorption Compared to Control*
4	37	37	60	1 **
	37	42	60	1.14
	42	42	60	2.78
	37	37	20	0.97
	37	37	90	2.20
40	37	37	60	1 **
	37	42	60	1.50
	42	42	60	2.32
	37	37	20	0.79
	37	37	90	2.75
400	37	37	60	1 **
	37	42	60	1.35
	42	42	60	1.61
	37	37	20	0.98
	37	37	90	2.56

* (% Dose Absorbed)/(% Dose Absorbed in Controls) calculated independently for each dose
** Control conditions for each dose. Note that these are based on the % of applied dose absorbed, which decreases with increasing dose.
The % dose absorbed under control conditions are 7.69% for 4 μg; 1.91% for 40 μg; and 0.46% for 400 μg.

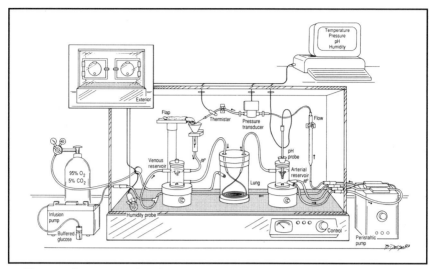

Figure 4. Schematic of perfusion chamber used in isolated perfused porcine skin flap (IPPSF) experiments.

To study these phenomena in a true in-vitro model, the isolated perfused porcine skin flap (IPPSF) was developed in this author's laboratory. The IPPSF is a single-pedicle, axial-pattern tubed skin flap based on the superficial epigastric artery of the ventral abdomen of weanling swine. Two tubed skin flaps (Stage One) are first created on the pig using reconstructive surgery techniques.[28,29] Two days later, in a separate procedure, the artery is cannulated on each flap and then transferred to a temperature- and humidity-regulated isolated organ perfusion chamber specifically designed for this purpose (Figure 4). This chamber allows the effect of altered temperature and varying relative humidity on compound absorption to be experimentally addressed.

By raising two flaps from each individual animal, a control preparation is available to assess experimental variables. A bicarbonate-buffered (pH=7.6) Krebbs-Ringer perfusate containing albumin is oxygenated (95% O_2/5%CO_2) and pumped through the IPPSF at an average flow of 3-7 ml/min/100g and a pressure of 30-70 mm Hg. Physiological concentrations of albumin are included because of the need to maintain a perfusate oncotic pressure sufficient to maintain capillary flow. Since many lipid soluble compounds are also bound to plasma proteins in vivo, the presence of albumin facilitates absorption. Viability of the preparation is assessed hourly throughout a permeation experiment by assessing arterial/venous glucose utilization. The stability of this parameter over the course of an experiment can be seen in Figure 5. The ability to monitor tissue viability is a major attribute of the IPPSF since cutaneous toxicity of a penetrating compound may be directly assessed.

The percutaneous absorption of compounds is assessed by topically applying chemical (or transdermal delivery device) on the surface of the IPPSF and monitoring venous effluent for absorbed compound. Figure 6 depicts a typical

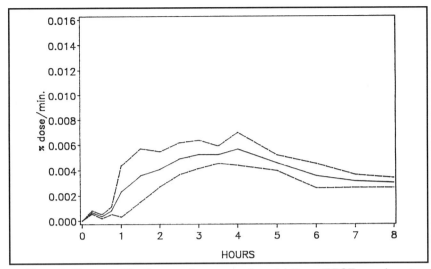

Figure 5. Glucose utilization over the course of an eight hour IPPSF experiment (mean ± SD, n = 145).

venous efflux profile for a topically applied penetrant. Through pharmacokinetic analysis of the venous efflux profile,[30,31] the rate and extent of compound penetration and absorption can be assessed. When data collected in 8-hour IPPSF studies are extrapolated to predict 6-day in-vivo absorption and compared to actual results, the correlation is r=0.97. This system and the structure of the pharmacokinetic models used are fully described elsewhere.[32]

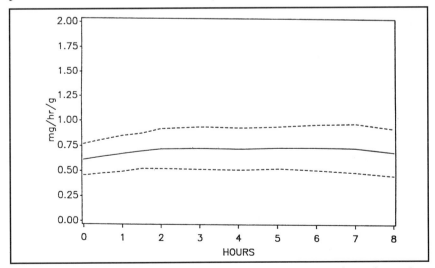

Figure 6. Cutaneous efflux profile of topically applied lindane (40 µg/sq.cm.) in the IPPSF. Mean ± SD.

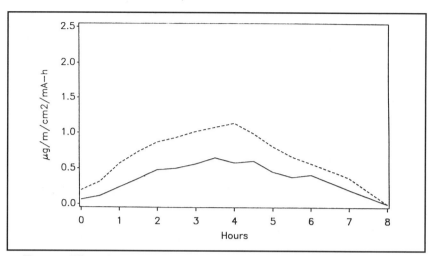

Figure 7. Effect of co-iontophoresis of the vasodilator tolazoline (broken line) on enhancing transdermal lidocaine flux (solid line = lidocaine alone) in the IPPSF

Studies conducted in this model demonstrated the importance of vasomodulation on percutaneous absorption. When lidocaine hydrochloride was administered by iontophoresis, flux dramatically increased with addition of the vasodilator tolazoline (Figure 7). Adding the vasocontrictor norepinephrine decreased flux compared to lidocaine alone.[32,33] The rate of percutaneous absorption of caffeine, a compound with vasodilatory activity, was also affected in individual IPPSFs where cutaneous caffeine concentrations were sufficiently high to enhance their own flux.[30] Studies such as these using in-vitro models which process an intact microcirculation clearly demonstrate the importance of using a model system with response comparable to that in-vivo.

These studies support the idea that percutaneous absorption can be modulated by alterations in cutaneous blood flow. The primary mechanisms responsible for altered blood flow would be changes in environmental temperature or pharmacological manipulation. However, dermatologic disease conditions may also alter resting blood flow, as evidenced by the erythema associated with some conditions. Any stimulus which causes the release of inflammatory mediators would be expected to alter vascular perfusion and/or capillary permeability, thus providing the mechanism for altering penetration and/or absorption. As was demonstrated with caffeine, if the compound being absorbed is inherently vasoactive, its cutaneous flux may also be affected. The inherent vasoactive properties of corticosteroids are what allows their penetration to be assessed by the vasoconstrictive assay (skin blanching).[34] Studies with nicotinate absorption further demonstrate the importance of a compound's vasoactivity.[35]

An important phenomenon which merits further study is the apparent inverse relation seen with vasomodulation between the amount of drug which enters capillaries and that which remains in the skin. The most important use of vasomodulation may be to regulate the fraction of penetrated dose which remains in the skin for local effect.

Skin Biochemistry

The lipid composition of the epidermis is a major determinant of compound permeation through skin. Elias has formulated a model of epidermal structure which intersperses proteinaceous corneocytes in an extracellular lipid matrix.[36] The primary pathway for chemical penetration through the stratum corneum is through these lipid-containing intercellular spaces. The biochemical composition of the lipid matrix is species dependent. Lipid conformation and corneum morphology may also play an important role in determining penetration of compounds.[37] Porcine skin is very similar to human skin in respect to physical properties (phase transitions) reflecting lipid composition.[38] Topical application of solvents results in solvent partitioning into this matrix, which alters its composition.

It is the partitioning of a compound from the application site into the lipid matrix and the corneocytes which determines the rate and extent of compound penetration. Factors which alter the lipid composition of this pathway thus alter the kinetics of permeation. A primary mechanism of action for many penetration enhancers may be their effects on this lipid pathway. One postulated mechanism is that some enhancers may increase lipid fluidity thereby decreasing barrier function. Williams and Elias should be consulted for a more complete review of these concepts.[39]

The lipid composition of skin can be experimentally manipulated through the use of topical delipidizing solvents or systemically through manipulation of the diet. A decreased barrier function has been demonstrated in essential-fatty-acid-deficient rodents.[40] Additionally, some strains of laboratory rodents have genetically deficient lipid metabolism resulting in skin of abnormal lipid composition which could likewise show altered barrier function. The same affect may be seen in certain dermatologic or possibly nutritional deficiency conditions in man.

Cutaneous Biotransformation

Recent studies have indicated that cutaneous metabolism may be an important component for permeation of some chemicals.[41-45] It has become clear that various factors influence the amount of chemical which, after penetrating the stratum corneum, is absorbed intact or as a metabolite due to epidermal biotransformation. Both phase I and II metabolic pathways have been identified. Some studies have indicated that the extent of cutaneous metabolism influences the overall fraction of topical compound absorbed.

Factors which may influence the fraction of penetrated chemical metabolized include the rate of permeation of parent drug, the residence times of parent drug and metabolite in the epidermis, the inherent activity of epidermal enzymes, the partitioning characteristics of the parent drug and metabolite, and the anatomical location of the enzymes. Details of the experimental design used to assess cutaneous metabolism (e.g. tissue viability, vehicle, receptor solution composition) may also have a dramatic effect on the results obtained. For compounds which undergo first-pass cutaneous metabolism, prior systemic (e.g. dietary) or topical exposure to enzyme inducers, inhibitors, or competing substrates could significantly affect the metabolic profile seen.

Topical parathion-absorption studies conducted in the IPPSF demonstrated a significant first-pass metabolism which was blocked by prior treatment with a cytochrome p-450 inhibitor. Extent of metabolism was also affected by occlusion, which also changed the fraction of parathion metabolized to paraoxon or p-nitrophenol.[46] First-pass metabolism also explains why the subsequent systemic disposition of a topically-applied drug may be different from that seen after parenteral administration. In the case of a compound such as parathion which does not possess inherent anticholinesterase activity, cutaneous metabolism to the biologically-active paraoxon would increase the systemic exposure to an active compound. However, extensive metabolism by the liver inactivates paraoxon. In contrast, if parathion were absorbed as the parent drug, the liver would instead now activate the drug to paraoxon. Thus, depending on the metabolic sequences involved, a first-pass cutaneous metabolism could either potentiate or reduce the systemic toxicity of a compound.

In an in-vivo study comparing the percent of absorbed dose which is excreted in pig urine or feces after either topical or intravenous dosing, the urine/fecal ratio was significantly different for a number of compounds.[47] This would suggest that, for certain compounds, collection of urine alone to monitor in-vivo percutaneous absorption may be erroneous, even if parallel parenteral studies are conducted to determine the fraction of dose excreted in urine. Obviously, the resulting pharmacodynamic profile of a transdermal drug may also be different from parenteral dosing if the systemic disposition is route dependent.

The effect of enhancers (chemical or iontophoretic) on the cutaneous metabolism of topically-applied drugs has not been fully addressed, nor has the effect of dermatologic conditions. For example, the role of epidermal bioenergetics on the capacity of these cells to metabolize drugs via the cytochrome p-450 mixed-function oxygenase system has not been addressed, nor has the effect of substrate depletion on cutaneous conjugation reactions been defined. This is particularly important since the skin predominantly utilizes relatively inefficient anaerobic glycolysis for basal energy needs. A great deal of additional research is required before the importance of these factors on an individual compound's permeation profile can be assessed.

Summary

The preceding overview of the effects of altered cutaneous biology on the permeation of topically-applied agents illustrates the complexity of the in-vivo situation. Most in-vitro studies are limited to studying the effects of single variables on the rate of penetration of model compounds. However, as can be appreciated by this brief overview, numerous factors may interact to determine the overall rate of permeation. Very different patterns of cutaneous permeation will result if these independent factors are competing, additive or synergistic. Theoretically, in order to precisely predict the rate of permeation of a compound in a specific individual, all of these factors would have to be taken into consideration.

Fortunately, for most compounds studied, the problem is simplified because of the rate-limiting role that the stratum corneum plays in compound absorption. However, even in these "simple" cases, extrinsic variables may influence stratum corneum permeability in-vivo and confound the ability to predict absorption in a specific individual. For example, interactions with coadministered chemicals (e.g. detergents, cosmetics, household pesticides) may affect a compound's permeation.

The quantitation of the extent and variability of permeation is often a multivariate problem. This is especially true for compounds which are either metabolized by the skin, penetrate through nonlipid pathways, are dependent on the rate of cutaneous blood flow, are administered by active delivery systems (e.g. iontophoresis), or are administered to individuals with abnormal skin. The problem has been circumvented in many transdermal drug delivery systems by making the drug delivery device, rather than the skin, the rate-limiting process. Obviously, this solution is irrelevant to problems in dermatotoxicology.

The solution to these problems would be facilitated by the development of pharmacostatistical approaches which couple dermatopharmacokinetic models of permeation with individual estimates of biological variability. The classification of dermatological disorders on the basis of their effects on model compound permeation would provide a foundation on which these models could be constructed. If noninvasive estimates of biological function (e.g. LDV blood flow, TEWL) were simultaneously measured, a basis for utilizing these "permeation classes" to predict individual compound absorption would be available.

Before this level of quantitation is ever achieved, one should at least appreciate that a myriad of biological factors could potentially affect topical chemical permeation. This should lead to a realization that inter-individual variability in chemical permeation is but another example of biological diversity which can never be eliminated but can be explained. By partitioning this variability into defined categories correlated to biological attributes, the process of predicting permeation on a population basis will be improved, and those groups of individuals at risk to excessive chemical permeation may be defined.

Modification of Skin Permeation by Solvents

By Joel L. Zatz, PhD

While we often speak of the application of various materials (such as drugs or cleansers) to the skin, it is understood that the active ingredients are not at full strength. Most often, they are contained in a preparation or device, or, as in the case of soap, diluted with water before application. The vehicle serves as a means of conveniently applying a compound and controlling its concentration. Whether intended or not, the vehicle also plays a major role in determining the rate of uptake and penetration through the skin.

That the activity of topically applied medicaments can be modified by vehicles has been known for some time. For example, in 1933 it was shown that the germicidal effects of phenol could be obtained when that compound was applied to the skin in a cream base, but not a fatty base.[1]

The purpose of studying the mechanism of solvent effects on skin permeation is to be able to predict the direction in which changing the solvent will alter permeation without having to do the experiment each time. However, even in the absence of a definitive understanding of solvent effects on a molecular level, it is possible to devise empirical rules that are useful formulation guides.

It has been known for many years that certain solvents, such as dimethyl sulfoxide (DMSO), can break down the skin's resistance to transport. This solvent, and others that are equally damaging to the barrier are not currently used in the U.S., although at least one pharmaceutical product containing this solvent has reached the market in Europe. Although some description of DMSO and other highly interactive solvents will be given, the bulk of our discussion will focus on solvents more likely to be encountered in skin products and treatments.

Categorizing mechanisms

Solvents can act on several levels and simultaneously modify permeation in different ways. By dividing these effects into categories, we attempt to devise a scheme that aids understanding and makes it possible to organize much of the data in the literature in a rational way.

For most substances in most vehicles, the stratum corneum represents the skin's principal barrier to transport. This is another way of saying that passage through the stratum corneum is usually the slowest (or rate-limiting) step. However, in rare instances, the rate-limiting step may be located in the vehicle rather than in one of the skin layers. It is always useful to determine which of the steps in the sequence of transfers leading from the vehicle through the skin is the slowest; this is the one that determines the overall rate. Modification of the permeation rate requires alteration of one or more of the parameters involved in the slow step. Formulation changes that influence only the other (fast) steps in the process will not have a noticeable effect. Having sounded this alert, we will concentrate on the usual situation in which stratum corneum transport is rate-limiting.

It is possible to divide solvent effects into three categories. In the first group we place a solvent's physicochemical characteristics such as surface tension and rheology. Rheology is particularly important if vehicle transport is rate-limiting, but when diffusion across the stratum corneum determines the permeation rate, differences in vehicle viscosity have no significant effect. Surface tension of the liquid is one of the major factors determining the degree of contact with the skin surface and therefore the effective area through which permeation occurs.

The second category is driving force or difference in chemical potential across the stratum corneum. This has also been referred to as the "push" effect.[2] Since the concentration of substances in the blood and lower skin tissues is frequently very small, the concentration in the outer surface of the skin determines the gradient across the membrane. This may be expressed as the product of a skin/vehicle partition coefficient and the concentration within the vehicle. As will be described below, it is sometimes useful to think in terms of permeant activity within the solvent when making comparisons between different vehicles.

In contrast to the first two categories, which represent non-interactive solvent effects, the third category is driven by solvent-skin interactions which modify the structure and/or integrity of the stratum corneum. Since the extent of interaction depends on the makeup of the membrane as well as the nature of the solvent, effects of this type can be classed as "membrane-specific." The changes in horny layer properties result in an increase or decrease in the rate of permeation through the skin ("pull" effect). A variety of solvent-skin interaction mechanisms is possible, and defining them is an active area of current research.

Contact with the skin surface

The area of contact between a solid surface and applied liquid depends on a variety of factors, including the extent of wetting, usually expressed in terms of a contact angle, and the degree of surface roughness. The contact angle can be measured directly, and several theories have been proposed by which that angle can be calculated if the solid and liquid involved are relatively simple substances whose properties are well defined.

The stratum corneum presents a complex surface because it is chemically heterogeneous and has numerous irregularities (such as pore openings and ridges). Sebum is deposited continuously on the surface, along with the products of intercellular lipid metabolism; sweat glands also empty their contents. Various surface-active compounds that are present because of secretion, excretion and cell breakdown affect the angle of contact that liquids make with the skin surface.[3]

Contact angles of water droplets on viable human skin provide an indication of the ease of wetting. Measurements of such contact angles were reported by Ginn et al.[4] Although there was considerable variation between subjects, the contact angle on skin washed with soap and water was generally greater than 100°. A contact angle of 0° represents perfect wetting. If the contact angle approaches 90°, wetting is very poor and a considerable amount of air, which separates the liquid and solid, may be entrapped, particularly when the surface is highly irregular, as is the case with skin. This tendency of normal stratum corneum to shed water droplets is in contrast to its ability to imbibe water and swell.

Using acetone-water mixtures as probe liquids, the critical surface tension (γ_c) for human skin was determined[3] to be approximately 27 dyn/cm. This value, which is slightly less than that for polyethylene, is another indication that skin has a "low energy" surface and is difficult to wet.

The value of the critical surface tension indicates the tendency of liquids placed on the skin to spread. Liquids whose surface tension is less than the γ_c value for skin (such as alkanes and lower alcohols) spread spontaneously while liquids with high surface tension (such as water and glycerin) remain as discrete droplets. (The high contact angles observed with water droplets have been mentioned.) Wetting of skin by aqueous liquids is improved by the inclusion of surfactants or water-miscible organic liquids of low surface tension.

When semisolid products are smoothed over the skin surface, the mechanical disturbance may exceed the yield value and cause them to liquify, thus promoting contact with the skin. Whether air is totally displaced by the preparation depends on the surface energy of the semisolid and its viscosity as well as the mechanical energy expended. By increasing contact with the skin surface, rubbing may serve to increase skin uptake. When maximal absorption is desired, total contact of skin and applied product is essential, because permeation is proportional to the amount of skin surface area covered.

Multiphase skin products usually contain surface-active agents that function in a variety of ways, depending on the intent of the product. These additives improve wetting of the skin surface. In addition, many surfactants are capable of interacting with the horny layer and promoting the permeation of compounds present within the formulation.

Stratum corneum hydration

It is generally accepted that most substances are absorbed through the stratum corneum more rapidly if this tissue is in a hydrated state rather than in its usual dry state. Measurement techniques and many of the factors influencing stratum corneum moisture content were recently reviewed.[5] The stratum corneum water content is a function of relative humidity and temperature. It does not seem to vary with age and season, although the physical appearance of the skin surface may. Transepidermal water loss values are not necessarily a sensitive indication of the hydration level of the horny layer.

One of the few studies to actually measure the water content of stratum corneum as well as its effect on permeation was recently reported.[6] The authors worked with a laminated membrane consisting of excised human stratum corneum sandwiched between layers of silicone membrane; this was designed to prevent soaking of the skin in the vehicle. Salt solutions were chosen to control water activity and the water content in the stratum corneum could be maintained at a desired predetermined level. The flux of nitroglycerin, a hydrophobic compound, increased marginally when the stratum corneum water content was raised from 17.5 to 34%. However, a substantial increase of flux was noted when water content was further increased to 49%.

Vehicles and skin patches can increase hydration directly (by providing water) or indirectly (by occluding the skin surface, thus reducing the rate of water transpiration to the outside). Water then accumulates in the stratum corneum instead of passing through to the atmosphere. A totally water-impenetrable covering, such as metal foil or certain plastic/metal laminates, is most effective. The outer layer of transdermal drug devices is composed of an impenetrable barrier to prevent the loss of volatile compounds and, at the same time, increase the water content of the stratum corneum. Among the usual dermatologic vehicles, petrolatum is the most occlusive.[7] In general, ointments are more occlusive than creams, while lotions and powders offer little resistance to moisture transport.

Unless the skin is literally soaked in water, the application of aqueous vehicles is not likely to have a significant effect on hydration of the stratum corneum. Water evaporates quickly from simple solutions or suspensions, especially when present in a thin layer on the skin surface. However, more complex vehicles may hold some water in contact with the skin for a longer period of time. For example, if a finite quantity of a hygroscopic substance remains on the skin surface, its water content will approach equilibrium with the ambient humidity.

Permeant-solvent affinity

The degree of affinity between the permeant and solvent system represents one of the major factors controlling permeation through any membrane, including skin. It should be considered whenever comparisons are made between vehicles. Several approaches have been developed to estimate the contribution to skin permeation made by permeant-solvent affinity. The starting point for all of these is the concept of diffusion through an inert membrane.

The relation for steady-state flux, J, is given by Fick's first law, Equation 1,

$$J = PC_v = \frac{K D C_v}{l} \qquad \text{(Equation 1)}$$

in which P is the permeability coefficient, K is the stratum corneum/vehicle partition coefficient, D is the diffusion coefficient within the membrane, C_v is the vehicle concentration (in solution) and l is membrane thickness. We assume that all of the skin's resistance to penetration resides in the stratum corneum and that the vasculature (or, in the case of an in-vitro experiment, the receptor) is a perfect sink.

According to Equation 1, if we compare permeation from two solvents containing the same concentration of a drug, the permeation rate is proportional to the partition coefficient. While there are techniques for measuring uptake by pieces of stratum corneum, the results are sometimes difficult to interpret because of the heterogeneous nature of the tissue. Many investigators have utilized an organic solvent, such as isopropyl myristate or octanol, in place of stratum corneum to obtain an indication of K for substitution in Equation 1. This is workable if the vehicle is aqueous, but not if it is an organic liquid.

In 1960, Higuchi showed that Equation 1 could be transformed into Equation 2,

$$J = \frac{D\alpha}{l\gamma_s} \qquad \text{(Equation 2)}$$

in which α is the activity of the permeant within the vehicle and γ_s is the activity coefficient in the stratum corneum.[8] For a group of noninteractive solvents, γ_s should be a constant. If a saturated solution is defined as the reference state, then α at any concentration can be approximated by the ratio of concentration to solubility, C_v/S. Again, for noninteractive solvents, D and l are constant, so that the flux depends solely on α.

For a given solvent at saturation, dissolved permeant is in equilibrium with excess solid. Since the activity of the solid is unity, that is also the activity of the dissolved material. For the same reason, all saturated solutions of the same compound have the same activity (unity) and, provided that membrane-specific interactions do not intrude, all saturated solutions of the same compound should exhibit the same flux. (This statement relies on having the various saturated solutions in equilibrium with the same excess solid material. The existence of solvates and nonequilibrium crystal forms can complicate the situation.)

To illustrate the principle, it is useful to perform separate experiments on simple polymer membranes. Work with model membranes permits us to try out theoretical ideas before applying them to complex biological systems. It can also be used to define the locus of action of a solvent; comparison of data through polymer and skin membranes allows us to decide whether the solvent effect results primarily from a change in vehicle activity or a membrane-specific interaction.

The permeation of several parabens through polydimethylsiloxane membranes containing silica filler from various noninteractive solvents (water, polyols and water-polyol mixtures) has been reported.[9] Horizontal (2-chambered) diffusion cells were utilized. To minimize solvent gradients, the receptor fluid was matched to the donor in each case. Examination of the permeation data, plotted in Figures 1 and 2, shows that, for each paraben, the steady-state flux from saturated solutions was independent of the solvent within experimental error. It is noteworthy that, in the best solvent (polyethylene glycol 400), the solubility of methylparaben is about 100 times that in the poorest solvent (water); nevertheless, the flux values are the same.

In parallel experiments, the uptake of methylparaben by the membrane was evaluated and values of the partition coefficient were obtained. Corresponding values of the diffusion coefficient were calculated from a rearrangement of Equation 3:

$$J = \frac{K D \phi_1 C_v}{l\tau} \qquad \text{(Equation 3)}$$

In this equation, ϕ_1 is the volume fraction of polymer in the membrane and τ is membrane tortuosity. As expected for a group of solvents that do not interact with

Zatz

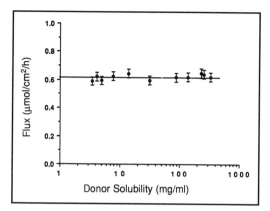

Figure 1. Steady-state flux of methylparaben from saturated solution in water and polyols (polyethylene glycol 400, propylene glycol, glycerin) and water-polyol mixtures through polydimethylsiloxane membranes. (Reproduced from Reference 9 with permission of the copyright owner.)

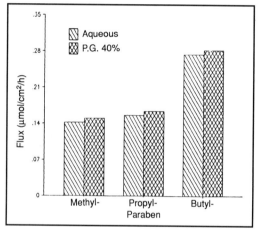

Figure 2. Effect of donor composition on steady-state flux from saturated aqueous and 40% propylene glycol systems through polydimethylsiloxane membranes. (Reproduced from Reference 9 with permission of the copyright owner.)

the membrane, the calculated diffusion coefficients were the same for all the solvents mentioned. The partition coefficients varied, but the amount of methylparaben sorbed from saturated solutions in the various solvents was the same. (The product of K and solubility was a constant.) The same result was obtained with the other parabens.

A reduction in concentration below saturation reduces the driving force for permeation. This can be interpreted as a reduction of α. Figure 3 shows an example from Reference 9. The steady-state flux of methylparaben is linearly related to the percent saturation.

The relationships described above make it possible to predict steady-state flux values for any solute concentration in a wide range of solvents in which solvent/membrane interactions do not play a significant role. The only pieces of information required are the solubility (S) of the permeant in the solvent of interest and the results from a single experiment performed using a reference solvent. The procedure is as follows:

1. Obtain the flux value (J_s) from a saturated solution in a reference solvent.

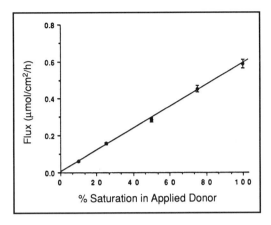

Figure 3. Steady state flux of methylparaben through polydimethylsiloxane membranes as a function of aqueous donor concentration expressed as a percent of saturation. (Reproduced from Reference 9 with permission of the copyright owner.)

2. Use Equation 4 to estimate the desired result in any solvent:

$$J_{predicted} = J_s \frac{C_v}{S} \qquad \text{(Equation 4)}$$

If we assume that the same permeant concentration will be utilized in a series of solvents, a, b and c, then J_s and C_v in Equation 4 are constant and it follows that

$$J_a S_a = J_b S_b = J_c S_c \qquad \text{(Equation 5)}$$

The permeation of a compound from a given solvent is thus inversely related to its solubility.

The approach stated in the preceding paragraph is of general utility. However, it must be applied with caution to permeation through skin because the horny layer is anything but inert. All, or nearly all, solvents left in contact with the skin surface will cause modifications of one kind or another which also affect permeability. The role of a particular solvent is therefore a function of both its interactions with the stratum corneum and noninteractive effects which can be related to solvency within the vehicle.

Nevertheless, activity adjustment within the vehicle is a viable component of formulation optimization. As an example, Barry et al.[10] reported a clinical and bioavailability study in which a cream base containing different concentrations of the same corticosteroid were compared. Both formulations were suspensions; they were saturated with respect to steroid. Both were also equivalent in terms of bioavailability and therapeutic response.

Calculations based on solubility parameter

Since membrane permeation is a function of both skin/permeant and solvent/permeant interactions, an effort has been made to model absorption through skin by quantitating these interactions using solubility parameters. The philosophy and some results were described by Sloan in a recent review.[11] Many of the assumptions made in carrying out the calculations are the same as those described above. These include the hypothesis that stratum corneum is a noninteractive membrane. The applicability of Equation 1 is also assumed.

The experimental procedure in Sloan's work utilized saturated solutions containing the same drug in various solvents which were therefore at maximum activity. Furthermore, after conducting a permeation experiment (through excised hairless mouse skin) a standard theophylline solution was applied to the same membrane. Flux values for this standard were then compared with previously obtained data through untreated skin. Significant differences indicated compromise of the skin barrier by the initial exposure. While deterioration of the horny layer, when it occurred, could usually be attributed to attack by the solvent, there were some instances in which the drug compound itself was responsible. This was the case with salicylic acid.

To perform the calculations, it was necessary to assign a value for the solubility parameter to the membrane. A frequent tack taken with polymeric membranes is to measure membrane swelling in the presence of a variety of solvents. Maximum solvent uptake occurs when the solubility parameter of the solvent matches that of the membrane. This technique is not possible with stratum corneum which is capable of sorbing large quantities of water despite the fact that it behaves as a lipophilic barrier. Instead, a solubility parameter value of 10 was inferred from previous data of skin permeation of alkanoic acids. (This value is typical of a slightly polar material. Hydrocarbons have values of about 7 to 9; water is 23.4.)

Sloan[10] used the following equation to calculate the theoretical partition coefficient ($K_i^{s,v}$) when drug solubility was small.

$$\log K_i^{s,v} = \frac{[(\delta_i - \delta_v)^2 - (\delta_i - \delta_s)^2]V_i}{2.3RT} \qquad \text{(Equation 6)}$$

V_i is the drug's molar volume; δ is solubility parameter and the subscripts, i, v and s refer to drug, vehicle and stratum corneum, respectively. The only quantity in the equation that varies if the same solute is placed in different solvents is the first term in the numerator. By inspection of Equation 6, matching the solubility parameters of solute and solvent (leading to high solubility) produces a minimal stratum corneum/solution partition coefficient, while making the two solubility parameters different (reduced solubility) leads to an increase in the partition coefficient. This is the same conclusion as that reached from an analysis of Equation 2.

Tables I and II are based on data for two compounds taken from Sloan's chapter. The product of the theoretical partition coefficient and solubility, S, represents the theoretical maximal concentration gradient, the driving force for permeation across the membrane. These values, shown in Tables I and II are not identical; they depend on the particular solute-solvent combination. For example, 6-mercaptopurine in propylene glycol has a value of 0.47 while the same solute in formamide has a value of 3.46, roughly 7 times greater.

If the effective barrier thickness remains constant and the drug diffusion coefficient is also unaffected by the solvent, the skin flux should be simply proportional to the gradient across the membrane. If these assumptions hold, the ratio of flux to theoretical gradient for a given substance applied in a variety of solvents should be constant. While approximately so for a group of systems shown in the tables, ratios for octanol and isopropyl myristate exhibit values significantly

Table I. Comparison of experimental flux through hairless mouse skin and theoretical concentration gradient of 6-mercaptopurine.				
Solvent	d_v $\sqrt{cal/cm^3}$	$k_i^{s,v} \cdot S$ (mg/cm³)	Flux, J ($10^3 \cdot$ mg/cm²h)	Ratio $\dfrac{J}{k_i^{s,v} \cdot S}$
Oleic acid	7.6	0.111	0.043	0.39
Isopropyl myristate	8.5	0.027	0.6	0.22
Diethyltoluamide	10.0	5.05	3.2	0.63
Octanol	10.3	0.163	18.6	0.011
Methoxyethanol	12.1	1.51	0.75	0.5
Dimethyl formamide	12.1	2.20	3.8	1.7
Dimethyl sulfoxide	13.0	3.32	2.1	0.63
Propylene glycol	14.8	0.470	0.093	0.20
Ethylene glycol	16.1	0.329	0.1	0.30
Formamide	17.9	3.46	1.5	0.43
Water	23.4	978	0.36	0.00037

(Data from Reference 11)

Table II. Comparison of experimental flux through hairless mouse skin and theoretical concentration gradient of theophylline.				
Solvent	d_v $\sqrt{cal/cm^3}$	$k_i^{s,v} \cdot S$ (mg/cm³)	Flux, J ($10^3 \cdot$ mg/cm²h)	Ratio $\dfrac{J}{k_i^{s,v} \cdot S}$
Isopropyl myristate	8.5	0.817	41.2	50
Octanol	10.3	1.12	547	490
Dimethyl formamide	12.1	3.62	17	4.7
Propylene glycol	14.8	0.486	1.54	3.2
Ethylene glycol	16.1	0.890	1.94	2.2
Formamide	17.9	1.37	3.69	2.7

(Data from Reference 11)

higher than the other solvents suggesting a specific effect on the barrier. This is in accord with the observation that treatment with these solvents caused an elevation in the flux of the theophylline standard, indicating membrane damage.

Assessing solvent-skin interactions

As pointed out in the previous section, permeant-solvent affinity always plays a role in defining the contribution of solvents to skin permeation. In addition, nearly all vehicles applied to the skin are capable of altering the character of the stratum corneum to some extent. These interactions, which are specific in that they depend on the nature of the membrane, alter permeability. Several kinds of interaction may be envisioned, all operating simultaneously. A basic factor in permeation is stratum corneum hydration. The use of water as a vehicle increases hydration, but other, water-miscible solvents may dehydrate the horny layer, thus decreasing permeation. Vehicles that are good solvents for skin lipids, such as methanol and lower hydrocarbons, probably extract lipids when permitted to remain in contact with the skin, thereby facilitating permeation. More subtle effects, including modification of the structure of the intercellular lipids in the stratum corneum, may be induced by solvents that are themselves well absorbed into this layer. Such modifications usually result in an increase in the penetration rate through the skin.

Given that just about any solvent will exert some effect on the horny layer, it is of interest to separate the role played by these interactions in permeation from the nonspecific solute-solvent interactions described above. Several methods for doing so will be described.

Maintaining constant donor activity

One approach that has been taken is to design experiments so as to compare solvents under conditions of equal thermodynamic activity, so that any differences in flux may be ascribed to interactions with the membrane. A reasonable reference point for such studies is the saturated solution.

Once again, it is convenient to study a simple membrane and then attempt to apply the same principles to the more complex situation. Figure 4, which contains data from our laboratory, shows the flux of two parabens through polydimethylsiloxane membranes from saturated alkanol solutions.[12] Shown in the same figure are the data for water. It is apparent that the flux of both parabens is much higher when the solvents are alcohols rather than water. This, in itself, is an indication that the alkanols interact with the membrane. (If no interactions occurred, the flux values should have been identical with those from aqueous solution.) Further evidence is provided by the fact that the membrane swells in the presence of the alkanols and that the degree of swelling correlates with the relative flux.[12]

A physical model has been developed to explain the effect of alcohols on permeation through polydimethylsiloxane membranes.[13] The alcohol is imbibed into the membrane, creating clusters within which other substances can dissolve. The membrane concentration of solutes is thus much higher than if alcohol were not present. This leads to an increase in the effective partition coefficient, and therefore (as stated in Equation 1), an increase in the flux. The apparent diffusion coefficient is unaffected.

The relationship between paraben concentration and steady-state flux from 1-propanol solutions is shown in Figure 5. The curves are unusual in that the flux rises with concentration, reaches a peak and then decreases. This complex behavior may be explained by recognizing that the driving force for membrane transport is the product of concentration and partition coefficient. Each of these factors changes simultaneously in opposite directions as the solute concentration is increased. When the paraben concentration is low, a concentration increase

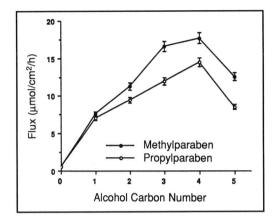

Figure 4. Influence of primary alcohols on paraben flux through polydimethylsiloxane membranes. The zero-chain homologue is represented by the corresponding aqueous system. Key: ☐ propylparaben; ■ methylparaben. (Reproduced from Reference 12 with permission of the copyright owner, the American Pharmaceutical Association.)

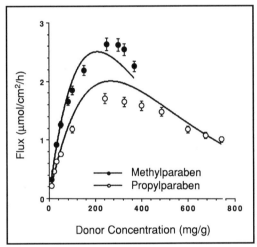

Figure 5. Steady-state flux profiles for methylparaben and butylparaben through polydimethylsiloxane membranes from solution in 1-propanol. The points are measured values; the lines are calculated values. (Reproduced from Reference 13 with permission of the copyright owner, the American Pharmaceutical Association.)

produces a nearly proportional increase in the driving force (concentration gradient). But very high solute concentrations cause a reduction in the alcohol activity; less alcohol is imbibed into the membrane and, as a consequence, there is a decrease in the relative paraben concentration within the membrane. Figure 5 contains theoretical curves, calculated from independently determined alcohol sorption data. (Details of the calculation are provided in Reference 13.) The agreement is good, showing that the factors involved have been accounted for.

As described in the previous paragraph, the use of saturated solutions allows comparisons to be made at equal solute activity, but the effect of high solute concentrations on solvent activity complicates the picture. One approach in such cases, is to work at low solute concentrations (so that solvent activity is maintained constant) and then calculate a normalized flux, J*, by extrapolating the data to saturation using Equation 7.

$$J^* = J \frac{S}{C_v} = PS \qquad \text{(Equation 7)}$$

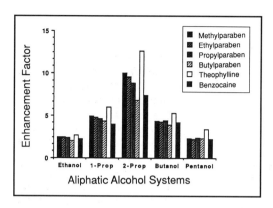

Figure 6. Alcohol enhancement factors through polydimethylsiloxane membranes for six solutes. (Reproduced from Reference 14 by courtesy of Marcel Dekker Inc.)

J* provides a means of comparing solvents under conditions of equal solute and solvent activity.

Frequently the effect of different solvent treatments is quantitated through an enhancement factor, usually a ratio of flux following a given treatment to a reference flux value. For solutes applied to polydimethylsiloxane membranes in alcohol solution, the enhancement factor may be defined as the ratio of J* for a given solvent to J* for a reference, in this case methanol.

Data for six solutes in six solvents are presented in Figure 6.[14] Flux values were obtained for a donor concentration of 10 mg/g. Although the enhancement factors vary from system to system, the relative ranking of the solutes from alcohol to alcohol is the same. It is clear that the effect of membrane interaction is greatest for 2-propanol, followed by 1-butanol, 1-propanol, 1-pentanol, ethanol and finally methanol, whose value is defined as unity.

The donor concentrations utilized in the paraben study covered a broad range because of the high solubility of parabens in alcohols (up to about 700 mg/ g). Donor concentrations in skin studies are usually much lower; typical drug concentrations in marketed products are kept as low as possible to minimize cost and reduce the risks associated with product misuse. Under most usual conditions, skin studies generally exhibit linear flux-concentration profiles.

We have evaluated the permeation of methylparaben and theophylline from several common solvents through dermatomed excised fuzzy rat skin.[15] Methylparaben flux was a linear function of propylene glycol and propanol concentration over the entire concentration range, up to saturation. Therefore, in this study, it was feasible to compare data for saturated solutions directly.

The values for methylparaben flux are shown in Table III. They range from a low of 0.055 μmol/cm²/h for polyethylene glycol 400 to a high of 9.1 μmol/cm²/h for methanol, a ratio of about 150. The values for theophylline are collected in Table IV. On a solvent by solvent basis, these values are substantially lower than for methylparaben. Nevertheless, if the two sets of values are compared (Figure 7), a consistent pattern is observed. Despite the differences in solubility and absolute permeability, the solvents line up in the same rank order. Flux values from polyethylene glycol 400, glycerin and dimethylisosorbide vehicles are less than

Table III. Methylparaben solubilities and permeation data

	Solubility @ 37°C		Flux (μmol/cm^2/h)	
Solvent	(mg/cm^3)	n	Mean	95%C.I.[a]
PEG 400	330	9	0.055	0.049 $\leq \mu \leq$ 0.061
Glycerin		6	0.11	0.094 $\leq \mu \leq$ 0.12
DMIS		6	0.16	0.14 $\leq \mu \leq$ 0.18
Propylene Glycol	260	6	0.55	0.49 $\leq \mu \leq$ 0.61
Water	3.5	12	0.67	0.60 $\leq \mu \leq$ 0.73
1-Propanol	360	6	0.68	0.61 $\leq \mu \leq$ 0.76
Ethanol	380	6	1.36	1.1 $\leq \mu \leq$ 1.6
Methanol	470	6	9.1	7.7 $\leq \mu \leq$ 10
Average Lag Time $\pm$ Standard error (h)		93	3.3 $\pm$ 0.1	

[a]Confidence Interval

Table IV. Theophylline solubilities and permeation data

	Solubility @ 37°C		Flux (μmol/cm^2/h)	
Solvent	(mg/cm^3)	n	Mean	95%C.I.[a]
PEG 400		9	0.011	0.011 $\leq \mu \leq$ 0.012
Glycerin		5	0.014	0.012 $\leq \mu \leq$ 0.016
DMIS		6	0.029	0.024 $\leq \mu \leq$ 0.033
Propylene Glycol		6	0.044	0.032 $\leq \mu \leq$ 0.057
Water		12	0.13	0.12 $\leq \mu \leq$ 0.14
1-Propanol	4.1	6	0.21	0.17 $\leq \mu \leq$ 0.25
Ethanol	4.8	6	0.29	0.27 $\leq \mu \leq$ 0.32
Methanol	8.4	6	0.65	0.54 $\leq \mu \leq$ 0.75
Average Lag Time $\pm$ Standard error (h)		56	1.5 $\pm$ 0.1	

[a]Confidence Interval
(Data from Reference 15)

that from water. Ethanol and methanol enhance permeation in comparison to water. Propylene glycol varies, depending on solute, from about 1/3 the value for water to almost the same value. Similar results were obtained in an earlier, less extensive study of benzocaine permeation through hairless mouse skin.[16]

Other studies confirm that penetration from saturated solution in propylene glycol is no better than from water under infinite dose conditions. Compare, for example, flux values for 6-mercaptopurine through hairless mouse skin (Table I). Similar results were obtained for estradiol through excised human skin.[17]

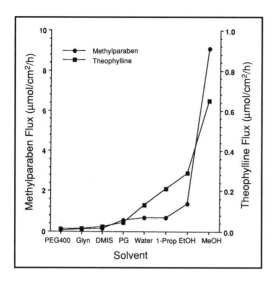

Figure 7. Average solute flux from saturated donors. (Reproduced from Reference 15 with permission of the copyright owner.)

Calculated vs. measured permeability

One way to gain an appreciation for the role of specific interactions with the skin is to estimate permeability characteristics under idealized or theoretical conditions and then compare them with real data. An example cited in an earlier section is the finding that solute permeability from octanol and isopropyl myristate were much greater than expected when compared to calculated values of partition coefficient.[11] The pattern found in the flux/theoretical concentration gradient ratio for a single permeant in a series of solvents permits a ranking of solvents in terms of their interaction with the skin barrier.

Returning to Table II, the flux/gradient ratios for propylene glycol, ethylene glycol and formamide with theophylline differ by only about a factor of two. The same is true of 6-mercaptopurine in the same solvents (Table I). This suggests that the three solvents mentioned exhibit about the same degree of interaction with the stratum corneum.

The ratio for water with 6-mercaptopurine is unexpectedly low (Table I). This is apparently due to the very high value calculated for the theoretical gradient. DMSO and diethyltoluamide (which increases the skin penetration of a variety of compounds)[18] have the same ratio. Data for these three solvents were reported with only one permeant[11] and further information is needed.

Kedir et al. described another method for using partition coefficients calculated from solubility parameters to separate the thermodynamic activity in the vehicle (the "push" contribution) from changes in resistance of the barrier.[2] The authors compared ratios of calculated partition coefficients for two solvents with the corresponding experimental flux ratios. If these ratios are similar, then push effects account for any differences in flux; deviations in the ratios are ascribed to changes in membrane resistance. Data for theophylline in a group of alkanoic acid vehicles disclosed that propionic acid increased drug flux through an interaction with the skin.

Dual membrane comparison

Roberts and Anderson described a technique for identifying the approximate magnitude of interactions between solvents and skin utilizing parallel experiments through skin and another, inert membrane.[19] The same solution (containing the same concentration of the same solute) is applied to both membranes and flux values are compared. The authors showed that the permeation ratio (permeability coefficient through skin/permeability coefficient through polyethylene) is independent of the permeant's thermodynamic activity if both membranes are inert. On the other hand a higher than expected ratio indicates the existence of an interaction between the solvent and skin. As mentioned above, no solvent is completely inert toward skin so that the ratios provide an index of relative alteration of the stratum corneum's barrier properties.

In the reported study, the authors measured the penetration of phenol through excised rat skin and polyethylene film; the latter was assumed to be inert toward all of the solvents. The same solutions, at fixed phenol concentration, were applied to both membranes in parallel. Some data from this study are contained in Table V.

Several solvents, liquid paraffin, arachis oil and glycerin, which might be expected to exhibit minimal skin interaction, had a skin/polyethylene ratio of about 2. The ratio for water and ethanol, both of which affect the stratum corneum to a greater extent, was approximately 4. Dimethyl formamide and dimethyl sulfoxide had much higher ratios, 11 and 18, respectively, in line with their known tendency to disrupt the stratum corneum.

A simple comparison of rat skin flux values or permeability coefficients does not provide the same information as the flux ratios. For example, phenol flux from water was about 10 times that from dimethyl sulfoxide (Table V), despite the fact that the latter disturbs the membrane barrier to a much greater extent. This is due to the fact that dimethyl sulfoxide is a better solvent for phenol, so solute activity was substantially lower in dimethyl sulfoxide than water. The

Table V. Permeability of phenol through two membranes and their ratio.			
Solvent	Polyethylene permeability coefficient (cm/min • 10^3)	Rat skin permeability coefficient (cm/min • 10^3)	Flux ratio (skin/polyethylene)
Liquid paraffin	0.5	1	2
Glycerin	0.005	0.010	2
Arachis oil	0.014	0.029	2
Water	0.044	0.19	4
Ethanol	0.004	0.016	4
Dimethyl formamide	0.002	0.022	11
Dimethyl sulfoxide	0.001	0.018	18

(Data from Reference 19)

greater escaping tendency of phenol from the water system overshadowed the degree to which the two solvents altered membrane properties.

Using similar reasoning, it is possible to apply the membrane sandwich method[6] to the study of solvent effects on skin penetration. The sandwich consists of two silicone polymer membranes bonded by silicone adhesive to an enclosed human stratum corneum membrane. The steady-state flux through the composite membrane is a function of the resistance of all three layers; there may also be a contribution from stagnant solvent layers at the membrane's boundaries. A separate experiment is used to measure solute permeability through the silicone membrane by itself. This is subtracted in an appropriate manner from the value for the composite membrane to yield data for the stratum corneum.

A group of solvents can be ranked in terms of its relative effect on barrier properties by performing the experiments described in the previous paragraph since the polymer permeation data reflect noninteractive contributions to flux while the composite responds to both noninteractive and interactive effects. The major advantage of this setup is that the stratum corneum is not macerated in solvent. However, it is limited to solutes capable of diffusing through the polymer membrane rapidly enough so that the major portion of the composite membrane's resistance resides within the stratum corneum. Also, the solvents should not cause swelling of the silicone polymer (in other words, this polymer should be inert toward the solvents). Finally, the solvents themselves must permeate the polymer membrane to reach the stratum corneum inside at approximately the same concentration.

Extrapolation to saturation

Several of the comparative techniques described in earlier sections rely on comparisons of saturated solutions. As has been mentioned, there may be drawbacks to the use of saturated solutions when the solubility is very high, as shown by the data for paraben permeation through polydimethyl sulfoxide membranes. Concentrations at saturation are likely to exceed those used in practice and the cost of solute used in preparing the solutions may be prohibitive,

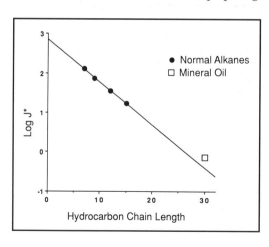

Figure 8. Effect of hydrocarbon chain length on normalized flux, J^*, of caffeine through hairless mouse skin.

particularly if radioactively labeled solutes are used. An alternative to the use of saturated solutions is to work at moderate concentrations and estimate the saturation flux, $J*$ using Equation 5.

The effect of a series of hydrocarbon solvents on permeation of caffeine through excised hairless mouse skin is shown in Figure 8.[20] $J*$ values were used as a basis of comparison to eliminate the effect of solvency. It is apparent that lengthening the hydrocarbon chain reduces the interaction with the horny layer. Interestingly, the logarithm of $J*$ is a linear function of hydrocarbon chain length.

The value for mineral oil is plotted on the same graph. Mineral oil is a mixture; its average chain length was estimated to be 30. Using this value, the data for mineral oil fall close to the line for the other hydrocarbons (Figure 8).

Finite dose studies

In the literature on solvent effects, most of the data are based on in-vitro studies performed under infinite dose conditions in which the membrane is immersed in a relatively large volume of applied material. Leaching of skin components into the donor may be exaggerated. With aqueous or largely aqueous solutions, the stratum corneum is completely hydrated. Steady-state data obtained from infinite dose studies is particularly convenient for mathematical treatment and is usually relevant to studies of transdermal delivery. However, the exposure to large amounts of solvent is often not typical of the usual dermatological or cosmetic application.

In such cases, it is possible to perform in-vitro studies using a finite dose application (described in some detail in the first chapter). Since the applied volume is small and the system is left open to the atmosphere, changes in vehicle composition and drug content can take place. Quite often, the permeation profile is complex and comparisons are made at single time points.

We can immediately anticipate a difference in the effect of vehicles containing large percentages of water and other volatile solvents. There will be significant losses of such materials shortly after application to the skin if an occlusive covering is not applied. Furthermore, even substances not normally considered very volatile, such as propylene glycol, may evaporate over time because the applied layer is thin and has a relatively large surface exposed.

Data for estradiol permeation through excised human skin from a number of solvents applied as a thin layer suggested that specific skin interactions were more important than thermodynamic activity.[21] Penetration was best from DMSO and several glycols. Those solvents that were themselves good penetrants seemed to produce the highest drug flux. From their data, $J*$ for propylene glycol is about 15 times that for glycerin, which, in turn, is 5 times that for polyethylene glycol 400. This is the same order as followed in the previously described work with fuzzy rat skin[15] although the relative values differ.

Penetration of two drugs, metronidazole and estradiol, as well as propylene glycol itself, from solvent mixtures was a function of glycol content.[22] There was essentially no difference in the penetration rate of the three compounds between a vehicle consisting of pure glycerin and one composed of a 50:50 mixture of glycerin and propylene glycol. With only propylene glycol as solvent, penetration was maximal for all three compounds. Excellent correlation between the permeation data for metronidazole and propylene glycol from a variety of vehicles was observed.

When complex vehicles are applied to the skin, some components evaporate while others become more concentrated. Coldman et al. showed that certain mixtures of a volatile and a nonvolatile component could result in high penetration rates when applied under finite dose conditions.[23] This was ascribed to the formation of supersaturated solutions on the skin surface. It should be noted that the nonvolatile components used in this study were propylene glycol and isopropyl myristate, two compounds that are interactive toward skin.

Penetration-enhancing solvents

Although several solvents have been identified as modifying the skin barrier thus permitting increased penetration of other substances, the mechanism(s) responsible are still under investigation. DMSO is perhaps the best known and most widely studied of these solvents. Kurihara-Bergstrom et al. summarized proposed mechanisms for the action of DMSO and provided further information using excised hairless mouse skin as a model.[24] The penetration rate of several alkanols was evaluated from vehicles containing DMSO and water. There was little effect of the vehicles on the skin barrier at DMSO levels up to 50%. At higher concentrations, the barrier became progressively impaired, and the amount of material leached by the donor from the skin increased. The data at high DMSO concentrations were consistent with protein denaturation and the damaging effect of cross solvent flows with water as receptor. The maximum effect was noted with pure DMSO; methanol, the most polar of the permeants used, exhibited the largest increase in permeability. Differential scanning measurements show that DMSO in high concentration lowers the temperature for peaks ascribed both to lipid and protein regions within the stratum corneum.[25]

The penetration pathway of mercury and nickel salts through nude mouse skin was altered by pretreatment of the skin with DMSO, dimethyl formamide and dimethyl acetamide.[26] The metal ions were found almost exclusively in the intercellular regions, but with solvent pretreatment, they also accumulated in the basal stratum corneum cells. This was attributed to frank damage to the horny layer. Later work with human skin confirmed some aspects of this picture, particularly the predominance of intercellular concentration of mercuric chloride within the stratum corneum.[27] However, DMSO treatment did not alter cell distribution of the salt although it did increase the rate of penetration.

It is well known that ethanol and other alcohols increase skin penetration provided that they remain in contact with the skin by application in a closed system. Studies of lipid extraction and nicotinamide penetration following pretreatment (for up to six hours) of hairless mouse skin with a series of n-alkanols, C_2 to C_{12}, were recently reported.[28] Skin uptake of alkanols increased with chain length but nicotinamide (and alkanol) penetration reached a maximum with hexanol and then declined. Lipid extraction by the alkanols was demonstrated and this form of membrane damage was taken to be the major effect in hairless mice. It was recognized that human skin might behave somewhat differently.

In contrast, there was no evidence of membrane damage in a study of the effect of ethanol on penetration of a lipophilic compound, estradiol, through a human skin sandwich flap model.[29] The permeability coefficient, P, was decreased tenfold when the compound was applied in 95% ethanol as compared to phosphate-buffered saline. Apparent partition coefficients were measured using human stratum corneum discs and the excellent correlation between P and K suggested that there was no change in diffusivity. The decrease in P in the presence of ethanol is in line with the increase in solubility (activity effect). However, the relative increase in solubility due to alcohol was much greater than its effect on K; when saturated estradiol solutions were compared, the flux was 1000 times greater from a saturated alcohol solution as from buffered saline.

Another study from the same laboratory focused on an ionic permeant, sodium salicylate.[30] Following infinite dose application to excised human cadaver skin, P values for both salicylate ion and ethanol increased with ethanol content in the vehicle, reaching a maximum value at a concentration approximately 60%; values at ethanol concentrations of 95 or 100% were lower. Salicylate uptake by stratum corneum was unaffected by ethanol content up to about 60% but decreased significantly at high ethanol levels. Another difference was in the times required to reach steady state; these were about 14 hours for ethanol concentrations up to about 60% and 40 hours for the very high concentrations. In this case, unlike the situation with estradiol, there was no correlation between P and K. Conclusions as to mechanism were highly tentative. Spectroscopic data suggested that protein conformational changes and/or lipid extraction might be involved.

Liu et al. described the effect of relatively low ethanol concentrations on diffusion and metabolism of estradiol in hairless mouse skin.[31] Their in-vitro experiments were conducted in horizontal diffusion cells in which both sides, donor and receptor, had the same ethanol content. Under these (nonphysiologic) conditions, the metabolism of estradiol was severely reduced even at 2% ethanol, and further reduced at higher ethanol levels. There was a slight concomitant increase in estradiol flux that was essentially independent of ethanol concentration. The data were consistent with a model in which enzyme activity resided within the basal area of the epidermis.

Data obtained with the same ethanol content on both sides of the membrane (symmetric configuration) were compared with an arrangement in which the donor contained various ethanol concentrations while the receptor consisted of water (asymmetric configuration).[32] Excised human skin was used in these experiments in which the ethanol concentration ranged up to 75%. In the asymmetric configuration there is an ethanol gradient through the membrane, so that enhancement effects vary depending on distance from the outer surface. Furthermore, because of lower concentrations in deep membrane sections, the influence of ethanol is much less when water is the receptor than when the receptor composition matches that of the donor. As an example, the estradiol flux from 50% ethanol was about 0.165 $\mu g/hr/cm^2$ in the asymmetric configuration and more than ten times that value in the symmetric configuration.

An interesting observation was that higher ethanol concentrations resulted in increases in both the flux of estradiol and ethanol itself.[32] A theoretical analysis suggested that there was an increase in diffusion coefficient of both substances with elevation of the ethanol concentration. Model calculations showed that drug enhancement and solvent enhancement were not necessarily linearly related.

Several studies have noted that diethylene glycol monoethyl ether (Transcutol®, Gattefossé) can increase skin penetration of various drugs. Rojas et al. measured morphine penetration through hairless rat skin from vehicles containing diethylene glycol monoethyl ether (DGME) alone and in combination with other solvents.[33] Of the various combinations used, DGME by itself exhibited the highest solubility as well as the lowest flux. However, several ternary systems yielded flux values that were higher than expected strictly on the basis of solubility behavior. Enhancement in skin uptake was judged by comparing relative values of skin/vehicle partition coefficient with corresponding reciprocal solubility data.

The effect of propylene glycol on the skin has been debated for some time. Application of propylene glycol to hydrated skin (under infinite dose conditions) is, in general, no more effective in promoting penetration than is water and it does not alter lipid structure.[25] However, propylene glycol appears to be a potent solvent when placed in contact with dry stratum corneum[22] and also works well in combination with many nonpolar surface active molecules to lower skin resistance. The use of solvents in combination with surfactants will be considered briefly in the next section; further discussion of surfactants will be found in the next chapter.

Solvent influence on surface-active penetration enhancers

Oleic acid and other fatty acids have been shown to increase the absorption of drugs and other substances. The effect of these molecules depends on the medium; propylene glycol is a preferred solvent in terms of skin penetration, although it has a tendency to be irritating to the skin in high concentration. The surface-active molecules that can be so effective in the presence of organic solvents are largely inactive when applied in water. For example, the resistance of hairless mouse skin to lidocaine penetration was hardly affected by polysorbates (nonionic surfactants) applied in vehicles containing propylene glycol and water if the glycol content was 60% or less.[34] However, at 80% propylene glycol, lidocaine absorption was enhanced approximately threefold. The enhancement was observed in both finite dose and infinite dose experiments.

A recent report described the effect of four solvents (sometimes combined with several proposed enhancers) on penetration of acyclovir through excised hairless mouse and rat skin.[35] Saturated solutions of the drug were used to maintain the same activity level within the vehicle. Some data from the paper are given in Table VI.

There is some difference in the values obtained for the various solvents, with isopropyl myristate producing the highest penetration. What is even more significant is that the effect of the enhancer Azone® was highly dependent on the solvent used. The largest effect was found with propylene glycol, the most polar of the solvents utilized. In fact, there was an inverse relationship between solvent polarity (quantitated through the solubility parameter) and acyclovir penetration in the presence of Azone.®

One consideration in this work is the partitioning of the vehicle components into the skin. Since Azone® is a lipophilic substance, its partitioning would be

Table VI. Penetration of Acyclovir through excised hairless rat skin.

| Solvent | Mean Percent Acyclovir Recovered from Receptor | |
	Solvent only	Solvent plus 0.1M Azone®
Propylene glycol	1.3	54
Ethanol	2.2	24
Isopropanol	3.1	4.8
Isopropyl myristate	3.4	2.4

(Data from Reference 35)

expected to be greatest from the most polar solvent although measurements of donor composition at the end of the experiment did not provide unequivocal support of this idea.

Another recent report investigated the effect of myristic acid on oxymorphone penetration through excised human skin from several solvents.[36] The solvents tested included propylene glycol, ethanol and polyethylene glycol 400. Data for systems containing excess drug are summarized in Table VII.

Solvent polarity does not appear to be the important factor here. The combination of propylene glycol and myristic acid produced the highest flux. Despite the higher drug flux from ethanol than propylene glycol plus the fact that ethanol is itself a better skin penetrant than propylene glycol, addition of myristic acid to an ethanol vehicle did not have a remarkable effect.

Researchers described the effect of oleic acid (0.25%) on piroxicam penetration through human and hairless mouse skin from ethanol-water.[37] Penetration was quite low from a vehicle containing no ethanol. As with the previous study,[36] steady-state flux from a vehicle containing only ethanol and oleic acid (no water) was not impressive. Maximal enhancement values of approximately one order of magnitude with human skin, two orders of magnitude with hairless mouse, were obtained at ethanol concentrations of about 40 to 50% by volume. Parallel changes in lipid-related DSC transition temperatures were observed,

Table VII. Penetration of Oxymorphone through excised human skin.

| Solvent | Mean Flux ($\mu gcm^{-2}h^{-1}$) | |
	Solvent only	Solvent plus 10% myristic acid
Propylene glycol	1.1	94
Ethanol	13	19
Polyethylene glycol 400	—	0.7

(Data from Reference 35)

suggesting that microscopic disruptions in the extracellular lipid due to oleic acid are responsible for the increase in flux.

The data published thus far suggest that the solvent must itself penetrate the skin if combinations with surface-active compounds are to effectively increase skin permeation. However, it is the combination of solvent, surface-active agent and permeant that must be considered rather than these agents separately. While it is clear that such combinations are effective in promoting skin permeation, the mechanisms involved have not yet been worked out.

Summary

In the literature on skin permeation effects from different solvents, many of the discordant data can be reconciled by taking the three major solvent effects into consideration. Poor wetting can result in incomplete contact with the skin surface. This problem is most likely to be encountered with viscous vehicles having high surface tension. The presence of surface-active substances, whether from the formulation or the skin, helps to improve wetting.

Flux depends on the permeant activity as well as changes in skin structure resulting from interaction with the vehicle. Simple relationships often allow us to calculate the effect of changing concentrations in a given medium. Empirical comparisons at equivalent permeant activities provide information on the consequences of interactions with the horny layer. We have reached a point at which it is often possible to anticipate the direction in which permeation values will be affected by a change in solvent. However, additional fundamental data leading to more detailed elucidation of the mechanisms involved would clearly be useful.

Chapter 7

Modification of Skin Permeation by Surface-Active Agents

By Joel L. Zatz, PhD

Surface-active agents are widely used in skin products to serve a variety of functions. Consequently, there is great interest in interactions of surfactants with the stratum corneum, especially those interactions that might modify the skin's resistance to molecular diffusion. Ideally, we would want to have mechanistic information that would provide an understanding of the processes involved. Failing that, empirical relationships with predictive value would be valuable.

The complexity of the multiphase systems commonly used as dermatological and cosmetic vehicles makes it difficult to get the type of detailed information desired. For one thing, surfactant molecules are distributed in the bulk phases as well as the interfaces that separate them. In addition, the formation of aggregates (micelles or vesicles) can change the extent of interaction with drug molecules or other solutes and modify the driving force for permeation. The large number of possible interactions usually precludes obtaining data of fundamental significance directly from investigations on complete formulations. Instead, most studies have focused on relatively simple prototypic solutions and dispersions which serve as models for the more complex systems used in the drug and cosmetic industries.

This review summarizes the recent literature about the influence of surface-active substances on permeation. It is not limited to compounds used commercially as surfactants, but includes other amphiphiles that may interact with the stratum corneum to influence its barrier properties.

Multiple mechanisms and study design

In many studies, drug penetration is measured from solutions containing a fixed drug concentration and various surfactants. Even in such relatively simple systems, several mechanisms may operate simultaneously to influence permeation. Any interaction that reduces permeant activity, such as complexation or micellar solubilization, also reduces the driving force for diffusion. One can imagine a situation in which a surfactant solubilizes an active substance and, at the same time, reduces stratum corneum resistance. The first effect would tend to lower penetration rate while the second would raise it, so that the end result might be lack of any difference between a drug solution containing no surfactant and a solution in which a surfactant was included. If the purpose of the study is simply to obtain empirical information on skin delivery from particular compositions, then the study design described above is fine. On the other hand, if its purpose is to evaluate the alteration of stratum corneum properties by a series of surfactants, it is first necessary to normalize surfactant-permeant interactions.[1]

Normalization can be accomplished by adjusting permeant activity to unity or some other consistent value in all of the systems undergoing comparison. The usual reference point is the solution saturated with respect to permeant (activity = 1), provided that solubility does not require an excessive concentration. While it is true that solubilization and other molecular interactions take place in a saturated solution, the concentration of free permeant molecules available for diffusion is unaffected. Thus, saturated solutions may be compared unambiguously as a means of measuring surfactant-skin interactions.

Another experimental approach involves pretreatment of the skin for a specified period of time by a solution containing the surface-active agent, followed by application of a model permeant in a standard preparation, usually a simple solution. It is assumed that pretreatment exerts no effect on the physical-chemical properties of the subsequently applied solution; the thermodynamic activity of the permeant is therefore unaffected. Differences in permeation behavior reflect changes in stratum corneum structure due to the pretreatment. However, a lengthy pretreatment time may accentuate leaching of skin components. It is important in such experiments to utilize a control to account for changes in the membrane due to hydration.

Nonionic surfactants

Nonionic surfactants are widely used in dermatologic and cosmetic products because of their relatively low irritation potential. Much of the literature through 1986 regarding the effect of surfactants (including nonionics) on skin resistance to permeation was summarized in the review by Walters.[2] Several examples of penetration enhancement in aqueous solutions by nonionic surfactants were given; it is apparent that nonionics interact with the skin, either by penetration and incorporation into the stratum corneum or by extraction of intercellular lipids. However, it should be noted that the degree of enhancement is relatively small, in most cases no more than a factor of two.

The relative effect on skin barrier properties is a function of surfactant chemistry. Among polyoxyethylene alkyl ethers, enhancement of methyl nicotinate penetration across hairless mouse skin was maximal from surfactants with a 12-carbon hydrophobe and polar head group containing 10 to 14 ethylene oxide units.[2] This is in contrast to the anticipated penetration order of the surfactants themselves. (However, it should be noted that most data involving drug systems were obtained in aqueous or partially aqueous media. On the other hand, in absorption studies of surfactants, organic liquids are frequently used to apply the compounds to the skin surface.)

Nishiyama et al. reported the percutaneous absorption of surface-active compounds based on lauryl alcohol.[3] The surfactants in ethanol solution were applied in vivo to the skin of hairless mice. Some of the results are compiled in Table I. Lauryl alcohol itself was absorbed to a significant extent during the 4-hour exposure. The incorporation of one to three ethylene oxide units into the molecule resulted in an increase in the extent of absorption. Further ethoxylation produced a dramatic decrease.

Table I. Total absorption following 4-hour exposure of lauryl alcohol derivatives (1.38 mmole) in ethanol (25 ml) on the skin of hairless mice in vivo.	
Mean number of ethylene oxide units/molecule	Total percent absorbed
0	46
1	56
2.6	61
6.4	28
10	5

(Data from Reference 3)

The influence of a series of polyoxyethylene nonylphenols on benzocaine penetration through hairless mouse skin was investigated.[4,5] The outcome depended on whether the permeant (benzocaine) was dissolved or present in excess as a suspension. The outcome also depended on surfactant hydrophilic chain length and concentration. With aqueous benzocaine solutions, the addition of polyoxyethylene (15) nonylphenol reduced steady-state flux, essentially in proportion to surfactant concentration. It was also noted that flux was inversely related to the length of the polyoxyethylene chain. These results suggested that the reduction in benzocaine flux was a function of the extent of solubilization within surfactant micelles. An additional piece of evidence supporting this idea was obtained by estimating the "free" benzocaine concentration in various surfactant solutions from solubilization studies. A plot of flux against free benzocaine concentration was linear, in agreement with the notion that alterations in permeant activity accounted for all or most of the observed changes in flux.[3]

Since the amount of benzocaine present in solution was not sufficient to saturate the vehicle, the compound was distributed between the aqueous bulk and sites within micelles. It is reasonable to assume that the penetration of micelles into the stratum corneum is negligible as they are much larger than monomeric species. Thus, drug molecules anchored to the micelles remained in the vehicle while only those in free solution were available for diffusion. The concentration of diffusible drug depended both on the tendency to enter micelles and on the number of micelles present.

As a follow-up to the work cited above, benzocaine compositions similar to those utilized were prepared with one difference: the benzocaine was present at a concentration well beyond that needed to saturate the various formulations.[4] In such circumstances, the actual solubilities differ from one vehicle to another, but the free benzocaine concentration would be the same. The steady state flux from these suspensions was unaffected by differences in surfactant concentration or polyoxyethylene chain length, confirming the lack of any significant effect of surfactant-skin interaction on drug permeation.

The role of solvent in modulating the interaction of nonionic surfactants with skin was explored in a study of lidocaine permeation.[6] The study investigated the flux of lidocaine through excised hairless mouse skin from solutions containing various concentrations of propylene glycol (40, 60 and 80% w/w) and polysorbates. Under infinite dose conditions, the surfactants had little effect on lidocaine flux except in solutions containing the highest propylene glycol concentration. The same trend was noted following a finite dose application.

In another study, the extent of hydrocortisone penetration following finite dose application increased as the propylene glycol concentration was raised.[7] Penetration enhancement was correlated with polysorbate hydrophobic chain length at 40 and 60% propylene glycol, but not at the highest concentration, 80%. With infinite dose administration, enhancement of hydrocortisone flux by polysorbate 20 and 60 was observed at both propylene glycol levels tested (40 and 80% w/w). The penetration curves for solutions containing the surfactants are similar at both propylene glycol levels. However, the penetration rate of hydro-cortisone is much lower from solutions with the higher propylene glycol content, so that the increase in penetration is greater in systems containing 80% propylene glycol. Apparently, nonionic surfactant molecules are more active in the presence of high concentrations of propylene glycol. This may be related to an increase in the critical micelle concentration in the presence of propylene glycol.[5]

Kadir et al. reported that diethyleneglycol lauryl ether enhanced the penetra-tion of theophylline and adenosine across excised human skin.[8] The surfactant, at a concentration of 20% in a vehicle based on propionic acid, resulted in a two-to three-fold increase in drug flux. Analysis of the experimental data suggested that the enhancement was due to an increase in thermodynamic activity within the vehicle, a "push" effect.

Fatty acids, alcohols and amines

The effectiveness of long-chain acids and alcohols in enhancing the epidermal penetration of a model lipophilic compound, salicylic acid, was reported by Cooper.[9] When binary mixtures of either oleic acid or oleyl alcohol and propylene glycol were applied to the skin, the degree of enhancement was maximized from compositions of approximately equimolar proportions. Pure fatty acid or alcohol had no effect on skin permeability. Among several fatty acids studied, those with unsaturated fatty chains caused the largest increase in penetrant flux.

The presence of a nonaqueous solvent is critical to the activity of fatty amphiphiles as penetration enhancers. In general, propylene glycol has been most effective of the various solvents tested. See the previous chapter for further discussion on the role of solvents in combination with amphiphilic vehicle components.

A recent paper summarized the alteration by oleic acid of biophysical measurements on stratum corneum.[10] Differential scanning colorimetry of isolated human and porcine stratum corneum yielded several peaks. The peak at the highest temperature (~95°C) was not affected by lipid extraction and was not thermally reversible, suggesting that it was due to a protein. The peak at approximately 65°C was thermally reversible and was abolished by lipid extraction, suggesting that it was due to lipid constituents.

FTIR absorbance spectra contained peaks due to symmetric and antisymmetric C-H stretching, ascribed to fatty chains of lipids.[10] The magnitude of these peaks was reduced by lipid extraction. Raising the temperature causes peak broadening

Table II. Perturbation of biophysical measurements and relative flux of salicylic acid through porcine skin.

Fatty acid	IR Frequency Shift (cm^{-1})	DSC T_m Shift (°C)	Flux Ratio[a]
none	-	-	1
octadecanoic	-0.7	-0.5	0.9
trans-9-octadecenoic	0.6	0.5	1.9
cis-9-octadecenoic	1.2	3.0	2.9
cis-6-octadecenoic	0.2	1.5	0.6
cis-11-octadecenoic	1.3	5.0	4.2

[a]Ratio of salicylic acid flux from saturated ethanolic solution containing 0.15 M fatty acid to that of saturated ethanolic solution (Data from Reference 11)

(but not a change in magnitude) and a shift in the peaks to higher frequencies. Over a range of temperatures and using porcine skin, the antisymmetric stretching frequency was linearly correlated with the permeability coefficient of tritiated water.

The FTIR frequency shift and DSC temperature shift resulting from skin treatment with various fatty acids in ethanolic solution were compared with changes in the flux of salicylic acid through dermatomed excised porcine skin.[11] These shifts were quite small in magnitude (Table II). The largest shifts as well as the greatest flux enhancement were obtained with cis-11-octadecenoic acid. Effects with octadecanoic acid (saturated) were negligible. Trans-9-octadecenoic doubled the flux despite a minimal influence on the biophysical parameters. The data suggested that the effective cis-fatty acids acted by a subtle disruption of the arrangement of the intercellular lipids.

Attenuated total reflectance FTIR measurements were performed in humans in vivo on the ventral forearm.[10] The antisymmetric stretching frequency shift in the presence of oleic acid (in a propylene glycol vehicle) reached a maximum value of 3 to 4 cm^{-1} regardless of exposure time. Although the same limiting effect was noted following application of different oleic acid concentrations in ethanol, the concentration of oleic acid within the skin continued to increase approximately in proportion to its concentration in the vehicle.

The stratum corneum concentration of a model penetrant, 4-cyanophenol, was also followed by the same technique.[10] Skin levels measured in situ were always lower when 5% oleic acid was included in the vehicle than when it was absent. Measurements over time suggested that penetrant loss from the skin was also more rapid in the presence of oleic acid.

Measurements using deuterated oleic acid provided further information on the interaction between oleic acid and stratum corneum lipids.[12] At temperatures below approximately 60°C there was no significant impact of oleic acid on the symmetric stretching frequency ascribed to skin lipids. This contradicts the notion that macroscopic fluidization of skin lipids is responsible for the penetration-enhancing effect of oleic acid. The authors instead propose a heterogeneous lipids model: oleic acid becomes part of the "fluid" region and increases the number of defects that permit other molecules to pass through.

In a wide ranging study, Aungst et al. evaluated the effect of three saturated fatty acids and dodecylamine, all at a concentration of 0.5 M in propylene glycol, on the skin penetration of six drug compounds.[13] The drug compounds were applied to excised human skin in saturated solution as an infinite dose. Three proposed mechanisms by which the amphiphilic compounds might influence drug permeation were evaluated:

1. increased vehicle solubility;
2. increased partition coefficient; and
3. barrier disruption.

Barrier disruption was not measured directly, but it was inferred when the other mechanisms could not account for changes in permeability. In most cases, the effects of the fatty acids (capric, lauric and a branched-chain decanoic) on flux and permeability coefficient were nearly equivalent. Table III contains some information extracted from the paper.

Penetration enhancement of benzoic acid, the compound in the group which traversed the skin most rapidly in the absence of any additive, was insignificant.[13] The increase in flux of methotrexate and indomethacin in the presence of dodecylamine could be accounted for on the basis of increased solubility, since the P ratio was about unity. Lauric acid had no effect on methotrexate. In the other cases, at least part of the mechanism for increased flux involved a decrease in effectiveness of the stratum corneum barrier.

Several observations made in the course of these experiments involved the effect of other vehicle components on penetration of the solvent, propylene glycol. As might be anticipated, the addition of lauric acid or dodecylamine at a concentration of 0.5 moles/l markedly increased the flux of propylene glycol through the skin. An unexpected result was that incorporation of methotrexate at saturation (54.1 mg/ml) in a vehicle containing dodecylamine completely negated the increase in propylene glycol flux. This is in line with the lack of methotrexate enhancement by dodecylamine.

Table III. Changes in solubility, human skin flux and permeability coefficient of six drugs by lauric acid and dodecylamine in a propylene glycol vehicle.

Permeant	Lauric Acid			Dodecylamine		
	S Ratio[a]	J Ratio[b]	P Ratio[c]	S Ratio[a]	J Ratio[b]	P Ratio[c]
Naloxone	2.2	38	17	0.22	6.9	31
Testosterone	1.3	5.5	4.1	0.41	2.6	6.3
Benzoic acid	1.0	1.3	1.3	0.92	1.6	1.8
Indomethacin	1.5	100	67	18	15	0.85
Fluorouracil	0.56	59	110	5.1	380	75
Methotrexate	1.3	1.4	1.1	20	19	0.92

[a]Ratio of solubility in vehicle containing fatty acid to control
[b]Ratio of flux from vehicle containing fatty acid to control
[c]Ratio of permeability coefficient from vehicle containing fatty acid to control
(Data from Reference 13)

Azone and related compounds

Azone® (1-dodecylazacycloheptan-2-one) is a commercial compound designed to increase the skin permeation of both lipophilic and polar compounds. Various studies have shown that combinations including Azone® at concentrations below 10% enhance skin permeation, particularly from a vehicle containing propylene glycol or ethanol.[14]

Guinea pig skin was used as an in-vitro model to study the mechanism of enhancement of Azone® and related molecules.[15] The skin was pretreated with either ethanol or an ethanolic solution of the enhancer (3% v/v). Twenty-four hours after this application, a standard solution of the drug was applied and its penetration measured. Azone® pretreatment resulted in an increase in both skin levels and throughput relative to the controls in every case, except for the compound with the highest octanol/water partition coefficient, butylparaben. Curiously, ethanol pretreatment lowered skin penetration of this compound; Azone® increased the skin content slightly, but significantly reduced the amount reaching the receptor. Analysis of the penetration data suggested that the major effect of Azone® pretreatment was on drug partitioning, while the diffusion coefficient was little changed.

In lipid-related peaks obtained by differential thermal analysis, Azone® and its homologues cause a shift to lower temperatures.[16] The data were interpreted in terms of fluidization of the oriented intercellular lipid layers. Pretreatment of the skin with an Azone®-propylene glycol combination increased intercellular deposition of mercury following application of mercuric chloride.[17]

The effect of propylene glycol and Azone® treatment was a function of the skin hydration level. Using a sandwich technique (described in the previous chapter), Boddé et al.[17] showed that skin treatment of hydrated stratum corneum with propylene glycol did not by itself increase nitroglycerin flux, while the Azone® mixture increased flux marginally. With stratum corneum maintained at a lower moisture content, both of these treatments increased nitroglycerin flux by 4 to 5 times. Remarkably, there was little difference between the effects of the Azone® combination and propylene glycol alone.

Other uncharged amphiphiles

n-Decylmethylsulfoxide is the most active skin penetration enhancer among a series of alkyl methylsulfoxides. It is surface-active, lowering the surface tension of water to about 25 mN/m^{-1} and exhibiting a critical micelle concentration of approximately 0.005 M.[18] Using hairless mouse skin as a model, researchers measured the effect of this compound on skin penetration of two drugs from two simple vehicles.[18] The results were opposite to those previously obtained in studies of amphiphiles in that n-decylmethylsulfoxide was more effective in a solution based on water than in a solution based on propylene glycol.

Barry and Bennett compared several amphiphilic compounds with regard to their effect on the penetration of three compounds through human skin.[19] The compounds mannitol, hydrocortisone and progesterone were chosen as models for polar, semipolar and nonpolar drugs, respectively. Using an "in-vivo mimic" protocol, the addition of Azone®, oleic acid or decylmethylsulfoxide in propylene glycol markedly increased the penetration of mannitol over that from propylene glycol alone. Azone® and oleic acid (but not decylmethylsulfoxide) increased hydrocortisone flux. However, neither Azone® nor oleic acid affected the flux of progesterone, which had the largest oil/water partition coefficient of the compounds studied.

Hexamethylene lauramide pharmacokinetics following topical application was studied in a rat skin-flap model.[20] Skin concentrations were high, and an apparent steady state was established within about 6 hours following dosing. Co-administration with hydrocortisone in an experimental formulation resulted in a doubling (as compared to a control) of skin concentration of the drug along with larger increases in blood concentration. Several cyclohexanone and piperidone derivatives, which had previously been shown to increase percutaneous penetration of indomethacin, were evaluated in terms of rat skin damage.[21] All of the compounds caused both epidermal and dermal deterioration; however, the extent of damage did not necessarily correlate with penetration enhancement potential within this group of compounds.

Zwitterionic surfactants

Ridout et al. recently described a study of nicotinamide flux through hairless mouse skin following pretreatment with several surfactants for 16 hours.[22] All of the surfactants except for N,N-dimethyl-N-dodecylamine oxide increased nicotinamide flux relative to that following pretreatment with a buffer solution. Some of the data are collected in Table IV. Although dodecylbetaine was itself absorbed through the skin to a much greater extent than hexadecylbetaine, these two compounds affected nicotinamide flux in the reverse order. The authors related the greater flux enhancement by the C_{16} compound to its smaller critical micelle concentration, suggesting that leaching of stratum corneum lipids played a crucial role in the compromise of skin barrier function resulting from surfactant treatment.

Table IV. Effect of zwitterionic surfactant pretreatment on nicotinamide penetration through hairless mouse skin[a]			
Surfactant	Applied Concentration (mM)	Critical Micelle Concentration (mM)	Cumulative Nicotinamide Absorbed (%)
None	0	-	0.32 ± 0.26
Dodecylbetaine	16	1.6	5.1 ± 1.7
Hexadecylbetaine	5.4	0.014	33 ± 6.1
Hexadecyl propyl sulfobetaine	10	0.02	26 ± 6.6
N,N-dimethyl-N-dodecylamine oxide	10	0.02	0.71 ± 0.10

[a]Data from Reference 22

The weak penetration enhancement with N,N-dimethyl-N-dodecylamine oxide is somewhat surprising in view of a report by Takahashi et al.[23] who found that this compound effectively disrupted guinea pig stratum corneum. A mixture of N,N-dimethyl-N-dodecylamine oxide and sodium lauryl sulfate, 1:4, was most effective in causing stratum corneum cell fragmentation.

The greater response with the C_{16} betaine as compared to the C_{12} homologue is in contrast to previously reported data on charged surfactants. In most studies the finished formulation is applied to the skin and drug permeation is measured. It is possible that the pretreatment approach accentuates the extent of skin damage.

Anionic surfactants

The tendency for many charged surfactants to alter the structure of the stratum corneum is well known. Most of the earlier work on absorption of anionics and their effect on skin permeation of water and other compounds was summarized in a chapter by Black and Howes.[24] Soaps cross the epidermal barrier; Bettley showed that hydrophobic chain length profoundly influenced the in vitro permeation of potassium soaps through human abdominal skin.[25] The C_{12} homologue was absorbed to a much greater extent than either the C_8 or C_{16} member of the series; these results correlated with the tendency of the soaps to produce skin irritation.

Using an electrometric approach, Dugard and Scheuplein[26] studied the alteration of percutaneous water transport through excised human skin by three homologous series of ionic surfactants, two anionic and one cationic. Data are shown in Table V. It is apparent that within each series, the maximum change is found at a chain length of 12 to 14 carbon atoms. The C_{16} member of each family was less active in every case.

Chowhan and Pritchard evaluated several surfactants as penetration enhancers for naproxen, a nonsteroidal anti-inflammatory drug.[27] The drug was dissolved in aqueous gels at a 0.5% concentration. No effort was made to standardize drug activity in the vehicles, so the penetration data reflect both the noninteractive drug-vehicle effects as well as alteration in stratum corneum resistance due to the surfactant present. Some of the data are shown in Table VI.

Table V. Effect of hydrocarbon chain length and surfactant type on rate of change of epidermal electrical conductance[a]

Carbon Atoms	R-COONa (anionic)	R-SO$_4$Na (anionic)	R-NH$_3$Cl (cationic)
8	0.0	0.0	0.0
10	0.1	0.1	0.2
12	4.5	5.0	25.0
14	4.0	2.0	21.0
16	0.2	0.4	2.5

[a]Data from Reference 25

Table VI. Effect of surfactants on naproxen flux through excised human skin from 0.5% aqueous gels[a]

Surfactant	Surfactant Type	Relative Flux
None	-	1.00
Polysorbate 60, 4%	Nonionic	0.97
Hexadecylpyridinium chloride, 0.5%	Cationic	0.44
Sodium lauryl sulfate	Anionic	8.3
Sodium laurate	Anionic	2.5

[a]Data from Reference 26

Both sodium lauryl sulfate and sodium laurate substantially increased naproxen flux. Sodium lauryl sulfate was the more effective of the two anionic agents. This contrasts with their relative effect (at a concentration of 5%) on water permeation through excised human epidermis.[28] The decrease in flux with hexadecylpyridinium chloride relative to the control is surprising at first. It may be ascribed to the long chain length (C_{16}) and possibly micellar solubilization of the drug, although the latter was not investigated.

The data in Table VII illustrate how failure to account for variations in drug activity within the vehicle can be misleading. Benzocaine flux from a solution containing sodium lauryl sulfate was about three times that from a solution containing a nonionic agent, polyoxyethylene (15) nonylphenol. In the presence of a combination of the two surfactants, the flux was no greater than that with the nonionic alone, giving the impression that the interaction of sodium lauryl sulfate with the skin has been eliminated. In fact, it is the increased micellar solubilization that is responsible for the reduction in flux, a fact that is made clear by examination of the suspension data. While the combination of surfactants results in a slightly lower benzocaine flux than due to the anionic surfactant alone, it is clear that there is still some residual stratum corneum-surfactant interaction.

Anionic surfactants, but not cationics or nonionics, induce swelling in pieces of human stratum corneum.[29] As with water permeation enhancement (and skin irritancy), the maximal swelling within several homologous groups of anionics was produced by the C_{12} or C_{14} member of the series. Swelling induced by sodium lauryl sulfate (SLS) increased with surfactant concentration until the critical micelle concentration was reached, and then leveled off. Ethoxylation of this detergent reduced the extent of swelling, as did admixture with ethoxylates or amphoterics. It is well known that such combinations are also less irritating to the skin than SLS alone.

Lodén measured the simultaneous penetration through excised full-thickness human skin of tritiated water and ^{35}S-labeled SLS from simple solutions.[30] Cumulative penetration values were generally not linear with time and rates were estimated at different times from the data. Some results are presented in Table VIII. Variability in SLS flux was much greater than that for water. SLS flux increased with time and applied concentration, even well beyond the critical micelle concentration. The pattern for water flux, which was much greater than that of SLS, was

Table VII. Steady-state flux of benzocaine through excised hairless mouse skin from vehicles containing surfactants, each at 0.0227 M concentration

Surfactant(s)	Mean Flux of Benzocaine (mg h^{-1} cm^{-2})	
	Solution (1.26 mg/ml)	Suspension (5 mg/ml)
POE (15) nonylphenol (I)	0.025	0.097
Sodium lauryl sulfate (II)	0.088	0.32
I + II	0.018	0.26

different. At 0.1% SLS, an apparent steady state was reached. With higher SLS concentrations, water flux increased with time and then decreased due to depletion. There was no substantial difference in water penetration at 1% or 10% SLS.

The increasing SLS flux with concentration suggests strong interaction with the stratum corneum. It is possible that contact with the surfactant solution results in dissolution and leaching of stratum corneum components that could open pores within the membrane. Another contributory factor may be the high sorptive affinity of the stratum corneum for SLS.

Not all anionic agents are equally interactive with the skin. The effect of hydrophobic chain length on irritancy and skin permeability has been mentioned. In addition, it should be noted that families of anionic detergents have different irritation tendency, and would therefore be expected to modify skin permeation to different extents.

Cationics

Cationic surfactants have not been investigated extensively for their potential to modify skin penetration because of the potential for skin irritation. Some data for cationics have been quoted above, in the section on anionic agents.

Hirvonen et al. showed that the flux of three drugs across human skin was increased by pretreating the skin with liquid dodecyl N,N-dimethylamino acetate.[31] The drugs, indomethacin, propranolol and 5-fluorouracil, were ap-

Table VIII. Simultaneous SLS and water flux through full-thickness human skin[a]

SLS Conc. (% w/w)	SLS Flux: Mean ± SEM (μg cm^{-2} hr^{-1})		Tritiated Water Flux: Mean ± SEM (mg cm^{-2} hr^{-1})	
	9-12 hr	21-24 hr	9-12 hr	21-24 hr
0.1	0.8 ± 0.7	6 ± 8	3.0 ± 1.1	3.3 ± 1.1
1.0	52 ± 64	612 ± 787	10.2 ± 3.2	7.2 ± 1.1
10.0	886 ± 1020	8460 ± 11300	10.6 ± 3.4	7.8 ± 1.1

[a]Data from Reference 28

plied as saturated solutions in phosphate buffer. Tritiated water, as a marker of skin resistance, was added to the donor solutions. Some data are supplied in Table IX. The increase in water flux, though not proportional to that of the drug compounds, indicates that the skin barrier was compromised by exposure to the enhancing compound.

More recently, the effect of several cationic surfactants on lidocaine permeation through dermatomed human skin from six donors was investigated.[32] The formulations, gelled 5% lidocaine suspensions in a 1:4 propylene glycol: water vehicle, were applied under infinite dose conditions. pH was adjusted to 7.9. Both tritiated water and ^{14}C-labeled lidocaine penetration were monitored simultaneously. Since all of the formulations contained lidocaine in excess of its solubility, its activity, and therefore the driving force for penetration, was the same in all cases. Differences in skin permeation could therefore be attributed to various degrees of stratum corneum alteration.

To circumvent the problem of variation in skin properties from different donors, each piece of skin served as its own control in the experiments. Testing was performed by sequentially applying three formulations: a control containing lidocaine but no surfactant (C_1), a test formulation containing surfactant (F) and a second control (C_2). The skin was washed between applications. Each formulation remained in contact with the skin for 24 hours. When the control was repeatedly applied to the same piece of skin, there was no significant change in flux of either water or lidocaine over the entire treatment period (72 hours).

The function of the first control was to normalize the different pieces of skin, since the permeation properties of skin from each donor were different. The ratio of the flux from the test formulation to that of the control (F/C_1) was labeled the enhancement ratio, ER. It was computed and used as a measure of the effect of the surfactant on stratum corneum resistance. The flux ratio of the second control to the first (C_2/C_1) was an indication of the reversibility of stratum corneum alteration. As might be expected with an in vitro preparation, the two flux ratios were usually close in value, indicating the absence of any operative repair mechanism.

Figure 1 contains results for one of the surfactants, tetradecyl trimethylammonium bromide, at a concentration of 81 mM.[30] Following application of the test dispersion (at 24 hours) there is a sharp increase in penetration of both lidocaine and water. The flux remains high following application of the second control formulation at 48 hours.

The effect of surfactant concentration on skin resistance was weak. Generally, a tenfold increase in concentration produced a doubling of the ER value. The most complete surfactant series utilized was a group of alkyl trimethylammonium halides with chain length of 10 to 18 carbon atoms. Enhancement ratios for this series are shown in Figure 2. It is noteworthy that the pattern for both lidocaine and water is the same, despite the vast difference in polarity of these molecules. For both permeants, peak ER values were obtained with the C_{14} homologue, in general agreement with earlier work.

All of the data obtained in the study (with three groups of cationic surfactants) are utilized in Figure 3, which shows the excellent correlation between ER values for water and lidocaine. The question of whether lipoidal and polar

Table IX. Enhancement of skin penetration of drugs and water by dodecyl N,N-dimethylamino acetate[a]		
Drug	Drug Permeability Ratio	Water Permeability Ratio
Indomethacin	21	3.1
Propranolol	13	2.8
5-Fluorouracil	22	4.4

[a]Data from Reference 29

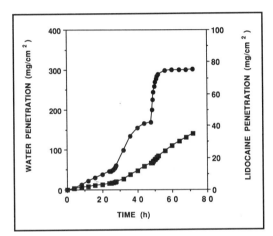

Figure 1. Cumulative amount penetrated through dermatomed human skin versus time following sequential application of control, test formulation (containing 81 mM tetradecyltrimethylammonium bromide), control, 24 hour applications. ■ lidocaine; ● water. (Reproduced from Reference 30 with permission of the copyright owner.)

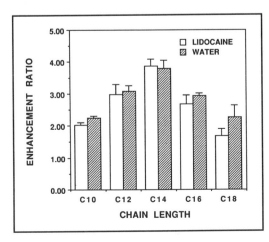

Figure 2. Enhancement ratios for lidocaine and water from 81 mM surfactant in 20% propylene glycol as a function of the alkyl chain length of members of the alkyl trimethylammonium halide series. Bars indicate SEM. (Reproduced from Reference 30 with permission of the copyright owner.)

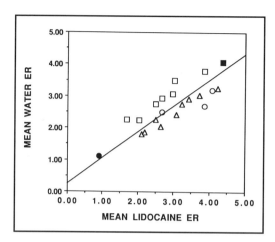

Figure 3. Correlation of water and lidocaine enhancement ratios through human epidermis in vitro. Key: ● control; △ alkyl dimethylbenzyl ammonium series; □ alkyl trimethylammonium series; ■ tetradecyltrimethylammonium bromide at pH 10.0; ○ alkyl pyridinium series. (Reproduced from Reference 30 with permission of the copyright owner.)

molecules follow separate pathways through the skin is a matter being debated at the present time. The relationship in Figure 3 suggests that the alteration in stratum corneum structure produced by cationic surfactants affects both molecule types to the same extent.

Conclusions

Surfactants are capable of altering skin transport by several mechanisms. Surfactant-permeant interactions, such as complexation and solubilization, generally reduce penetration rate if the permeant is totally dissolved. No reduction in penetration should occur by these mechanisms whenever the system is saturated with permeant. Interactions between surfactants and the skin usually result in an increase in penetration. Most nonionics exhibit negligible or weak effects on the skin in purely aqueous solution, but their interaction with skin may be more pronounced in the presence of other solvents, particularly propylene glycol. Ionic surfactants frequently increase skin permeation; there is a pronounced chain length effect, with peak effects within a series usually occurring at C_{12} or C_{14}. In at least one group of experiments utilizing cationic surfactants, flux enhancement of both a polar molecule (water) and a nonpolar molecule (lidocaine) was affected to approximately the same extent.

Optimization of the Skin Availability of Topical Products

By Joel A. Sequeira, PhD

Optimization can be defined as a process that results in the development of the "best" system or product.[1] In an industrial research and development environment, time constraints must be considered, so an "optimized" product is the best product which can be developed in a reasonable time period.

How can we clarify this definition as it pertains to drug treatment with a topical product? What is the end goal in the development of an optimized topical product? For all medications, the best product is one which delivers the drug molecule to the site of action and keeps it there for as long as it takes to achieve cure. This is an ideal situation. In reality we know this is very difficult to achieve for most dosage forms. With products designed for systemic delivery (e.g., orals, injectables, transdermals), the best dosage form is one which delivers therapeutic levels of drug to the body (most usually determined as blood levels), and maintains these levels relatively constant until therapeutic cure results. The end goal in developing an optimized systemic product is then easily definable, i.e., the dosage form should provide optimal blood/body levels of the drug candidate for the necessary time period.

Since the site of topical dosage forms is local, i.e., the skin, an optimized topical product is one which delivers the drug to the necessary skin site and achieves therapeutic local concentrations for as long as it takes to achieve cure or amelioration of disease symptoms. On the other hand, for sun care and cosmetic products, an optimized topical product is one which is formulated to leave the active ingredient on skin for as long as is necessary with minimal absorption into skin. And in today's world of super moisturizers and/or anti-aging products (skin wrinkle removers), ideal delivery of the therapeutic ingredient(s) may require delivery and localization into the stratum corneum and/or into the epidermis, thereby putting in question the regulatory status (drug or cosmetic?) of these products.

All definitions so far mentioned concentrate on optimizing the topical dosage form from an "availability" (and subsequent site clearance) or a "lack of availability" point of view. In reality, however, true optimization of a topical drug product must also include the following considerations in the optimization process:

- optimal stability profile
- lack of irritation/sensitization potential
- optimal esthetic characteristics
- timing.

Consequently, a broader definition of optimization of topical products or the end goal in developing an optimized topical product can be stated as "a product which is optimized from a topical availability (or lack of availability), stability, irritation/sensitization and esthetic viewpoints in the shortest time." This chapter is intended to provide the pharmaceutical/cosmetic scientist with a feel for the requirements, design, models and other factors necessary to develop an optimized topical drug or cosmetic product. It is not intended to provide a step-by-step development route since each drug or active ingredient has unique properties, and consequently a unique development pattern. Also, the last section of this chapter offers some further thoughts and discussion on the complexity of optimization as it pertains to topical products.

Optimization of Topical Availability

"Optimization" of topical availability is easily defined. But how is the process or optimal product measured? How are we to be sure that the product is optimized? The answers to these questions are difficult and some of the author's views are discussed later in this chapter. To complicate matters, the etiology of many topical ailments (psoriasis, acne, herpes, etc.) is unknown. Current therapy for these diseases is only ameliorative. Consequently, for drug products and cosmetic products looking to make drug-like claims, the "site of action" is not clearly established.

Except for a few superficial fungal infections, most topical agents have to permeate through the stratum corneum to reach the "site of action." (In the case of onychomycosis of the nails, the drug must achieve static/cidal concentrations of the drug not only in the nail but also the nail bed). This unfortunately is no easy task since the skin is an excellent protective barrier of the human body. To date, in spite of an extensive ongoing search, only a handful of candidates can be identified as having potential for transdermal delivery. Even fewer have so far been commercialized.[2] This reiterates that skin is a formidable barrier to the diffusion of foreign substances, drugs and toxins alike.[3] Also, compounds of different physico-chemical properties are hindered in different skin layers,[4-5] indicating that the skin is a complex, multifaceted membrane or barrier.

What is our objective in optimizing the availability of a topical product? For most ailments, our objective is to deliver therapeutic concentrations of the drug in and beyond the stratum corneum without significant systemic effects. For example, an optimal corticosteroid preparation is one which rapidly achieves and maintains therapeutic drug concentrations in the diseased skin site with no hypo-pituitary axis (HPA) suppression, until the inflammation or lesion is cleared. This assumes that the corticosteroid preparation is also optimally "cleared" or perhaps metabolized to an inactive, nontoxic metabolite after it exerts its local anti-inflammatory effect. In reality, all potent corticosteroids have some manifestation of systemic side effects and optimal delivery, i.e., efficacy with no side effects (systemic or local), is a challenge.

The skin's excellent barrier properties are a blessing to the cosmetic scientist whose objectives are generally the opposite of that of the pharmaceutical scientist. The objective of an optimized cosmetic product is to achieve little or no skin absorption of the "active" cosmetic ingredient(s) while the product adheres/binds to the upper layers of the stratum corneum. This is also a very challenging task. Although human skin is rather impermeable it has finite permeability for a wide variety of safe and harmful ingredients that are commonly used or required for ideal product performance.

Although we know what we wish to accomplish for topical products from an "availability" viewpoint, we do not have an easily accessible compartment, such as blood, to measure the delivery profile. Consequently, unlike the situation for certain systemic products whose therapeutic and toxic blood levels are known, it is difficult to set an objective or goal that a truly optimized topical dosage form must achieve. Even though the objective for an optimized drug or cosmetic product could be interpreted as being frustrating, herein lies the opportunity for a development scientist to explore unique methods and/or novel vehicles to develop the ideal "availability" profile for a topical product.

Knowing our objective or what we wish to accomplish, how can we quantify or measure the optimization of topical availability? Several approaches currently being explored can be grouped into two categories: preclinical methods and clinical methods.

Preclinical methods

All in-vitro and in-vivo test methods that do not involve testing in humans are preclinical methods. These are generally faster and less expensive than clinical methods. Depending on the drug candidate and available resources at the disposition of the development scientist some or all of the following methods can be used in the development of optimized topical dosage forms:

a. Theoretical physico-chemical approaches
b. In-vitro release rates
c. In-vitro diffusion methods
d. In-vivo animal models.

It is important to determine the physico-chemical characteristics of the drug before one begins to develop the right vehicle. Well-designed preformulation studies are necessary to determine all the parameters that affect drug permeation through skin and the compatibility of the drug with potential vehicle components.[6]

It is generally accepted that for most compounds skin permeation is described by the following equation as expressed by T. Higuchi:[7]

$$\frac{dQ}{dt} = \frac{PC_v D_s A}{h}$$

where: dQ/dt is the steady-state rate of penetration,
P is the effective partition coefficient of drug between skin and the vehicle,
C_v is concentration of dissolved drug in the vehicle,
D_s is the average diffusion constant of the drug in skin,
A is the area of drug application, and
h is the thickness of skin at the site of drug application.

Consequently, the key parameters that a development scientist can influence are the solubility and the partition coefficient. A good preformulation profile should measure the drug solubility in a variety of potential solvents and the partition coefficient in selected oil/water systems. Since the partition coefficient between solvents is meant to simulate the partitioning of the drug between the stratum corneum and the vehicle, attempts should be made to measure the partition coefficient using excised human stratum corneum and potential vehicles in a manner similar to the sorption experiments reported by Chandrasekaran et al.[8]

Poulsen[9] has shown the relationship between the solubility and partition coefficient of a corticosteroid in a co-solvent vehicle. His findings indicate that the maximum flux would be achieved when the product of the partition coefficient and the solubility is the highest.[9] However, this assumes that the dose applied is infinite and that no evaporation or other compositional change takes place. In reality, except for certain disease conditions requiring occlusion, the dose applied is finite and evaporation of vehicle components does occur.

T. Higuchi et al.[10] have shown how the thermodynamic activity can in fact be enhanced when the product has a volatile component in the vehicle. The factors and kinetics affecting finite dose applications have also been examined.[11,12] Several articles and texts are available which describe the thermodynamic parameters that affect the release and subsequent diffusion of drug through skin.[9,12,13,14,15] Additionally, with the advent of skin penetration enhancers the product could be formulated to affect the diffusion constant of the drug in the skin by altering skin permeability.

The development scientist has to balance thermodynamic considerations with the type of disease state the drug product is intended to treat. For example, a product to treat vaginal candidiasis may need superior spreading and substantivity to vaginal membrane as opposed to maximizing the vaginal flux rate. On the other hand, an antifungal drug molecule intended for the treatment of tinea pedis (sometimes a deep-seated fungal infection) may have to be formulated to achieve maximum skin flux. A topical steroid may work best in a vehicle which restricts skin flux to moderate values to avoid potential systemic side effects while still providing adequate drug leels at the skin receptor site(s). These are some examples of the considerations that are necessary to develop an optimized drug product.

The concerns of a cosmetic chemist, on the other hand, may necessitate that he use vehicles that "bind" the active ingredient within the formulation so as to minimize skin absorption and maximize residence of the product on skin.

In-vitro release rates: From first principles, the drug has to be released from the vehicle in order to be absorbed into the skin. Several methods and data analyses have been published in order to assess the release rates of drugs from topical dosage forms.[16,17,18,19] Two of the common problems or areas of contention with assessing release rates are the selection of the membrane and/or the medium into which the drug is released and measured. Since the medication is intended to be released onto skin, should the medium be water, octanol or one of intermediate polarity such as isopropyl myristate?

Also, is the product intended for ophthalmic, vaginal, general body surface, or cosmetic application? These factors should be taken into consideration before screening formulations to select ones with the highest, slowest or "optimal" active ingredient release patterns. If high, slow or sustained release rates are desired it is important to find out if the drug or active ingredient release rates are being facilitated or hindered by the formulation.

In general, it is important to verify if the release rates of drug or active ingredient out of the product corroborate or correlate with those predicted from theoretical considerations. Preferably, the release rates must also be used in conjunction with other methods such as skin diffusion or in-vivo animal model assessments. A paper by Ostrenga et al. serves to clearly demonstrate this point.[20] They showed excellent in-vivo vasoconstrictor activity with Fluocinonide ointments although the measurement of release rates showed no drug release from the preparations.[20] This was probably due to the fact that conditions on the skin surface were markedly different from those employed in the in-vitro model. Measurement of release rates are indeed helpful only if one has been able to demonstrate a positive correlation with clinical efficacy or topical availability as assessed by absorption or pharmacological activity.[9,21]

In-vitro diffusion methods: In-vitro diffusion methods utilize a barrier membrane to mimic skin as a barrier. By virtue of this fact, diffusion measurements are generally better than simple release rate determinations for the selection of the vehicle. The membranes selected range from simple synthetic materials occasionally impregnated with lipids to skin from various animals to human cadaver skin. [22-26]

One of the chapters by R. Bronaugh in this book serves as an excellent article reviewing the methodology and the various models that have been used to measure drug diffusion.[27] It is apparent from this article as well as the above referenced articles that the best in-vitro model for screening vehicles is the one which best correlates with clinical activity. When developing a topical product for a new, unique molecule without any prior information regarding correlation with clinical activity, the use of comparative diffusion rates in an in-vitro model to select a vehicle is risky. This is because there may not be a good correlation with subsequent clinical data. As we all know, incorrect vehicle selection results in large losses of time and money. It is generally recognized that, in lieu of a demonstrated correlation between in-vitro synthetic membrane or animal skin diffusion rates and in-vivo efficacy, human cadaver skin best approximates the "real" situation. However, most researchers working with human cadaver skin would agree that the variability observed for certain molecules makes it difficult to discriminate or select vehicles; the limited availability of skin supply further complicates matters.

Albeit the limitations, it is the author's opinion that measurement of in-vitro human skin diffusion rates allows one to optimize drug or active ingredient delivery into skin since there is methodology to investigate the localization of the drug in skin. This is particularly useful if, for a cosmetic product, one desires minimal diffusion into skin; or vice versa if one desires to maximize skin flux to reach deep seated skin or nail infections.

In addition, it is essential to know the eventual application of the dosage form, so as to select the appropriate diffusion cell, dose and other experimental conditions when screening vehicles utilizing skin diffusion. For example: does one use finite or infinite dosing? A single chamber or two-chambered diffusion cell? Expose the preparation to ambient laboratory conditions or use occlusion?

The methods are well described in R. Bronaugh's chapter.[27] However, lacking any clinical feedback, the decisions as to which diffusion model is appropriate are dependent on the dose, anticipated dosing frequency, the skin site and the disease state the drug is intended to treat. For a drug product dosed into the vaginal vault, measurement of in-vitro skin diffusion rates may be more appropriate if studied under occlusion as compared to exposure to ambient room temperature conditions. On the other hand, for an acne drug product applied primarily on the face, it is appropriate to expose the drug diffusion cell containing preparation to ambient laboratory conditions as opposed to occlusion.

Depending on dosing frequency one may need to use a finite dose application (simulating once a day) versus multiple or infinite dose application (simulating *t.i.d.* or *q.i.d.*). Since all of the in-vitro drug diffusion measurements are preclinical, it is good judgment to explore additional in-vivo animal models to confirm pharmacological activity and/or absorption, before recommending a final formulation.

In-vivo animal models: Animal models designed to screen vehicles range from those primarily used to assess drug absorption to those used to measure pharmacologic activity or activity in artificially induced infections.

It is not an easy task to screen vehicles by measuring drug or active ingredient absorption in an animal species. It could be time-consuming and expensive since assays for the active in biological fluids may have to be developed. These studies, usually referred to as ADME studies (absorption, distribution, metabolism and excretion) are usually employed after the formulation intended for commercialization has been selected.

ADME studies, usually conducted in rabbits, are primarily utilized to assess any systemic toxic effects of a topical product. Similar to the in-vitro situation, the relevance of in-vivo animal absorption data to select vehicles suffers the same limitations as discussed earlier. Since the product is intended for local use, the measurement of systemic drug levels serves only as an indirect indication of the local skin drug levels. ADME studies also help to confirm the lack of systemic absorption for certain cosmetic or suncare products.

An advantage of in-vivo animal absorption models is that one may observe the magnitude of local skin metabolism, a factor that may be totally overlooked if only in-vitro models are utilized. Depending on the extent of metabolism there is the possibility that a vehicle which alters skin metabolism may be selected. Recently, researchers have grafted human skin onto athymic mice in order to more closely simulate absorption through human skin in an in-vivo environment.[28] A still more sophisticated model called the "sandwich flap" has been reported.[29] This model allows one to assess absorption and metabolism through grafted human skin in live athymic mice.[29] Both these models[28,29] appear promising for assessing drug absorption through human skin using an animal species — although the latter[29] requires intricate surgery and may turn out to be too costly.

Another approach is to develop a lesion or infection which simulates the human disease state in animals. These animal models can then be used to screen the activity of various vehicles.

Animal models include the croton oil ear,[30] *P. ovalis* acanthosis,[31] rat paw carrageenan,[32] granuloma pouch[33] and reduction of UV-induced erythema[34] for anti-inflammatories; rabbit ear comedone,[35] sebaceous gland,[36] and rhino-mouse[37] models for acne; and infectious disease models such as the guinea pig dermatophyte and hamster vaginal candidiasis[38] models. These are just a few that are routinely used for activity screening.

In using these models for selection of vehicles, it is important to keep in mind the similarity (or lack of) between the implanted disease state in animals versus the actual disease in humans. For example, the psoriatic type lesions in the *P.ovalis* guinea pig model[31] lack a well-defined stratum corneum. Consequently, one has to interpret vehicle effects from such a model cautiously. On the other hand, due to a similarity of the disease state, the guinea pig dermatophyte model or the hamster vaginal candidiasis model[38] generally show a good correlation with clinical efficacy and are quite helpful in the selection of vehicles for such indications.

In the author's experience, pharmacological activity or disease models are generally quicker than "bioavailability" models to screen formulations. However, in addition to some of the earlier-mentioned limitations, many of these models do not discriminate between formulations at clinical dose levels. This is because quite often the doses intended for clinical use are on the plateau of the dose response curve measured in animals. Consequently, true vehicle effects in these models can only be assessed at a selected dose level which is identified only after characterizing the entire dose response curve — the selected dose level being one which is sensitive to vehicle changes. This does lengthen the vehicle screening process, but the alternative (having no knowledge of the shape of the dose response curve) is risky.

One of the major advantages of using animal "disease" models is that, apart from measuring a specific response such as "rate of kill" for the antifungal models or antimitotic activity in the anti-inflammatory models, one can also make "clinical assessments" on how the lesion or infection is responding to treatment.[38] This is very helpful to a formulation scientist who may discover that an "inert" excipient which does not aid drug diffusion may assist in lesion healing. In general, animal models are yet another tool to screen vehicles in the optimization process.

Clinical Methods

The methods described here refer to testing done in humans. These methods can be divided into three major categories by what they measure:

a. absorption,
b. pharmacological activity, or
c. clinical activity.

Methods assessing absorption: As mentioned earlier, for topical product development where the site of action is local, methods assessing drug absorption are indirect. They assess drug availability by measuring the systemic levels of the active ingredient. Despite this fact, absorption methods do provide guidance in selection of vehicles since systemic active levels generally reflect skin levels for the same moiety, assuming the well-accepted Fick's diffusion laws.

Dr. Bronaugh has described several methods used to assess drug or active ingredient absorption in humans for topical products.[27]

Absorption methods that would investigate levels of the active ingredient in the skin, preferably at the "site of action," are the ones that would be most useful. These methods are currently in investigational stages.

One of the limitations of using systemic absorption for vehicle screening of topical drug products is that drug absorption, usually assessed in healthy volunteers with intact skin, may be very different in healthy or disease states.[39] Consequently, using intact skin data one may select a vehicle which causes undesirable side effects in clinical use on barrier-compromised skin.

Methods assessing pharmacological activity: In the selection of an optimal vehicle, it is quite common to use a human pharmacological activity assay to assess drug activity. Vasoconstrictor assays for steroids,[40] wheal and flare assays for antihistamines,[41] and comedolytic activity for acne compounds[42] are a few of the models that are currently in use. These methods are faster and cheaper than clinical efficacy trials. They are generally easier to conduct since safety (toxicological data) requirements are less than those needed to conduct full-blown clinical trials.

Before selecting a model, it is imperative that one knows the correlation between pharmacological activity as assessed in the model and clinical activity. Cornell and Stoughton have demonstrated an excellent correlation between vasoconstrictor activity of topical corticosteroids and clinical antipsoriatic activity.[43] Although there may be risks in using the vasoconstrictor activity model[43] to assess the potency of different steroids (since there are exceptions to the rule), the model is excellent for screening vehicles containing the same steroid. One of the drawbacks of the vasoconstrictor activity model (and likewise other pharmacological activity models) is that certain formulation excipients may alter the response and mask true activity; hence the use of appropriate controls is essential. Alternately, the model(s) may not be able to assess the beneficial property of other formulation excipients and lead to improper vehicle selection.

Methods assessing clinical activity or product performance: This is the acid test for vehicle and/or product selection. However, it is the most expensive, lengthiest and the one requiring an appropriate degree of safety testing to be approvable by regulatory authorities. Historically, fine tuning a formulation or selecting between vehicles is seldom done at this stage since the regulatory requirements and costs for a new drug can be overwhelming. However, for certain reasons (such as projected market potential, any intended promotional claims, or lack of appropriate animal/human models), it is not uncommon in today's environment to use clinical assays to select or fine-tune formulations. The clinical test can be so designed that it not only answers a product development question but can also be a decision point to finalize the commercial product before initiation of full-blown Phase III clinical trials.

In order to shorten development times and reduce costs, formulation scientists together with their clinical colleagues have explored abbreviated clinical trials which in certain cases provide the same information as full-blown clinical investigations. These abbreviated clinical tests can be an ideal way of optimizing and finalizing the commercial product. One such example is a bilateral psoriasis test as demonstrated by R. Stoughton.[44]

This bilateral psoriasis trial is a fine discriminating assay for new corticoster-oids as well as different formulations of the same steroid.[44] The test has a high degree of statistical power. With a few patients (approximately 20-30) and a short application period (approximately 2 weeks) one can select between different formulations of a steroid having varying degrees of efficacy due to differences in topical availability. Most importantly, the test is a clinical efficacy measurement. Similarly, one can explore means of shortening the number of subjects and the length of treatment for assessing the clinical efficacy of other therapeutic agents so as to select the best or optimized dosage form in a clinical setting.

It can be easily appreciated that human testing is essential in assessing the attributes of a suncare or cosmetic product. Fortunately, since these are not drug products and require minimal toxicological screening, the evaluation of various vehicles is both rapid and relatively inexpensive.

Optimization of Other Parameters

Other major parameters involved in the development and optimization of topical products are:

a. Stability profile,
b. Irritation/sensitization potential,
c. Cosmetic properties, and
d. Timing.

These parameters are all important in the development of topical products. It is not the intent of this chapter to go into details of how to optimize a dosage form in each of the above categories. But since optimization would be incom-plete without due consideration of these factors, a brief discussion of each of these parameter's effects on topical proucts is presented.

Stability profile: In most cases, the age-old techniques of subjecting a product to accelerated temperature testing and/or adverse storage/shipping conditions to detect any physical, chemical or preservative instability work relatively adequately. These aging techniques and kinetic interpretations can help discriminate between formulations in a relatively short time.[45] Alternately, Wolfe and Worthington discuss the determination of product expiration dates from short-term storage at room temperature.[46]

Most topical products (creams, ointments, gels, lotions) by virtue of the fact that they are neither solutions (such as injectibles) nor solids (such as tablets) can manifest stability problems that are unique.

Consequently, the aging techniques used to screen topical products very often have to be tailored to the product to detect any peculiar instabilities and/or changes in rheological properties. For example, if due to availability or efficacy requirements a drug needs to be solubilized in a cream or ointment, special attention must be given to assuring oneself that the drug does not come out of solution on aging. This may take the form of accurate equilibrium solubility measurements of the active ingredient and polymorph(s), if any, and microscopic examination to confirm solubilization.

The longer the shelf-life and the wider the storage temperature tolerance for a product, the more advantageous it is to a manufacturer from a cost viewpoint.

These stability attributes are of a relative nature; consequently, optimizing a product from a stability viewpoint can mean obtaining the longest shelf-life and widest temperature storage label one can achieve in a short time period. In certain cases, formulation excipient selection and subsequent stability profile may be dictated by efficacy and/or topical availability requirements. However, in situations where equivalent efficacy is observed for several formulations, one has to take into consideration the comparative stability profile before selection of the final product.

Irritation/sensitization potential: Several animal models are available to assess the irritation and sensitization potential of topical products. Most of these have been described in books edited by H. Maibach[47] and Maibach and Lowe.[48] The models and protocols that are eventually selected clearly depend on the drug and the disease that one intends to treatment in the clinic or the intended claims desired of the product in commerce.

Even before initiation of a development project it is essential to confirm that the drug or active ingredient is not a sensitizer when delivered topically using an adequate animal model. After clearing this hurdle, a formulator needs to be aware of the irritation and sensitization potential of all the ingredients to be explored in the development of the topical product. This necessitates that the formulator must initiate adequate safety testing if he (she) intends to use a "new" excipient, before it is given due consideration as a vehicle component. This occasionally can escalate development costs, and the formulator has to weigh the advantages/disadvantages of using the new excipient.

Irritation/sensitization issues can sometimes become quite messy in a development program. It is best to clear these obstacles very early in development. Sensitization, if caused by the drug itself, is a problem that a formulator can do very little about. Irritation, on the other hand, is a response that the formulator can modulate by appropriate selection of vehicle components.

Consequently, it is essential that any potential irritation problems due to the drug or vehicle components be explored early. Historically, the rabbit has been the animal commonly selected and generally accepted by the FDA for irritation studies. It must be remembered that irritation data from a rabbit, like human data, can be variable. In selecting formulas (especially if the number of preparations is four or less) the author has found it most beneficial to divide the back into quadrants and to assess the irritation potential in the same rabbit. This sometimes allows the formulator to pick up subtle differences in the irritation potential whch may otherwise be missed due to inter-rabbit variability.

It is obvious that, if one has several formulations of equivalent availability and stability profiles, one would choose the formulation with the least potential for irritation and for sensitization. Oftentimes due to availability and/or stability constraints, the formulator may need to reduce or eliminate the irritation response observed in animals with a special or optimized vehicle. In this case, the formulator may wish to explore the addition of "inert" excipients which have "anti-irritant" properties as often touted by their manufacturers.

In today's competitive environment and especially in the cosmetic industry, it is very desirable for a topical product to make claims that indicate that the product is noncomedogenic and/or hypoallergenic. In these cases, the development chemist has to pay particular attention to the appropriate selection of inert excipients and their history of use. In addition, in order to make these claims on the label, the manufacturer has to undertake special additional studies in humans with his intended marketed preparation. These studies are often conducted against leading competitive products. The successful completion of these studies results in identifying an optimized product from an allergenic, irritation and/or comedogenic point of view.

Esthetic properties: Esthetic properties are quite important in the development of topical products since many of the therapeutic categories (psoriasis, acne, etc.) require long treatment periods and extensive body surface area application. Esthetic characteristics also depend on the therapeutic and/or product category: for acne, alcohol- or aqueous-based gels and nongreasy creams are preferred. In this case, emollient creams or ointments would be contraindicated. Likewise, if the intention is to develop a vaginal product, vehicle considerations and consequent cosmetic properties may be quite different from those intended for general skin application. For example, emolliency, occlusivity and diffusion may be some of the key criteria needed for product performance on skin. The latter may be less important attributes compared to spreading and substantivity for a vaginal product.

Apart from certain product requirements needed for special disease states or specific site applications, important consideration should be given to product rheology, ease of skin application and consequent product "feel" for all topical products.[49,50,51] If other considerations such as availability, stability, irritation and cost are not controlling, esthetic properties may decide which vehicle is selected.

Comparing the esthetic properties of topical vehicles can be quite a difficult task. Before one brings a panel of test volunteers together it is best to reduce the number of vehicles being screened to the minimum, preferably two. This is best achieved by bringing together a few experts and asking them to concentrate on specific properties, such as tackiness, ease of rub-in, lack of staining, afterfeel, etc. After one has reduced the selection of vehicles to the minimum one can then put a larger panel together to get a further opinion on the esthetic attributes of the base. Even at this time it is good to ask the panel to concentrate on specific product characterisics and to standardize the experimental design as much as possible, i.e., state the amount to be applied, specify skin site, and randomize the order of application. Last but not least for the drug products, it is advisable to solicit observations and comments from patients using the drug product in early clinical trials. This information from the potential end-users of the product may be invaluable since it could lead to early detection of a potential problem in commerce.

For reasons cited earlier, choosing the best vehicle from an esthetic viewpoint is important for topical products. For obvious reasons, it is important to engage the help of your marketing colleagues before selecting the eventual commercial product. To the chagrin of many a development scientist, too often a product is criticized by the marketing product manager just before commercialization. This situation can be avoided by good communications, proper planning and decision making.

For suncare and/or cosmetic products, the esthetic properties of the vehicle are of paramount importance. In these situations, it is best to use large panels of target consumers who would be heavy users of the particular product class in order to select the optimal vehicle. The protocols and controls employed in panel testing should also be judiciously selected in order to avoid any bias.

Timing: This parameter is well understood by most research and development personnel. Apart from extremely rare situations, the product is needed in the fastest time possible. The "ultimate-optimized" product is worthless to a marketing colelague if developed "too late." On the other hand, even though there can be substantial pressure on the formulator due to projected market needs, one cannot compromise essential product attributes to satisfy market timing needs. Consequently, it is important to carefully estimate the time needed to complete the development of an optimized dosage form so as not to cause "surprises" among your marketing and senior management staff. "Optimization" does not by definition include a time element. However, due to therapeutic and market needs one has to use good judgment in deciding when the development process is complete. Consequently, this necessitates the incorporation of a time element.

The Optimization Process

This chapter is not intended to "show" a formulator the right way to end up with an optimized product. Each drug or active ingredient is unique and requires a unique development plan. On the other hand, this chapter is meant to point out the critical parameters in the development of a topical product and how to balance these parameters to develop an optimized product. A key word in this optimization process is "balance."

The formulator has to balance optimizing each of the parameters to end up with the best product. In today's competitive commercial environment, all of the parameters discussed in the preceding section are important. It is difficult to attach a weighting system and say that one of the parameters is more important than the other. The topical availability, irritation and esthetic properties of a product were probably not as keenly investigated in the past as is the case today. If timing is critical, one of the parameters that is usually compromised is the esthetic property of the base. Another parameter that may be compromised due to time pressures is the stability shelf-life, since a shelf-life of approximately 24 months is considered adequate for product launch. On the other hand, optimizing the esthetic and irritation/sensitization properties of a suncare and/or cosmetic product may be the most important criteria for a cosmetic chemist.

How would one develop an optimized total product in today's environment with adequate funds and resources but not free from time pressures?

After determining the disease state(s) that the dosage form is intended to treat, one would embark on a good preformulation scheme. Apart from the usual studies in a preformulation protocol,[6] one would include the possibility that a skin penetration oenhancer may be needed to facilitate obtaining a desired optimal topical availability. Upon completion of the preformulation studies one would develop several formulations using all of the relevant thermodynamic principles referenced earlier. These formulations may be different in that they utilize different excipients or that they are different from a thermodynamic viewpoint or from the viewpoint of occlusivity and/or substantivity.

After identifying these formulations one would simultaneously explore the availability, stability and the irritation potential of the vehicles (assuming the drug has already been screened for sensitization in an appropriate model). Topical availability screening is best achieved using human cadaver skin and radiolabelled drug. After obtaining the desired in-vitro permeation profile(s) and/or optimal skin levels, it is best to confirm the topical availability utilizing an in-vivo animal or human model. The model to be used is usually dictated by the drug and the disease for which the product is being developed.

Hopefully, upon completion of the in-vitro/in-vivo availability studies, one has also simultaneously completed the stability and irritation screening. If one has been thorough and planned well, one usually ends up with two or three prototypes that may have to be fine-tuned for esthetic reasons and/or an improved stability profile.

These minor changes hopefully have no effect on the topical availability and irritation potential which have to be reconfirmed using the in-vitro or in-vivo model(s) used earlier. The fine-tuned formulations are now ready to be screened in the clinic. At this time it is best to confirm eshetic attribute acceptability and select one for the Investigational New Drug Application and clinical trial. The prototype(s) not selected can be kept as backups. Depending on the outcome of the clinical trial, the final product or a backup is selected for further evaluation.

For a cosmetic product, the emphasis during development would be more along the lines of optimizing the product from a skin compatibility (irritation, sensitization, comedogenicity) and esthetic viewpoint. Panel testing to optimize the esthetic properties and stability would normally precede the skin compatibility testing.

The above, rather simplistic, scheme did not include problem situations whch are usually encountered in every development program. These situations and their solutions obviously affect timing which is another of the parameters in the optimization process.

Is the Product Truly Optimized?

This is by far the most difficult question to answer for a topical dosage form. With the availability of hundreds of usable excipients and the advent of skin penetration enhancers it is nearly impossible to say that a product has been truly optimized from an "availability" or "lack of availability" standpoint. Besides, if one has used the state-of-the-art in optimizing the topical availability, is the product likewise optimized with regards to esthetic properties, stability profile, irritation potential, etc.?

It is perhaps comforting that if one has improved the topical delivery of a therapeutic an agent by adjustment of the vehicle, one has achieved a degree of optimization. The improvement could be such that one has enhanced the potency of a steroid from that of a moderate to a high potency category, or reduced frequency of dosing to once a day from two or three times a day. In the case of antifungals and acne compounds, where treatment are lengthy, optimizing the dosage form could result in a much-reduced treatment period. For Clotrimazole and Miconazole (two imidazole antifungals), proper selection of the vehicle and drug concentrations has resulted in shortening the treatment period for vulvo-vaginal candidiasis from seven days to three days, and most recently to a one day, single dose product (in the case of Clotrimazole).

Deep-seated antifungal infections and onychomycosis of the nails are examples of diseases where current therapy is lacking primarily due to lack of topical availability or lack of "the optimized dosage form." These therapeutic areas offer an ample challenge for improving or "optimizing" current topical dosage forms.

In the suncare field, novel vehicles have resulted in superior performance of the sunscreen product. For example, products have been formulated to be substantive to skin and offer protection from water wash-off while retaining their high sun protection factor values.

These are but a few examples of "optimized" topical products or areas which need optimization for ideal skin treatment.

Toxicological Aspects of Percutaneous Absorption

By Edward M. Jackson, PhD

This chapter will discuss elements of percutaneous absorption such as product type, use and exposure, differences between the various sites of exposure, the condition of the skin and enhancers of percutaneous absorption as well as applications to various product categories. Next we will review percutaneous absorption data on colors, preservatives and pesticides, fragrance ingredients, biologically and pharmacologically active ingredients and nitrosamines. The chapter concludes with a view of our current understanding of percutaneous absorption, the impact of this rapidly developing future of percutaneous absorption and the elaboration of some fundamental toxicological principles for interpreting the significance of percutaneous absorption data.

Everyone is aware that the skin allows passage to certain things: energy, water and other chemicals. This is really common sense. Energy comes through the skin in the forms of light and heat. We know that bathing, saunas, steam baths and humid climates are all ways in which water can enter or leave the skin. Chemicals can pass through the skin from environmental and occupational exposures as well as topical drug and cosmetic applications.

We sweat and experience cutaneous dehydration. Our skin regulates the loss of heat calories from our bodies. Oil exudes from pilosebaceous follicles. The nonwater components of sweat represent the loss of electrolytes. Water, energy and chemicals, then, enter and leave our bodies through the skin. (For a more complete discussion, see Reference 1.) The toxicity of a chemical when applied to the skin depends on the rate of its penetration as well as its inherent biological toxicity.

Biological Parameters

The biological parameters of percutaneous absorption are the anatomy of the skin, the physiology of the skin, and the actual condition of the skin.

The Anatomy of the Skin: Structurally, the skin absorbs materials through a dual membrane system perforated with shunts.[2] The first rate-limiting membrane is the stratum corneum of the epidermis. The second rate-limiting membrane is the epidermal-dermal junction or basement membrane. The various types of shunts are the pilosebaceous units and the ducts of the apocrine and eccrine sweat glands.

However, the skin is not the same all over the body in spite of these anatomical features. For instance, the periocular, scrotal and labial skin is notably lacking in dermis. Glabrous skin, such as the palms of the hands and soles of the feet, lacks the pilosebaceous units and therefore hair follicles. And the literature is replete with different percutaneous absorption rates for various skin body zones such as the back skin and forearm skin. Transdermal therapeutic systems (TTS) attempt to take advantage of these percutaneous absorption rates.

Finally, there is a difference among the various species of laboratory animals and man in reported rates of percutaneous absorption.[3-5] The literature in this area is clear only on two points: (1) there are definitely differences among the various species in terms of percutaneous absorption rates, and (2) the ranking of percutaneous absorption potential among these various animal species and man differs.

The Physiology of the Skin: The physiological aspects of the skin in percutaneous absorption are the metabolism of the penetrant by the skin and the removal of the penetrant from the skin via the vascular and lymphatic pathways of the circulatory system.

Skin is the site of extrahepatic metabolism for certain types of chemicals such as drugs and carcinogens, not to mention carbohydrates, lipids and proteins.[6] Once metabolized, these products are readily released from the skin and cleared by the vascular and lymphatic systems. If the penetrant is not metabolized, the vascular and lymphatic systems are still involved in actively clearing it from the surface of the skin.[7] In fact, the dermal capillary loop clearance potential is such that the rate of a penetrant's percutaneous absorption is not limited to its accumulation in the dermis.[8]

Metabolism isn't the only physiological function of the skin which has a major impact on the percutaneous absorption of a substance. Binding of the penetrant to protein in the skin is critical for the occurrence of certain responses, such as allergic contact dermatitis (ACD).[9] Here binding of the penetrant (called a hapten in ACD) to a cutaneous or serum protein is crucial to producing the hapten-protein carrier complex, termed a complete allergen, before induction can begin and cutaneous sensitization can result.

The question is often posed whether or not a penetrant is more readily available for systemic absorption via the cutaneous or gastrointestinal routes. The answer to this question is simply not known at this time. Parallel studies would help our understanding here, but the major difficulty would be the physiologies of cutaneous versus gastrointestinal routes of absorption and distribution.

Skin Condition: The actual condition of the skin can modify percutaneous absorption. Skin permeability is modified by disease, damage, loss, age, race, hydration, nutrition, exposure to topical products, and prior exposure to a given test material.

Diseased skin is damaged skin. It is modified through the process of inflammation which is clearly visible as erythema and edema and felt as pain and heat.[10] Whether the skin is diseased by a transient infection or a chronic condition such as acne or psoriasis, it is more penetrable by environmental, occupational or topical product exposures than healthy, normal skin. Diseased skin increases the potential for percutaneous absorption precisely because it is inflamed.

Another form of damaged skin is skin which has been breached by an epidermal break which may penetrate into the dermis, the subcutaneous layer or even the muscle tissue. Any cut or scratch, any crack or split from excessive dryness, opens us up to virtually instantaneous exposure through this cutaneous breach.

Skin which has been exposed to irritants, sensitizers, phototoxins, photoallergens, even demyelinating neurotoxins, is potentially modified in terms of percutaneous absorption. In fact, the cutaneous reaction of inflammation itself implies absorption of these physical, chemical or biological agents. Not only do the objective inflammatory responses of erythema, edema, pain and heat indicate percutaneous absorption, but so do the subjective responses such as stinging, burning and itching sensations. When these responses occur, percutaneous absorption has occurred through both of the rate-limiting membranes previously described.

Further, previous cutaneous exposures to such agents can modify percutaneous absorption. For example, the frequency with which the skin is exposed to a low-level irritant predisposes it for increased percutaneous absorption. Also the induction of an allergen can result, upon challenge, in an inflammatory response known as sensitization.

Skin which has been lost through injury or disease, obviously, exposes us to the surrounding environment. Here, of course, as in breached skin, percutaneous absorption is not the issue, rather it is a case of direct exposure to the material in question.

Hydrated skin also increases percutaneous absorption potential. The very fact that skin swells or plumps is itself a demonstration of increased water absorption which increases the partitioning of certain materials into the skin. There are differences between water uptake by skin and by hair. Water uptake by the keratin in corneocytes is a permeating phenomenon spreading out in all directions. Hair, on the other hand, swells longitudinally, lengthening the hair strand itself. Finally, the epidermal membrane or stratum corneum is more sensitive to water uptake than hair.[11]

Hydration of the skin occurs through bathing, sweating, being in an area of high humidity, occlusion or application of a film-forming product such as a moisturizer. Using a moisturizer after bathing is a way of putting moisture back into the skin and then, by applying a film over the skin, retarding moisture loss into the surrounding atmosphere. In this process, very little moisture comes from the moisturizer itself. But when bathing does not precede application of a moisturizer, there is some cutaneous water uptake from the moisturizer which competes to a slight degree with the more intense evaporation of the volatile water in the product from the skin.

Occlusion of the skin can result from wearing clothes, from patches in patch tests, from bandaging or treatment modes such as plasters or masks, or from application of oleagenous materials such as petrolatum.[1] Applying occlusive, oleagenous materials markedly decreases normal water loss from the skin, as does the wearing of tight-fitting (especially waterproof) clothes. The latter situation is not unlike a patch test, where physical occlusion of a test material increases not only the temperature of the skin but its humidity as well. In this way, the test material under the patch is driven into the skin through pressure and increased hydration, resulting in an exaggerated exposure to the test material. Plasters containing an active drug have long been used to enhance percutaneous absorption of that drug. Cosmetic facial masks are films cast upon the skin to enhance percutaneous hydration by occlusion. The cosmetic mask product, of course, does not contain drugs; rather it is simply a film-forming product which, after the solvents volatilize, leaves on the skin an occlusive film which is removed after a short period of time.

Both hydration and occlusion have increased the percutaneous absorption rate of certain materials. Topically applied drugs such as nicotinic acid,[12] salicylic acid[13] and aspirin[14,15] have all been shown to be enhanced in terms of absorption on hydrated skin versus normal skin. Fragrances under occlusion have further been demonstrated to have double or triple the percutaneous absorption rate of unoccluded fragrance materials.[16]

Inflamed human skin can be treated to reduce the inflammatory response, thereby reducing the increased percutaneous absorption potential and restoring the skin to its normal state. The best example of this has been the change of topical steroids from prescription status to over-the-counter drug status.[17] Hydrocortisone-containing creams are now readily available to the consumer. Physiologically, the hydrocortisone reduces the factors in the inflammatory process which increase the percutaneous absorption potential of the skin. As previously mentioned, these factors are vasodilation resulting in visible erythema and palpable edema. Topical steroids such as hydrocortisone reduce these factors through vasoconstriction of the dermal vasculature.

Much has been written about age as a factor in percutaneous absorption. However, a review of the literature can be succinctly summarized by simply stating that, in the main, skin is skin. There is a difference in the rate of percutaneous absorption between very young skin (probably neonatal skin) and very old skin (the skin of persons of very advanced age). Beyond that, the results in the literature are not indicative of any other differences in the percutaneous absorption rate of skin due to age.

Finally, race has been shown to be a factor in percutaneous absorption. Differences in the thickness of the stratum corneum varies between the Caucasian and Negroid races to such an extent that the thicker stratum corneum in the Negroid race may result in a slightly decreased percutaneous absorption rate for certain test materials.[18]

Chemical Parameters

The chemical elements of percutaneous absorption are the penetrant, the vehicle, exposure and chemical enhancers of percutaneous absorption.

The Penetrant: Several chemical aspects of the penetrant itself affect toxicology considerations. Obviously, the concentration of the penetrant in the product is crucial. Its chemical structure, molecular weight and reactive sites must also be considered. The partition coefficient of the penetrant in a given vehicle is also important when attempting to determine the availability of the penetrant for interaction with the skin. As an example of these physicochemical considerations of the penetrant, radiolabeled detergents in the form of alcohol sulfates, ether sulfates and alcohol sulfates with varying chain lengths have been studied in rat skin.[19] The results indicated low percutaneous absorption potential with varia-

Table I.	
Cosmetics (21 C.F.R. 720.4)	Primary Exposure
Baby products	Skin
Bath preparations	Skin, mucous membrane
Eye makeup preparations	Eye, skin
Fragrance preparations	Skin
Hair preparations (noncoloring)	Hair
Hair coloring preparations	Hair
Makeup preparations (not eye)	Skin, eye
Manicuring preparations	Nails, skin
Oral hygiene product	Mucous membrane, skin
Personal cleanliness	Skin, mucous membrane
Shaving preparations	Skin, eye
Skin care preparations	
(creams, lotions, powders, sprays)	Skin, eye
Suntan and sunscreen preparations	Skin, eye

tions in absorption occurring with the alcohol species, the chain length and the degree of ethoxylate. This demonstrates the impact of the physicochemical properties of the penetrant on the percutaneous absorption of a given material.

The Vehicle: A detailed treatment of the product vehicle has been reviewed elsewhere.[20] Again, we will mention only those aspects which impact directly on the toxicological considerations of percutaneous absorption.

There are several ways to describe product vehicles. For example, the legal definition of products known as cosmetics in the Food, Drug and Cosmetic Act[21] is somewhat helpful by itself, but even more helpful when we assess the primary exposure site for these types of products.[22]

Table I summarizes these legal product types with their primary exposure site. Eleven of the thirteen product types involve exposure to the skin or mucous membrane. The point is that there are several different types of formulations which must be considered when discussing vehicles.

From a pharmaceutical formulation perspective, vehicles can be one of the following types.

1. Emulsions
   —Oil-in-water (O/W) emulsions
       Pigmented   Nonpigmented
   —Water-in-oil (W/O) emulsions
       Pigmented   Nonpigmented
2. Suspensions and Gels
3. Solutions
   —Aqueous   —Hydroalcoholic
4. Physical Mixtures
   —Powders   —Waxes
5. Gases

The predominant emulsion type is the oil-in-water emulsion, where the dispersed phase is oil and the surrounding phase is water. The vast majority of vehicles and, therefore, consumer products, are the oil-in-water emulsion variety. Water-in-oil emulsions, where the water is dispersed in a surrounding medium of oil, are far less common as a vehicle or product type, although cold cream remains the oldest and most common example of this type of emulsion system.

In either type of emulsion system, the oil and water are held together by applying physical energy and using chemical emulsifiers, which have hydrophilic and lipophilic ends, to bind both the oil and water. Viscosity-increasing agents can be used as emulsion stabilizers.

Solids which coat the dispersed phase can be used to aid in emulsification. For example, iron oxides, talc and titanium dioxide can all help emulsify a system in addition to providing color and coverage in the finished product.

Suspensions and gels consist of solid particles suspended in a liquid or semiliquid phase. Ointments are good examples of suspensions. Many toothpastes are gels.

Solutions are either aqueous or hydroalcoholic solutions, but both consist of a solute dissolving in a solvent: one chemical dispersed in another, each in its molecular form. Toners, cleansers, colognes and perfumes are good examples of vehicles or products which are true solutions.

Physical mixtures are represented by various types of powder products and wax products. Loose or pressed facial powders, dusting powders, and eye shadows are physical powder mixtures. Lip balms, eye shadow pencils and lipsticks are examples of wax mixtures.

Toxicologically, pharmaceutical formulations can be ranked according to their impact on percutaneous absorption as follows:

Emulsions > Solutions > Suspensions and gels > Physical mixtures

Emulsions tend to be more difficult to successfully patch test, from a safety testing viewpoint. Less difficult are solutions. Physical mixtures are the easiest to patch test. In the case of emulsions, the oil phase increases skin hydration, leading to increased percutaneous absorption. With solutions, the solvent can be primarily responsible for increased percutaneous absorption rates.

Before concluding this section on the product vehicle, mention should be made of the actual manufacture of products. A product's characteristics can be significantly altered in the progression from a bench formulation in beaker-size quantities, to the process scale-up in drum-size quantities, to actual plant manufacture in 1,000 to 10,000 gallon vessels. These alterations include not only its marketable properties, but its physicochemical composition and toxicological qualities as well. For this reason, a manufacturer must physically, chemically and toxicologically insure that the bench product and plant-manufactured product are virtually the same. This is the basis of an effective quality control program.

Exposure: The third chemical parameter of percutaneous absorption is exposure, whether it be environmental, occupational or product-related. For purposes of clarity, we will limit our discussion on exposure to topical products.

Exposure is dependent on both product type and product purpose. Topical drug products are either prescription or over-the-counter (OTC) drug products.

Prescription drugs tend to be prescribed for more serious disease states or conditions. OTC topical drug products are generally intended for self-diagnosed and self-treatable conditions. Their use can go on for a much longer period of time than that of the prescription drug product, increasing the exposure to the active and the vehicle. The contact time for any topical drug product is dependent upon a relatively fixed or prescribed time period, until the condition subsides enough to discontinue use. Exposure is, therefore, generally measured in days.

Cosmetic products, on the other hand, are used daily. Contact time for some products can be as long as 8-12 hours at a time. The consumer can be repeatedly exposed to them over many years. The difference in exposure for a cosmetic versus a drug product can therefore be enormous.

Although it is possible that such continued and chronic use can lead to problems, the overwhelming facts are that—as a product category—cosmetics truly have an impressive safety record. No other topical product type is used more frequently, and in such varied combinations with other products, than cosmetic products. Fewer reactions occur with cosmetic products under these multiple and prolonged exposures than with all other topical products combined.

Loss of topically-applied products diminishes exposure and therefore percutaneous absorption. This, of course, applies to both drug and cosmetic products. In a recent study on the percutaneous absorption of minoxidil,[23] 53-57% of the applied dose was calculated to have been lost through friction (rub-off onto hands, wearing apparel and bed clothes), evaporation and rinse-off.

Since minoxidil was applied in a simple vehicle where maximum saturation did not occur, the actual percutaneous absorption of this active could be higher. But the fact remains that there can be huge losses of product, which can markedly reduce the potential for percutaneous absorption of a given test material.

Household products represent acute exposure measured in minutes, certainly no longer than hours. Such product exposures are really more unintended—often accidental—than intended. But this does not mean that percutaneous absorption is not possible under these circumstances. While the exposure time may be limited, the chemicals in such products can be harsh chemicals, often requiring dilution before actual use. At full strength, they are capable of driving percutaneous absorption, or causing it to occur at a much faster rate.

In summary, a consumer product ranking for exposure based on time can be expressed. For these product categories:

cosmetics > OTC drugs > prescription drugs > household products

where relative lengths of exposure can be, respectively, years, months, days or weeks, and hours.

A ranking of risk from exposure to topical products must be adjusted with information about the ingredient of concern and the vehicle ingredients. This type of ranking gives the reverse order from the product ranking:

cosmetics < OTC drugs < prescription drugs < household products

Enhancers: Percutaneous absorption can be enhanced either chemically or physically. Although the literature lists various chemicals which have been demonstrated to enhance percutaneous absorption, these lists can be summarized as either solvents (which dissolve a solute down to its molecular species and can also dissolve to some degree the rate-limiting stratum corneum of the epidermis) or surfactants (which simultaneously accommodate both hydrophilic and lipophilic moieties).[8,19,24,25] Even chemicals where the mechanism of action is not known can be placed in one of these two general chemical categories. An example of this is Azone® (1-dodecylazacycloheptan-2-one), which acts like a surfactant.[26]

Physically, there are numerous ways to enhance percutaneous absorption.[27] We have already discussed the unintended effects of occlusivity from clothing or patch testing. Intentional enhancement by physical means can be accomplished through friction such as massage.[8] In addition, there are other physical means which can be utilized when formulating a product for a specific purpose.

To these should be added two processes which fall neither under biological nor chemical parameters. In a way, they are a combination of both. One method is to intentionally inflame the skin, either subclinically or clinically, thereby enhancing percutaneous absorption, by adding a selected ingredient to a vehicle or formulating a vehicle in such a way (i.e. by adjusting pH or formulating it with a soap) to produce low-grade inflammation. This is simply another way of saying inflammation presupposes percutaneous absorption and, therefore, can itself be used to enhance percutaneous absorption.

Finally, the simple application of heat before, during or after application of the product can alter the percutaneous absorption rate of a material.

Toxicological Aspects of Percutaneous Absorption

There are four elements to consider in assessing the toxicological aspects of a chemical exposure. They are the chemical, its presentation to the skin, the dose of (or exposure to) the chemical, and the amount of chemical actually absorbed percutaneously. This section will apply an understanding of these elements to actual exposures to chemicals both topically in products and environmentally.

Preservatives: Preservatives are important to topical products, whether they be drugs or cosmetics. These pharmacologically active materials extend the life and, therefore, the usefulness of the product, permitting continued use under nonsterile conditions. But, the presence of pharmacologically active materials in a topical product can pose a risk if these materials are absorbed through the skin.

Figure 1 lists three preservatives commonly used in topical products, together with their recommended concentration in the product.[25] All are broad-spectrum antibiotics, although phenoxyethanol probably performs a little better against Gram-negative than Gram-positive microorganisms.

If certain solvents or surfactants are used in an emulsion system using phenoxyethanol as a preservative, two safety considerations become apparent. First, phenoxyethanol penetration through the skin could be enhanced. Secondly, the use of the preservative in eye-area drug or cosmetic products could enhance the absorption potential due to the lack of supporting dermis in the periorbital skin. In short, materials tend to be more readily absorbed through the skin around the eye.

Preservatives			
Chemical name	Structure	% Recommended Product Concentration	Product Class
Phenoxyethanol	—O-CH$_2$CH$_2$OH	0.5 - 1.0	Mascaras Eye Shadows
N-(Hydroxymethyl)-N-(1.3-Dihydroxymethyl-2,5-Dioxo-4-Imidazolidinyl)-N-(Hydroxymethyl) Urea (Germal II™)		0.2 - 0.5	Creams and Lotions Pigmented Emulsions Powders
5-Chloro-2-Methyl-4-Isothiazolin-3-one and 2-Methyl-4-Isothiazolin-3-one (Kathlon CG™)		0.02 - 0.1 (Actives, 0.0003 - 0.0015)	Shampoos Conditioners

If diazolidinyl urea[a] is the preservative of choice in a topical product containing low concentrations of solvents or surfactants, the length of contact of such formulations with the skin must be considered. This could increase the penetration of the preservative through the skin. Body burden which should also be considered here, is cumulative in terms of the number of products containing this particular preservative that the consumer is exposed to.

The mixture methylchloroisothiazolinone/methylisothiazolinone[b] represents one of the more effective preservatives used in topically applied products as indicated by the extremely low concentrations which are used in topical products. This may be the reason why shampoos and hair conditioners are the majority of products which currently contain this type of preservative. Since these are rinse-off products, the potential enhancement of percutaneous absorption from solvent or surfactant components in either shampoos or conditioners has little impact.

Pesticides: We can be exposed to biocides not only in topical drug and cosmetic products, but in environmental situations as well. From the point of view of safe handling of chemicals, we are becoming increasingly aware that chemicals for specific uses, which have passed certain toxicological tests required by regulatory agencies, may require further testing to substantiate their true safety in use.

One serious example of this was the death of a farmer from the percutaneous

[a]Germall II, registered trademark of Sutton Laboratories
[b]Kathon CG, registered trademark of Rohm & Haas

absorption of the herbicide paraquat, which leaked from his backpack spraying apparatus.[28,29] One of the more startling aspects of this case report is that it was a fatality from paraquat exposure in uncompromised skin. However, the leak of the paraquat-containing solution from the backpack onto the farmer's shirt essentially made the garment into a closed patch, thereby enhancing paraquat penetration through the uncompromised skin and increasing its percutaneous absorption. The toxicological testing requirement of a regulated herbicide, therefore, may be less than adequate to substantiate actual safety of that herbicide for those who need to use it.

Fragrance ingredients: Fragrances are major additions to topical products because they are generally formulations of between 50-200 individual fragrance ingredients, and because they may include many biologically active ingredients.

The range of their biological activity is enormous. Their negative effects range from neurotoxicity, phototoxicity, and photoallergenicity to sensitivity and irritation. The photosensitizating potential of fragrance ingredients has recently been the subject of a major review.[30,31]

Fragrance chemicals pose the greatest hazard to consumers if not monitored by a review of the fragrance ingredients in a given fragrance, where that review tests the fragrance both in an appropriate vehicle and in the product itself. The latter has been a consistent practice of the various consumer product industries, but the former has unfortunately been relatively rare until recently. Ten years ago, few consumer product manufacturers had fragrance disclosures, since the fragrance industry's position was solidly based on the proprietary nature of their formulations.

Two things prompted a change. First, as the toxicological and dermatological literature began to report increasing cases of various types of dermatitis caused by fragrance ingredients, the responsibility for safety of consumer products began to be much more focused on the consumer product manufacturer rather than on the fragrance manufacturers. Secondly, the technological growth of analytical chemistry methods made it possible to chemically analyze fragrances into their component ingredients with a high degree of sensitivity and accuracy. Fragrance companies began to disclose their formulae on a confidential basis to the consumer product manufacturer.

Some examples of biologically active fragrance ingredients will serve to demonstrate the toxicological importance of screening out these materials. The discovery that acetyl ethyl tetramethyl tetralin (AETT) is a neurotoxin is perhaps the most sensational example of the toxicological effect produced by a single fragrance ingredient.[32,33] AETT has the potential to both demyelinate nerve fibers and discolor central nervous system (CNS) tissue (a blue color is elaborated after exposure to AETT). Such powerful effects can be serious if the stratum corneum and epidermal-dermal junction are breached.

The phototoxin 6-methylcoumarin (6-MC) is another interesting example because it raised the question of cross-sensitization with coumarin and other coumarin derivatives important for fragrance formulation. Coumarin is used extensively by the fragrance industry, but after additional testing it was shown not to have any photosensitization potential itself. However, many coumarin derivatives were demonstrated to be photosensitizers. As it turned out, 6-MC was demonstrated to be both a phototoxin and a photoallergen,[34] but another coumarin derivative, 7-methoxycoumarin, tested out as only a phototoxin.[35]

Musk ambrette (MA) was first discovered as a photoallergen in after-shave lotion and was originally thought to be reactive as a photoallergen because of the typical product vehicle (a hydroalcoholic solution) and special product uses (shaving, which strips away layers of the stratum corneum). However, numerous reports began to appear in the literature.[36-38] Now musk ambrette has been demonstrated to be a true photoallergen. It is even used as a positive control in animal tests designed to detect photoallergenicity.

Sensitizing fragrance ingredients do not always need to be removed for toxicological safety reasons. Their activity can be quenched or chemically neutralized from forming a true allergen or hapten-carrier protein complex.[39-43] There is also a dose-response relationship in cutaneous sensitizers; a low level of a given sensitizer can, therefore, be used in a fragranced product without eliciting the sensitizing effect this same chemical produces at either higher concentrations or through different exposures.

As for irritation-producing fragrance ingredients, it appears that cutaneous irritation potential can be reduced—by achieving chemical complexations of the irritant, by blocking the reactive cell sites, or by reducing to some degree the effect of the neat chemical.[10] The topic of anti-irritancy, that is, producing these effects on known irritants, has been extensively reviewed.[44-46]

Fragrance, then, must be carefully monitored, reviewed and tested before being cleared for use in consumer products because fragrance compounds contain numerous biologically active ingredients.

Biologically and pharmacologically active ingredients: Hexachlorophene was a widely-used bacteriocide in hospital hand cleansers and consumer products such as medicated cosmetics and baby powder during the 1960s. However, this bacteriocide was later demonstrated to be a neurotoxin.[47,48] The deaths of several infants in France were the result of a manufacturing error which resulted in the production of a baby powder containing over ten times the intended concentration of hexachlorophene in that product. Since the product was used under occlusive conditions (diapering), the high concentration of hexachlorophene coupled with what was, in essence, a closed patch enhanced the percutaneous absorption of hexachlorophene from the product, resulting in the death of the infants.

Although tragic, this incident clearly demonstrated the impact of manufacturing on the safety of a product. In addition, it demonstrates how an error can be compounded through mode of application for the consumer product.

Contaminants: Contaminants are materials not intentionally formulated into products. Some contaminants "come with the territory," so to speak, in that they are residuals of incomplete reactions from the actual manufacturing of a chemical. *para*-Toluidine is a contaminant from the manufacture of D&C Green No. 6; *para*-toluidine is also a known carcinogen. The toxicological question is: can D&C Green No. 6 be used safely in externally applied consumer products? Food and Drug Administration scientists concluded that applying the principle of *de minimis* was appropriate in this particular case, allowing the listing of this color for use in externally applied drugs and cosmetics in spite of its containing a trace amount of a known carcinogen.[49]

Not all contaminants "come with the territory" however. Nitrosamines are a class of chemicals which also are carcinogens of varying potency. They can be formed in situ when an amine-containing compound such as an ethanolamine (mono-, di-, or triethanolamine) is used in the same formulation with a nitrosating agent, such as the preservative Bronopol (2-bromo-2-nitropropane-1,3-diol). The result can be the in situ formation of a carcinogen in a consumer product such as cosmetics.[50] Percutaneous absorption of such a contaminated cosmetic product can occur and, furthermore, can be detected.[51]

The solution to this problem is two-fold: proper formulation and chemical monitoring of incoming raw materials as well as chemical monitoring of finished goods. The proper formulation means insuring that an amine-containing compound is not used in conjunction with a nitrosating agent. This will chemically preclude the formation of nitrosamine species in situ. Monitoring incoming raw materials for nitrosamines insures absence of any nitrosamine species from either the actual manufacture of the raw material in question or its treatment in preparation for sale, such as the addition of a preservative to the chemical. Finally, monitoring the finished goods to make certain there are no contaminants is the final step in the solution to preventing nitrosamine formation in consumer products.

Colors: In 1983, the Food and Drug Administration completed its review of an industry-sponsored two-year chronic feeding study on D&C Orange No. 17. They concluded from the data in this study that there was a carcinogenic potential in D&C Orange No. 17 and that it should be permanently delisted as a color.

The cosmetics industry took an extremely conservative approach. Through its trade association, the Cosmetic, Toiletry and Fragrance Association (CTFA), the cosmetics industry asked the FDA whether or not D&C Orange No. 17 could be used in externally applied cosmetics such as facial makeup, but not in products such as lipsticks that are subject to incidental ingestion. The reply from FDA was the expected request for additional data. The same question was raised by the CTFA as the FDA reviews of D&C Red No. 19, D&C Red No. 9 and FD&C Red No. 3 were completed.[37,8]

Percutaneous absorption data was generated on these four colors and is summarized in Tables II through V. The vehicles were chosen based on the principal constituents of certain products (for example, talc in blushers and mineral oil in lipsticks) plus various standard formulations (such as a wax-based blusher product or a standard oil-in-water emulsion product).

The data in these tables clearly demonstrates the infinitesimal amount of percutaneous absorption. Permitting use of externally applied cosmetics containing D&C Orange No. 17, Red No. 19, Red No. 9 or FD&C Red No. 3 should be safe, therefore, even assuming that these colors are truly carcinogenic in animals.

However, regulation is not just a simple question of good science and common sense. Unfortunately, a zero-risk approach to regulating carcinogens in foods, drugs and cosmetics has been written into the law in the form of the Delaney Clause. This has until recently prevented the FDA from either listing or delisting certain colors.

This use of percutaneous absorption data to demonstrate the safety of certain FD&C and D&C colors is destined to become a classic example not only in the percutaneous absorption literature but in the regulatory literature as well.

Table II. In-vitro percutaneous absorption of D&C Orange No. 17 through human skin[52]

Vehicle	% D&C Orange 17	% Dose Absorbed in 48 Hours
Mineral oil	0.6	0.0093
Castor oil	0.6	0.0032
Wax Blusher formula	0.6	0.0083
Talc	5.0	0.0001

Table III. In-vitro percutaneous absorption of D&C Red No. 9 through human skin[53]

Vehicle	% D&C Red 9	% Dose Absorbed in 48 Hours
Talc	5.0	0.022
Mineral oil	5.0	0.010
Castor oil	5.0	0.027
Wax Blusher formula	0.5	0.073

Table IV. In-vitro percutaneous absorption of D&C Red No. 19 through human skin[54]

Vehicle	% D&C Red 19	% Dose Absorbed in 72 Hours
Talc	0.5	0.073
Mineral oil	0.5	0.390
Castor oil	0.5	0.007
Oil-in-water emulsion	0.001	0.470

Table V. In-vitro percutaneous absorption of FD&C Red No. 3 through human skin[55]

Vehicle	% FD&C Red 3	% Dose Absorbed in 48 Hours
Mineral oil	1.0	0.003
Castor oil	1.0	0.002
Talc	1.0	0.0003
Ethanol/water(50:50)	0.1	0.134
Oil-in-water emulsion	0.1	0.040

Conclusions

It is challenging to consider whether or not there are any principles which can be drawn from our current state of awareness and knowledge about percutaneous absorption. A review of the percutaneous absorption literature on any given point reveals a kaleidoscope of facts, opinions and theories which do not necessarily point in any one direction. Be that as it may, we need to attempt to summarize our current knowledge and, further, we need to attempt to elaborate some general toxicological principles about percutaneous absorption at this time.

Current knowledge: The most impressive aspect of our current state of knowledge about percutaneous absorption is that toxicologists are becoming more aware of the skin as a route of dosing, and therefore, of the delivery of a test material in toxicological testing. The use of skin to provide systemic drug delivery has dramatically increased the awareness of the potential of toxicity.

This leads naturally to the need to compare the results of being exposed to the same test material through ingestion, inhalation or absorption through the skin. Currently, there is no body of comparative knowledge on the gastrointestinal and cutaneous absorption of the same test material. However, as we stated previously, such research is critical to understanding the risks involved in exposures from ingestion, inhalation or exposure to the skin.

Toxicologists once again are finding themselves in the situation that occurred when in-vitro mutagenicity testing gained such ascendency in cancer research over in-vivo carcinogenicity testing. The in-vitro percutaneous absorption tests are developing at a much faster rate than the in-vivo percutaneous absorption tests. Therefore, the data which is being generated tends to be based more on direct in-vitro sampling through human skin rather than on indirect in-vivo studies in animals. The fact that a test material penetrates skin is not enough to assess a risk, however. We must also know whether or not it is cutaneously metabolized. We need to know the target organ and tissues of the test material and its metabolites. None of this information is available from in-vitro tests, some of it is available with animal models and very little of it is available from tests conducted in humans. All of this is to say caution must be exercised in using percutaneous absorption data in estimating the risks of a cutaneous exposure to a given chemical.

Physiological principles of percutaneous absorption: Some attempts have been made to generate rules for percutaneous absorption.[56] These are worth summarizing here.

1. Percutaneous absorption appears to be governed solely by the principles of passive diffusion.
2. Although there are two rate-limiting membranes—the stratum corneum of the epidermis and the epidermal-dermal junction—the stratum corneum controls percutaneous absorption to a greater degree.
3. The reciprocal function of the stratum corneum is also its reservoir function. This gives unique pharmacokinetics to the effectiveness of external therapy through topically applied drug products.
4. The first area of product application may or may not be related to localization of the chemical in the epidermis. The penetrant's concentration in the vehicle and the application site as well as the state of cutaneous

hydration play important roles here.

5. Flux of a penetrant across the stratum corneum increases with the solubility and mobility of the permeant through the stratum corneum.
6. Molecular weight below 500 (5000 daltons) has no effect on percutaneous absorption. For such materials, partition coefficient and lipid solubility are more important.
7. Rapidly penetrating substances go directly through the cells of the stratum corneum.
8. After the initial application, flux through the remaining layers of the epidermis is greater than through the stratum corneum, and the concentration of the permeant decreases with each successive epidermal stratum.
9. Flow through dermal tissue proceeds at a faster rate than through epidermal tissue. Again, the concentration of the permeant decreases from the stratum papillae to the stratum basale of the dermis.
10. Although metabolism, binding to protein and accumulation in the epidermis and dermis play a role, they ultimately have little influence on the overall percutaneous absorption rate.
11. Total absorption by the vasculature (blood and lymph systems) results from absorption of a permeant into the epidermis and dermis.

In addition to these general rules, we propose the following as guidelines in interpreting percutaneous absorption data. They can be used to interpret percutaneous absorption data and apply these data to estimations of either risk or safety.

Mathematical modeling: Mathematical modeling is not a substitute for actual percutaneous absorption data.

As a corollary to this general principle, we would state that the validity of mathematical modeling varies in direct proportion to its relationship to the actual data. The further the mathematical modeling takes one from the data, the less value the mathematical modeling has in truly describing percutaneous absorption.

The gestalt principle of percutaneous absorption: Percutaneous absorption data must be reviewed against information on the biological condition of the skin and the chemical constituents or formulation aspects, such as: the ingredient of concern, vehicle, chemical enhancers, manufacturing and exposure. Only in this way can the estimation of risk, safety or meaning of the percutaneous absorption data be adequately assessed.

Toxicological risk from topical product exposure: In decreasing order of risk and increasing order of time of exposure, the ranking is:

Household products > Prescription drugs > OTC drugs > Cosmetic products

The relative increase in percutaneous absorption by formulation type is:

Solutions > Emulsions > Suspensions and gels > Physical mixtures

Emulsions (either O/W or W/O types) can influence percutaneous absorption more than any other type of formulation probably because the volatile components are driven off, leaving behind either a film or residue. Next come solutions, probably because of their solubility aspects, followed by suspensions and gels. Interestingly enough, physical mixtures such as wax products or powder products can occlude, but they do not appreciably influence percutaneous absorption.

In any rapidly-developing field such as percutaneous absorption, there comes a time when an island is needed in a sea of fast-developing facts and test methods. A line needs to be drawn. A benchmark needs to be made. We have attempted to do just that in this chapter on the toxicological aspects of percutaneous absorption. The application of this information and knowledge, these principles and guidelines, will test whether or not this exercise has contributed to the making of such an island.

Topical Application of Liposomal Preparations

By K. Egbaria, PhD and N. Weiner, PhD

Liposomal formulations, when applied topically, exhibit unique properties beneficial to a wide variety of cosmetic and pharmaceutical applications. They can encapsulate high concentrations of water and lipid soluble substances and facilitate their delivery into the skin while limiting their permeation into the central blood supply. Liposomes are biodegradable, nontoxic and can be prepared on a large scale. They also can be useful in the formulation of a large variety of ingredients (such as moisturizers, skin care agents, sunscreens, vitamins and tanning agents) in moisturizing creams, aftershave lotions, hair products and bath lotions.

Liposomes are microscopic vesicles composed of one or more lipid bilayers arranged in concentric fashion enclosing an equal number of aqueous compartments.[1] Various amphipathic molecules have been used to form the liposomes, and the method of preparation can be tailored to control their size and morphology. Drug molecules can either be encapsulated in the aqueous space or intercalated into the lipid bilayer; the exact location of a drug in the liposome will depend upon its physicochemical characteristics and the composition of the lipids.[2,3]

Liposomes have shown great potential as a drug delivery system. An assortment of molecules, including peptides and proteins, have been incorporated in liposomes, which can then be administered by different routes.[4-6] Due to their high degree of biocompatibility, liposomes were initially considered as delivery systems for intravenous use. It has since become apparent that liposomes can also be useful for delivery of drugs by other routes of administration.

Mezei et al.[7] reported that topical application of liposomal triamcinolone acetonide for 5 days resulted in a drug concentration in the epidermis and dermis four times higher than that obtained using a control ointment, while urinary excretion of the drug was diminished. Mezei et al.[8] compared also the deposition of topically applied gels of free and liposomally-entrapped triamcinolone in rabbit skin and found that application of the liposomal gel resulted in a concentration of triamcinolone acetonide approximately five times higher in the epidermis and three times higher in the dermis, than application of the free drug gel. The results of these studies suggested to them the inherent potential of liposomes as a selective drug delivery system for cutaneous application.

Vermorken et al.[9] tested the effect of topical application of dihydrotestosterone encapsulated in liposomes and as an acetone solution on the hamster flank organ.

These authors reported that the systemic absorption of dihydrotestosterone from the liposomal system was negligible, whereas significant absorption was observed from the acetone solution. Since they were only concerned with systemic absorption, they reported no advantages of the liposome system over the acetone solution in achieving the desired biological effect.

Ganesan et al.,[10] performing in-vitro diffusion experiments with hairless mouse skin using liposomal formulations, found that neither intact liposomes nor the phospholipid of which they are comprised diffuse across the skin into the receiver compartment of Franz diffusion cells.[4] They also reported that lipophilic drugs such as progesterone and hydrocortisone, which are expected to be intercalated within the bilayer structure of phospholipid multilamellar liposomes, passed through the skin with comparable facility to the free drug. The effect of application of liposomal progesterone in reducing the rate of hair growth in idiopathic hirsutism was reported by Rowe et al.[11]

Patel et al.[12] suggested that liposomes can be used for the sustained release of drugs into the epidermis when applied topically.[6] For example, when free and liposomally-entrapped ^{3}H-methotrexate was applied to the skin of nude mice, percutaneous absorption of drug was greatly reduced by liposomal encapsulation. Furthermore, the retention of ^{3}H-methotrexate in the skin was two- to three-fold higher from the liposomal formulation than from the solution, again suggesting a localization of the liposomes in the epidermis, where a sustained release of methotrexate takes place.

This chapter presents a review of topically-applied liposomal formulations, with emphasis on the evaluation of liposomal systems in a wide variety of animal models and human skin using both in-vivo and in-vitro techniques. The mechanism by which liposomes facilitate deposition of their lipid constituents and entrapped active ingredients into the skin and potential applications of topical liposomes in cosmetics and pharmacy are discussed.

Liposomes in cosmetics

Recently, a great deal of interest in the use of liposomes in skin gels or skin creams has been generated in the field of cosmetics. Vegetable phospholipids are widely used for topical applications in cosmetics and dermatology since they have a high content of esterified essential fatty acids, especially linoleic acid which is believed to increase the barrier function of the skin and descrease water loss within a short period of time after application.[13,14] Soya phospholipids or other vegetable phospholipids, due to their surface activity and their ability to form liposomes, are also an ideal source for possible transport of linoleic acid into the skin. Lautenschläger et al.[15,16] discussed the potential use of liposomes derived from soya bean phospholipids in cosmetics. They predicted that liposome technology offers great opportunities for several new cosmetic products and that cosmetic developers would now have to deal very intensively with questions of raw material selection, characterization of raw and finished formulations, and clinical safety of these unique formulations. They suggested that soya phospholipids in the form of liposomes satisfy many of these requirements.

Liposomes and Skin Humidity

The key ingredient which keeps the human skin soft and flexible is water. Skin, particularly the horny layer, performs a significant protective role by providing, in addition to mechanical protection, a barrier against extraneous substances. This function of the horny layer is dependent on its elasticity, determined by the content of fats and inorganic salts, as well as by the hydration state. Increasing the skin humidity leads to an increase in the skin's elasticity.

Skin humidity is regulated to a large extent by lipids in the skin's horny layer. This complex lipid mixture is oriented, at least in part, as a bimolecular leaflet.[17] Liposomes have been employed in cosmetics and skin care products for several years with great success. Few reports of the effects of liposomes on the humidity of human skin after topical application have been published.[18-20]

Artman et al. examined the effect of several liposomal formulations with varying compositions on the hydration of the skin using measurements of the capacitative resistance of the skin.[18] They applied three liposomal formulations with varying soya phospholipid composition topically, to the hairless inner forearm of ten normal subjects together with a control (physiological salt solution). A significant increase in skin humidity was observed only with the liposomal formulation containing the highest phosphatidylcholine (PC) content (80%). For this formulation, a 38% humidity increase was observed within 30 minutes of application. After three hours, the measured value was still 10% above the control value. Liposomal formulations with lower PC content (28%) showed only a slight increase in the skin humidity 30 minutes after application, and the baseline value was reached within one hour.

Oleniacz recently reported the use of liposomal formulations as skin moisturizers.[19] His patent claims that nonsubstantivity and loss of water migrating from the underlying tissues of skin are resolved by the use of liposomes. The liposomes are substantive to the skin and absorb water from the atmosphere. The topically applied liposomes share their entrapped water with the skin resulting in an increase of moisturization, softness and flexibility of the skin. The water binding capacity of normal stratum corneum reportedly drops sharply when damaged but is restored to acceptable levels after being treated with liposomes containing a humectant.[19]

The water binding capacity and occlusivity of liposomal formulations containing different sterols and humectants were also evaluated. The liposomal formulations were found to be very effective at 98% relative humidity, holding at least 4 times their weight of water. Comparisons of the in-vitro water binding capacity of untreated stratum corneum and stratum corneum treated with liposomes led to claims of a substantial increase (> 100%) of water capacity of the treated stratum corneum relative to its own untreated control. Finally, it was reported that treatment with liposomes reduced the degree of scaliness and roughness of the skin after a single 18-hour treatment.

Tagawa et al. studied the humectant effects of a cream containing hydrogenated lecithin liposomes with natural moisturizing factors (NMF) such as amino acids and sugars.[20] At 16% relative humidity, the application of this cream gradually increased the skin's moisture content, whereas at 40% relative humidity there was no effect. They postulate that the liposomally encapsulated NMFs were more effective due to their absorption into the skin.

Advantages of Liposomes

In the past decade, liposomal formulations have been extensively employed to enhance the efficiency of drug delivery via several routes of administration. In a number of instances, liposomal drug formulations have been shown to be markedly superior to conventional dosage forms, especially for intravenous and topical modes of administration of drugs. Recently, it has become apparent that liposomes may offer special advantages as a topical delivery system. The major advantages of topical liposomal drug formulations can be summarized as follows:

- In a manner similar to that of biological cells, liposomes can store water-soluble substances in their interiors and lipophilic and amphiphilic substances in their membranes, where they are positioned to be transferred to other membranes such as the skin.

- Most conventional vehicles are inefficient in their ability to deliver their active ingredient into the skin because of their failure to penetrate the horny layer. The bilayers of liposomes, on the other hand, efficiently penetrate the skin.

- Liposomal incorporation of drugs which readily penetrate the skin results in a decrease in systemic absorption compared to that resulting from topical application using conventional vehicles.

- Liposomal deposition into the stratum corneum results in a substantial reservoir effect.

- Liposomes are nontoxic, biodegradable and can be prepared on a large scale.

- Liposomes can provide a large "value added" to cosmetic products by encapsulating a variety of ingredients (such as moisturizers, skin care agents, sunscreens, vitamins and tanning agents) in moisturizing creams, cleansing creams, aftershave lotions, hair products and bath lotions.

- Liposomes, when applied topically, can be used to control the moisture content of the skin.

Mechanism of Liposomal Action

Experimental Materials: Cholesterol (CH), palmitic acid (PA), hydrocortisone (HC), cholesteryl sulfate (CS), bovine brain ceramides (CM), and HEPES free acid were obtained from Sigma (St. Louis, MO). Egg lecithin (PC) and phosphatidyl serine (PS) were obtained from Avanti Polar Lipids (Birmingham, AL). Lyophilized recombinant γ-interferon in vials was supplied by Genentech (South San Francisco, CA). ^{125}I-labeled lyophilized recombinant γ-interferon was obtained from New England Nuclear Corporation (Boston, MA). Lyophilized recombinant leukocyte α-INF in vials, each containing 18×10^6 IU of INF, 9 mg of sodium chloride and 5 mg of human serum albumin was supplied by Hoffman LaRoche Inc., (Nutley, NJ). α-Tocopherol (α-T) was obtained from Eastman Kodak (Rochester, NY). ^{14}C-PA, ^{3}H-HC, ^{3}H-CH, L-3-phosphatidylcholine and 1,2-di{1-[14]C} palmitoyl (^{14}C-DPPC) were obtained from Amersham (UK). All other chemicals were of analytical grade.

Liposome Formulations: Multilamellar liposomes (MLV) containing PC:CH:PS, referred to as "phospholipid-based" liposomes, at a mole ratio of 1:0.5:0.1 or containing CM:CH:PA:CS, referred to as "skin lipid" liposomes, at a weight ratio of 4:2.5:2.5:1 were prepared using the conventional film method.[1] Briefly, the lipid mixtures were dissolved in a 2:1 (v/v) mixture of chloroform and methanol. Trace amounts of ^{3}H-CH and ^{14}C-DPPC were incorporated in the phospholipid-based liposomes and trace amounts of ^{3}H-CH and ^{14}C-PA were added to the skin lipid liposomes. In all cases appropriate combinations of the radiolabels were chosen to provide a dual-labeled liposomal formulation. One percent of α-tocopherol (based on total lipid amount) was also added to the solvent mixture as an antioxidant. Appropriate amounts of drugs, if lipophilic, were also dissolved in the solvent mixture. The lipids, drug and markers were then deposited as a thin film in a round-bottom flask by rotary evaporation under nitrogen. The flask containing the lipid film was stored in vacuum overnight to facilitate removal of any residual solvents. The films were hydrated by the addition of an isotonic 0.05 M HEPES buffer, pH 7.4, with mild agitation at a temperature above the phase transition temperature of the highest melting component in the mixture. Water-soluble drugs and markers such as inulin were included in the buffer used for hydration of the lipid films. After the film was homogeneously dispersed, the mixture was bath-sonicated for five minutes and the suspension was stored at 4°C overnight before use in the diffusion experiments. The final concentration of lipids ranged from 5-50 mg/ml. All of the liposomal preparations were examined with a Nikon Diaphot Light microscope to evaluate liposomal quality and integrity. Additionally, the multilamellarity of the vesicles was confirmed by freeze fracture electron microscopy.

Large unilamellar vesicles (LUV) were prepared by a modification of the reverse-phase evaporation method of Szoka and Papahadjopoulos.[21] Appropriate amounts of the lipids, drugs, radiolabels and α-tocopherol were dissolved in 10 ml of a chloroform-methanol mixture (2:1 v/v). Five ml of 0.05 M HEPES buffer (pH 7.4) and enough additional methanol (up to 1.5 ml) were added to yield a clear solution after brief sonication. The organic solvents and a small amount of water were then removed under nitrogen at a temperature above the phase-transition temperature of the highest melting lipid component by using a rotoevaporator. Solvent removal was continued until all foaming ceased. The resulting liposomal suspension was stored at 4°C overnight before use in the diffusion experiments.

Dehydration/rehydration liposomes (DRV) were prepared by a modification of the method reported by Kirby and Gregoriadis.[22] Briefly, appropriate amounts of various lipids, drugs and radiolabels, contained in a flask, were dissolved in chloroform/methanol (2:1 v/v). The solvent mixture was removed using a rotoevaporator under vacuum at a temperature above the phase transition of the lipids. The resultant film was dried overnight in a desiccator to remove any residual solvent. An appropriate aliquot of 0.05 M HEPES buffer (pH 7.4) was then added and the mixture was hydrated at a temperature above the phase transition of the lipids for about an hour. Intermittent vortexing was required for complete hydration. The resultant dispersion was then dehydrated at 50°C under vacuum using the rotoevaporator. When the liposomal suspension became very viscous, an amount of water, equivalent to that removed, was reintroduced into the viscous suspension. The rehydrated liposomes were then allowed to equilibrate for about 45 minutes at a temperature above the phase transition temperature of the lipids. The dispersion was then stored at 4°C overnight before use in the diffusion experiments.

Diffusion Experiments: Full-thickness hairless mouse, pig and hairless guinea pig skins were excised from the fresh carcasses of animals and were used immediately after removing subcutaneous fat. Full-thickness human skin was obtained at autopsy and used immediately after removing subcutaneous fat. The skin was mounted on a Franz diffusion cell with a nominal surface area of 2 cm^2 and a receiver compartment having a 7 ml capacity (Crown Glass, Somerville, NJ). The epidermal side of the skin was exposed to ambient conditions while the dermal side was bathed by a 0.05 M isotonic HEPES buffer, pH 7.4. The receiver solution was stirred continously using a small Teflon-covered magnet. Care was exercised to remove any air bubbles between the underside of the skin and solution in the receiver compartment. The temperature of the receiver was maintained at 37°C. Following mounting of the section of skin, 200 µl of the test formulation were applied to the epidermal surface. A smaller amount of formulation was found to be insufficient to ensure uniform spreading across the entire exposed surface of the skin in the cell. A minimum of three cells was used for each formulation and duplicate experiments were carried out using sections of skin from different skin specimens for each formulation. All experiments were carried out with nonoccluded donor compartments. At predetermined time periods, the experiments were stopped and the diffusion setup was dismantled for assay of radiolabeled drug and lipids.

Assay of Radiolabeled Markers: Upon dismantling, the donor compartment of the cell was rinsed carefully five times with 0.5 ml HEPES buffer, pH 7.4. The skin was then removed and rinsed twice with 3.0 ml of the same buffer. The washing procedure was found to be sufficient to remove >99% of the formulation when determined at time zero. All washings were collected and assayed for radiolabel. Following the rinsing procedure, the skin patch was mounted on a board and a piece of adhesive tape (Scotch Magic tape, 810, 3M Commercial Office Supply Division, St. Paul, MN), 1.9 cm wide and about 6 cm long, was used to strip the skin. The tape was of sufficient size to cover the area of skin that was in contact with the formulation. Several strippings were carried out for each specimen and each strip was analyzed separately for radiolabeled drug and lipid. The number of strippings carried out were as follows: 9 for mouse skin, 20 for guinea pig and pig skin and 25 for human skin. The amount adhering to the stratum corneum surface was determined by analysis of the first two strippings and the amount in the deeper stratum corneum was determined by analysis of the remaining strips. The amount of drug and lipid penetrating the deeper skin strata was determined by analysis of the remainder of the stripped full-thickness skin. The remaining skin, and the receiver compartment solution were also assayed for drug and lipid. Assay of the donor, skin rinse and receiver solutions were carried out after addition of about 15 ml of Ecolite + (ICN Biomedical, Inc., Irvine, CA) to each system. The tape strippings and remaining skin were assayed as follows: Each sample was placed in a combustion-cone and burnt in a tissue oxidizer (Model 306 Packard Oxidizer, Packard Instrument Co., Downers Grove, IL). The separated radionuclides were then assayed using a scintillation counter.

Validation of the Stripping Procedure

In order to determine if treatment of skin with formulation affects the stripping procedure, we carried out in-vitro diffusion studies using hairless mouse skin with incorporated radioactive ^{14}C-glycine. When glycine is injected intraperitoneally, the turnover time for its incorporation into the skin has been reported to be about four days, at which time the cumulative glycine uptake in the skin is at a maximum.[23]

Briefly, 0.5 ml isotonic phosphate buffer (pH 7.4) containing 5mCi ^{14}C-glycine was injected intraperitoneally into each mouse. The animals were sacrificed on the fifth day and the skin of each mouse was excised and cut into four pieces. Each piece was weighed and exposed to one of the following four procedures: (i) no treatment (control); (ii) treatment with isotonic HEPES buffer, pH 7.4, for 24 hours in a Franz diffusion cell; (iii) treatment with the phospho-lipid-based liposomal dispersion for 24 hours in a Franz diffusion cell; and (iv) treatment with the skin-lipid-based liposomal formulation for 24 hours in a Franz diffusion cell.

Following each of the treatment procedures the diffusion cell was dis-mantled, the skin rinsed (as described previously) and allowed to dry. Each piece of skin was then mounted on a board and stripped as described previously. Each of the strippings was then analyzed for ^{14}C-glycine using a tissue oxidizer.

Vesicle charge and permeation effects

The effect of liposomal charge on in-vitro permeation into hairless mouse skin was evaluated recently in our laboratories using positively- and negatively-charged phospholipid multilamellar liposomes. Liposomes containing phosphatidylcholine:cholesterol:stearylamine at a mole ratio of 1:0.5:0.1 were prepared using the conventional film method as previously described.[1] For experiments testing the incorporation of liposomal bilayer lipids into the various skin strata, trace quantities of ^{14}C-DPPC and ^{3}H-CH were included in the formulation.

The data shown in Table I indicate that application of positively-charged liposomes resulted in almost twice the amount of lipids deposited in the deeper layers of the skin compared to application of the negatively-charged liposomes, suggesting that mixing and interaction of the liposomal bilayers with the stratum corneum bilayers was more extensive with positively charged lipo-somes. However, it should be pointed out that the application of formulations containing stearylamine results in marked irritation.

Table I. Distribution of liposomal bilayer lipids in various strata of hairless mouse skin 24 hours after in-vitro application of negatively-charged (PC/CH/PS) and positively-charged (PC/CH/SA) MLV.

	(PC/CH/PS)	MLV	(PC/CH/SA)	MLV
Distribution	^{3}H-CH	^{14}C-DPPC	^{3}H-CH	^{14}C-DPPC
Total donor compartment	20±4	20±4	9±3	9±3
Stratum corneum surface	54±11	53±11	48±17	49±16
Deeper stratum corneum	22±12	22±8	40±14	36±12
Deeper skin strata	3±0.3	3±1	3±2	3±2
Receiver	0.03±0.03	0.024±0.02	0.18±0.10	0.023±0.02

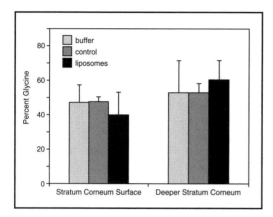

Figure 1: Adhesive tape stripping profiles of ^{14}C-glycine from hairless mouse skin after the following treatments: (i) control (untreated skin) t=0 hr; (ii) liposomal for 24 hr and (iii) isotonic buffer solution, pH 7.4, for 24 hr (n=3).

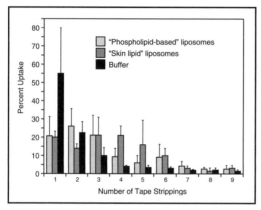

Figure 2: Adhesive tape stripping profiles of ^{14}C-glycine 24 hr after in-vitro topical application of: (i) phospholipid-based liposomes; (ii) "skin lipid" liposomes and (iii) isotonic buffer solution, pH 7.4 (n=5).

Results

Figure 1 shows the distribution of incorporated glycine label in various strata of hairless mouse skin after 24 hour treatment with liposomal formulations and buffer solution. Figure 2 shows the distribution of glycine label in the first ten strips of hairless mouse skin treated with liposomes and buffer solution. The near-identical profile for the two liposomal systems and the buffer-treated skin indicates that liposomal treatment for 24 hours does not induce any significant alterations in stratum corneum integrity compared to a 24-hour buffer treatment. More importantly, the results imply that the stripping technique is just as valid for skin samples treated with liposomal formulations as for those treated with aqueous solutions.

The 24-hour in-vitro uptake of HC from various formulations upon topical application to hairless mouse skin is shown in Table II. It is evident that the total amount of HC associated with the skin is significantly greater for the liposomal system than for the aqueous solution. It is also observed that the percent HC found in the receiver is much lower for the liposomal formulation.

Table III shows the distribution of α-interferon in various strata of hairless guinea pig skin at 24 hours after in-vitro application of (a) "phospholipid-based"

Table II. Distribution of hydrocortisone (HC) (expressed as percent formulation applied ±S.D.; n=3-5) in various strata of hairless mouse skin 24 hr after in-vitro topical application of hydrocortisone-containing formulations onto full-thickness skin.

Formulation	% HC in total stratum corneum	% HC in deeper skin strata	% HC in the receiver	% HC in combined donor cell and skin washings
Aqueous solution	44.37±7.20	1.06±0.10	23.71±4.68	31.28±12.08
PC:CH:PS-MLV	78.93±6.85	1.94±0.80	1.56±0.47	16.91± 1.20
PC:CH:PS-DRV	70.99±4.06	1.02±0.58	1.88±0.34	26.10± 3.72
PC:CH:PS-REV	74.79±3.08	1.18±0.12	2.53±0.47	22.08± 2.73

LUV and DRV, (b) "skin lipid" LUV and DRV and (c) an aqueous solution. The total amounts of α-interferon found in the skin and especially in the deeper skin strata indicate that liposomal formulations greatly enhance the deposition of drug compared to the aqueous solution.

Table I shows the distribution of liposomal bilayer lipids in various strata of hairless mouse skin 24 hours after in-vitro application of negatively-charged and positively-charged liposomes. It is also clear from the results in Tables that the composition, charge and concentration of lipids as well as the method of liposomal preparation have a major effect on the efficacy of drug deposition.

Figures 3-5 show the distribution of γ-interferon and TGF-α in different strata of human cadaver skin and mouse skin, respectively, at various times after topical in-vitro application of a liposomal formulation and an aqueous solution. It is also clear from the results in Figures 3-5 that the liposomal preparation greatly enhances the deposition of drug as compared to the aqueous solution.

Figure 6 shows a comparison of the distribution of retinoic acid in various strata of hairless mouse skin when applied in-vitro as a liposomal suspension

Table III. Distribution of interferon (expressed as percent formulation applied ±S.D.; n=3-5) in various strata of the skin 24 hr after in-vitro topical application of interferon-containing formulations onto full-thickness skin.

Formulation	% IFN Surface Stratum Corneum	% IFN Deeper Stratum Corneum	% IFN in Deeper Skin Strata	% IFN in Combined Donor Cell and Skin Washings
Aqueous solution	8.5 ± 4.2	8.5 ± 7.1	0.6 ± 0.1	74.0± 0.2
EL:CH:PS-LUV	46.1 ± 4.2	38.3 ± 2.1	2.6 ± 1.5	8.9± 2.8
"Skin Lipid"-LUV	5.5 ± 1.5	62.6 ± 5.5	4.5 ± 2.5	17.7± 5.1
"Skin Lipid"-DRV	6.6 ± 1.9	58.6 ± 7.9	9.6 ± 2.6	15.4± 3.0
CM:CH:CS-DRV	7.4 ± 2.0	53.9 ± 8.5	12.8 ± 3.5	17.8± 1.5

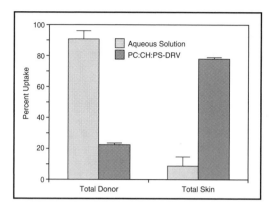

Figure 3: Comparison of the 24 hr in-vitro uptake of γ-interferon from phospholipid-based DRV and from aqueous solution in various strata of human cadaver skin.

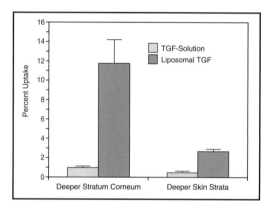

Figure 4: Comparison of the 24 hr in-vitro uptake of TGF-α from phospholipid-based MLV and from aqueous solution in various trata of hairless mouse skin.

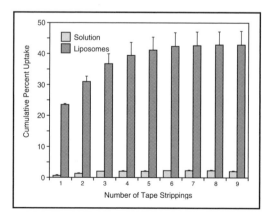

Figure 5: Comparison of the 24 hr in-vitro uptake of TGF-α from phospholipid-based MLV and from aqueous solution in various strippings of hairless mouse skin.

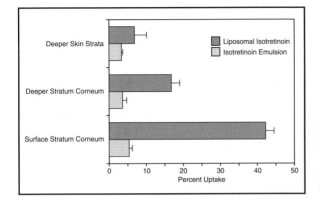

Figure 6: Comparison of the 24 hr in-vitro uptake of ^{3}H-isotretinoin from "skin lipid" MLV and from an emulsion in various strata of pig skin.

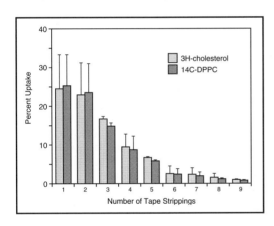

Figure 7: 24 hr in-vitro uptake of ^{3}H-cholesterol and ^{14}C-DPPC from positively charged phospholipid MLV in various strippings of hairless mouse stratum corneum.

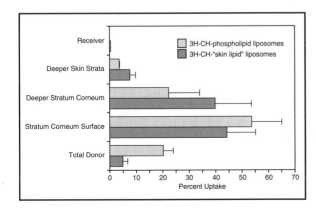

Figure 8: Comparison of the 24 hr in-vitro uptake of ^{3}H-cholesterol from "skin lipid" MLV and from phospholipid MLV in various strata of hairless mouse skin.

and as an emulsion. The amount of drug associated with the stratum corneum and in the deeper skin strata is substantially higher for the liposomal system compared to the emulsion.

A plot of the percent uptake in the stripped layers of hairless mouse stratum corneum of dual lipid label after 24 hours of in-vitro treatment with positively-charged phospholipid liposomes is shown in Figure 7. Plots of the percent cumulative uptake in the various strata of hairless mouse skin of lipid label after 24 hours of in-vitro treatment with negatively-charged phospholipid liposomes and "skin lipid" liposomes are shown in Figure 8. In all cases, a mass balance of >95% was achieved after the donor compartment and the skin rinses were taken into account.

Discussion

Although the use of liposomal drug formulations for topical application has been steadily increasing, few studies have been undertaken in an attempt to explain the mechanism by which liposomal entrapment improves drug transfer into the skin. Most of the in-vitro and in-vivo studies, to date, have been concerned with the extent of percutaneous (systemic) absorption. However, the treatment of many dermatological diseases by topical application is expected to be more efficient if a significant concentration of the drug is retained in the living epidermis and dermis.

It has been demonstrated convincingly in several in-vitro studies that the percutaneous absorption of a drug is severely and dramatically retarded after topical application of liposomal drug formulations as compared to their absorption from solution.[24-26] The use of topically-applied liposomal formulations as a means to provide adequate systemic levels of drugs would therefore be counterproductive.

The ability of the stratum corneum to act as a reservoir of drug transport through the skin was amply demonstrated by Rougier et al.[27] They reported that the absorption of a variety of drugs through the skin was proportional to the amount of drug recovered in the stratum corneum following 30 minutes topical application. Although in-vitro diffusion studies with Franz cells allow the prediction of percutaneous absorption of drugs from various topical formulations with great precision, no evident correlation exists between the extent of percutaneous absorption and local action of the drug, especially when liposomal formulations are employed. Therefore, in order to accurately estimate the potential effectiveness of liposomal formulations in alleviating local skin conditions, it would be necessary to determine drug levels in the deeper layers of the skin such as the epidermal/dermal junction and the dermis itself.

Several methods can be used to determine drug levels in the dermis. Separation of the epidermis by heat or enzyme treatment and dermatome sectioning have been widely used.[28,29] A simple method commonly employed is the stripping technique, which has been shown to provide accurate estimates of drug deposition within various strata of the skin.[30]

The stripping method using adhesive tape has also provided a few clues to the mechanism of liposomal action on transfer of drug into skin. The structure and composition of stratum corneum has been the subject of several excellent papers and reviews by Elias et al.[31-33] Very briefly, the stratum corneum of humans, mice and pigs has been shown to be devoid of phospholipids. The lipid composition is rather nonpolar in nature and consists primarily of ceramides (40%), cholesterol (25%), fatty acids (25%) and cholesteryl sulfate (10%). These lipids are termed "skin lipids" and are arranged in bilayer sheet structures that fill the intercellular space in the stratum corneum. The primary pathway to the transport of water and other drugs is believed to reside mainly in these bilayer structures. The removal of these bilayer sheets either by solvent treatment[34] or by successive tape stripping[29] increases the permeability of water, suggesting a decreased barrier function.

The stripping technique was used in our laboratories to investigate the deposition of drugs and lipids in various strata of skin after topical application of liposomal formulations and conventional formulations such as solutions and emulsions. The results with glycine-incorporated hairless mouse skin in-vitro studies (Figures 1 and 2) indicate that the amounts of glycine found in the stratum corneum strippings after liposomal treatment were similar to those found with buffer treatment and with untreated controls. These experiments revealed that the stripping method adopted is valid even for 24-hour diffusion experiments wherein degradation of the stratum corneum as well as the epidermal-dermal junction due to extensive hydration effects may affect the nature and extent of the layers stripped.

The distribution of drug and liposomal lipid label in the various strata of skin application of liposomes in in-vitro studies revealed the following major trends:

- The amount of drug obtained in the deeper skin strata after stripping of the stratum corneum (and possibly the epidermis) at 24 hours was generally 3-4 times higher from liposomal formulations than from solutions or emulsions (Figures 3-6).

- The uptake and distribution of retinoic acid from emulsion having an emulsifier composition similar to the lipid composition of "skin lipid" liposomal formulation is markedly reduced (Figure 6). This finding suggests that, for efficient drug transfer to occur, the lipid structure in the vehicle must be a bilayer configuration.

- The amount of drug in the deeper skin strata depends on the concentration of lipids used. For example, twice as much α-interferon was found in the dermis with a 15 mg/ml "skin lipid" liposomal system as opposed to a 50 mg/ml phospholipid-based system containing the same concentration of interferon (Table II). This can be explained based on the dilution effect in terms of a lower drug-to-lipid ratio at the higher lipid concentration.

- The ratio of radiolabeled lipids of the liposomal preparation was essentially maintained throughout the stratum corneum layers (Figure 7). This strongly suggests a molecular mixing of the liposomal bilayers with those of the stratum corneum bilayers.

- The method of preparation of liposomes affects their ability to transfer or deposit drugs in the deeper skin strata. A comparison of "skin lipid" LUV with "skin lipid" DRV interferon formulations in in-vitro studies with hairless guinea pig showed that DRV are twice as effective as LUV in depositing interferon in the deeper skin strata (Table II). Similar differences between LUV and MLV ciclosporin-A formulations were observed with both "skin lipid" and phospholipid-based liposomal formulations in in-vitro human skin studies.[35] These findings indicate that the lamellarity of the liposomes as well as the extent of bilayer-drug interation play a crucial role in the liposome-aided transfer of drug into the deeper skin strata.

• The in-vitro results are reasonably consistent with in-vivo efficacies of the various liposomal and conventional formulations tested.[36] The agreement of the in-vitro results with in-vivo effects suggests that the stripping technique can be used to accurately assess formulation efficiency.

A significant fraction of the applied liposomal formulation is found in the strippings of the stratum corneum. This stratum corneum-associated liposomal formulation could be the result of several interrelated phenomena. One scenario involves the applied liposomal drug suspension, upon dehydration, being transformed into lipid bilayer structures that adhere or bind strongly to the surface of the skin. Such binding may occur between liposomal lipid bilayers and corneocytes or between liposomal and stratum corneum bilayers. The adhesive strength appears to be quite high judging from the inability of simple rinsing procedures to dislodge a significant portion of the applied liposomal lipids. The 'surface' liposomal lipid bilayers containing drug provide a drug reservoir allowing sustained release of the drug, especially small lipophilic drugs such as hydrocortisone (Table I), across the stratum corneum into the dermis and blood vasculature. The sustained activity of liposomal hydrocortisone activity observed by Jacobs et al. and of liposomal tetracaine by Mezei et al. may have been the result of such a "surface reservoir" effect. The liposomal lipid bilayers formed on the surface after dehydration present an additional and substantial barrier to drug diffusion. It is possible, therefore, to control drug release into and across skin by controlling the amounts of applied liposomal lipids.

A second scenario involves the liposomal lipid bilayers, after dehydration, interacting with the stratum corneum bilayers, perhaps by a fusion mechanism. The superior efficiency of "skin lipid" liposomal formulations compared to phospholipid-based liposomal systems in both in-vitro and in-vivo studies were interpreted in terms of the greater ease of "molecular mixing" of "skin lipids" with the stratum corneum lipids. This was argued to be a reasonable assumption since "skin lipid" liposomes were prepared using lipid components similar to those found in the stratum corneum.[37] The glycine experiments also provide strong support for the contention that liposomal lipids are intimately associated with the stratum corneum bilayers. It must be pointed out however, that the high degree of mixing may be the result of a weakening of the stratum corneum's integrity caused by the exaggerated hydration inherent in in-vitro diffusion cell studies. In-vivo experiments were therefore carried out with several liposomal formulations in order to assess these factors.

The mechanism by which liposomes allow deposition of or transfer drug into the deeper skin strata of the dermis is at present not completely resolved and is beyond the scope of this chapter. It is clear, however, that liposomes are extremely efficient in aiding the translocation of large hydrophobic drugs such as ciclosporin-A and of hydrophilic drugs such as interferons and growth factors into skin strata associated with lymph and blood supplies.

Transdermal Drug Delivery

By Gary W. Cleary

At first glance a transdermal patch may look like a simple enough device, but actually, it's a very complex drug delivery system. Every transdermal device has to make the drug available so that it will permeate through the skin at the specific rate necessary to provide the desired therapeutic results. The device must adhere well to the skin yet be easily peeled away, be cost effective, and be esthetically acceptable to the physician and patient. Once a device is developed, there is still a series of barriers within the skin that has to be overcome for the drug to reach the systemic circulation (see Figure 1, pg. 223). The process by which a transdermal system is developed and manufactured is also highly complex. A deliberate project plan which addresses all these factors is required at the outset of a project if a successful transdermal delivery system is to be realized.

Several drugs have now reached the marketplace in the transdermal dosage form. This chapter will attempt to focus on integrating some of the more critical considerations in delivery system design, drug release mechanism, adhesiveness, and manufacturing, as well as how transdermal products have contributed to drug therapy.

It takes a team of people from several distinctly different scientific disciplines to bring all the knowledge to bear that is needed to develop an optimal transdermal design. This includes areas of biological sciences (skin physiology and toxicology, biophysics, clinical pharmacokinetics and pharmacodynamics), physical and chemical sciences (pharmaceutics, adhesive and material sciences, analytical chemistry), engineering (bioengineering, process engineering, product characterization) and regulatory expertise (FDA regulations, quality control and assurance, environmental and safety). Figure 2 illustrates the diversity of sciences that are needed. Of course to entertain an electrical approach (iontophoresis) to transdermal drug delivery would require an additional set of disciplines in electrical engineering and bioengineering.

The Product Profile

Before beginning a transdermal system development program, one must consider what the final transdermal product is to achieve; that is, develop a "product profile" that describes essential characteristics of the system to be designed. Once the performance criteria are determined, attributes of the delivery system can be listed to provide direction to the formulator or "system designer." A typical product profile will describe the following:

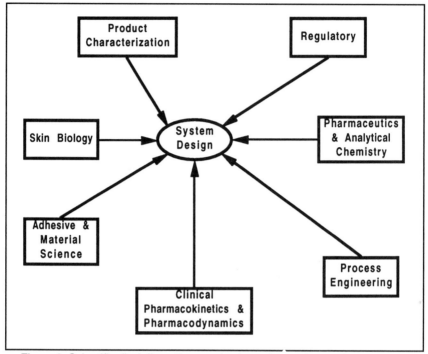

Figure 2. Scientific disciplines that need to be an integral part of transdermal development.

- physical characteristics of the system (e.g. size, shape, thickness, construc tion, amount of the drug, color, flexibility)
- functionality (necessary rate of release through the skin, rate of release from the system, degree of adhesion to the skin, length of time to adhere on the skin site, method of applying system to the skin, and similar considerations)
- patient demography (young, elderly, ambulatory, bed ridden)
- degree of irritation tolerance by patient
- cost to patient, third party payers
- medical rationale and intended indications (blood level and its profile, acute or chronic therapy, pharmacodynamics)
- required profit margin
- feasibility to manufacture (efficiency)
- availability of raw materials
- patent requirements (infringement, prior art)
- impact of regulatory environment

This list serves as a roadmap for the formulator that keeps the development on track. It entails more than just physical characteristics, but how to have the transdermal system release drugs at proper rates, cross the barrier layers of the skin and finally achieve the therapeutic effect. Compromises are constantly being made in order to achieve the final product.

Table I. Pharmacokinetic and physical/chemical data

	M.W. (Daltons)	pKa	m.p. (°C)	log K (o/w)	Perm. Coeff. (cm/hrx10³)	Cl$_T$ (L/h)	V$_D$ (L)	t$_{1/2}$ (h)	Oral Bioavail. (%)	Efficacious Blood Level (ng/ml)
Scopolamine[1]	303	7.8	59	1.24	0.5	67.2	98	2.9	27	.04
Clonidine[1]	230	8.2	140	0.83	35	13	147	6-20	95	0.2-2
Nitroglycerin	227	—	13.5	2.05	20	966[2]	231	0.04	<1	1.2-11
Estradiol	272	—	176	2.49	5.2	615-790	4.8	0.05	—	.04-.06
Fentanyl[1]	337	8.4	83	2.93	10	27-75	280	3-12	—	1
Nicotine	162	6.16 10.96	<-80	—	3	77.7	182	2	30	10-30

[1]Base form of drug
[2]Following prolonged infusion

Selecting Suitable Drug Candidates

Aside from carefully reviewing the medical rationale, the system designer can do some preliminary screening by studying the drug's physicochemical and pharmacokinetic properties. A thorough understanding of the drug's physical chemistry is vitally important when formulating a transdermal system. Generally, drugs with high lipid solubility permeate the skin at greater rates.[1,2] Drug crystallinity, or melting point, influence permeability. The lower the melting point, the greater the drug's ability to permeate the skin.

Information gained from studying the drug's pharmacokinetic properties is also valuable in estimating its potential as a transdermal candidate. Using parameters related to a drug's distribution in the body such as volume of distribution (V_d), area under the curve (AUC), clearance rate (Cl_T), therapeutic blood level (C_p or C_{ss}), biological half-life ($t_{1/2}$), the system designer can get an estimate of the skin flux rate and size of the transdermal system necessary to achieve an efficacious blood level. For example, Table I presents those parameters that can give a rough idea of what level of skin flux (J_{skin}) is needed to achieve a therapeutic blood level. J_{skin} can be calculated as follows:

$$k_o = J_{skin} = C_{ss} \times Cl_T$$

where k_o is the input rate to achieve a steady state blood level (C_{ss}).

Fentanyl base (a narcotic analgesic) can be used as a typical example of how to evaluate drug as a potential transdermal candidate. Pharmacokinetically, it has a clearance rate Cl_T = 49 L/h, and C_{ss} = 2 ng/ml for the therapeutic blood level.[3] To achieve a therapeutic blood level, skin flux, J_{ss}, would have to be 2 ng/ml x 49 L/h = 98 mcg/h. For a 50 cm² transdermal patch, the flux rate through skin would have to be about 2 mcg/cm²-h. A review of the literature shows that this rate has been achieved in an in vitro human skin permeation study.[4] Fentanyl also has a relatively low melting point and molecular weight, moderate hydrophobicity, and high partition and permeation coefficients. Thus, from the data gathered in Table I, fentanyl's physical chemistry and pharmacokinetic profiles show that it is a reasonable candidate[1,3,4] (see Table I). This has been borne out by the recent FDA approval of a fentanyl transdermal system(Table II).

Table II. Transdermals currently marketed worldwide			
Drug	mg/day Delivered	Active Area, cm^2	Total Area,cm^2
Nitroglycerin[a]	2% ointment	variable	variable
Nitroglycerin[b,c]	2.5-10	5-20	53-93
Nitroglycerin[b]	2.5-15	5-30	5-30
Nitroglycerin[d]	5-10	8-16	30-50
Nitrogylcerin[e]	2.5-10	5-20	7-27
Nitroglycerin[f]	5-10	16-32	16-32
Nitroglycerin[g]	5-15	10-30	42-62
Nitroglycerin[h]	—	—	—
Nitroglycerin[i]	2.5-15	3.3-20	3.3-20
Isosorbide dinitrate[j]	11	50	50
Scopolamine[e]	0.5mg/3 days	2.5	2.5
Scopolamine[k]	—	—	—
Clonidine[l]	0.1-0.3	3.5-10.5	3.5-10.5
Progesterone[m]	gel	variable	variable
Estradiol[e]	0.05-0.1	10-20	19-35
Estradiol[m]	.06% gel	variable	variable
Nicotine[e]	7-21	10-30	10-30
Fentanyl[n]	0.6-2.4	10-40	—

[a]Several companies
[b]Key Pharmaceuticals
[c]This patch, Nitro-Dur I, has been replaced
    by an improved patch, Nitro-Dur II
    (now known as Nitro-Dur).
[d]G.D. Searle
[e]Ciba-Geigy
[f]Wyeth

[g]Bolar, others
[h]Nichiban/Nippon/Taiho
[i]3M Riker
[j]Yamanouchi
[k]Myum Moon Pharm
[l]Boehringer-Ingelheim
[m]Besins-Iscovesco
[n]Janssen Pharmaceutica

Skin Properties

The skin influences transdermal delivery through its control of the transport of drug across its barrier layers, the adhesion of a transdermal system, and by providing a warning system for the body by regulating against xenobiotics entering the skin in the form of irritation and sensitization. None of the factors that contribute to these influences are mutually dependent phenomena between the drug, system composition and skin. The biological, chemical and physical properties of the drug, skin and formulation influence the ability of the transdermal system to deliver the drug on a continuing basis.

Skin permeation studies. Diffusion studies can be used to determine if a drug candidate can transit the skin from a simple solution or suspension in a liquid or prototype solid polymer. There are a multitude of designs for diffusion cells as illustrated in Figure 3, each cell having its own merit. Films, membranes, or skin may be mounted and tested in either a horizontal or vertical position.

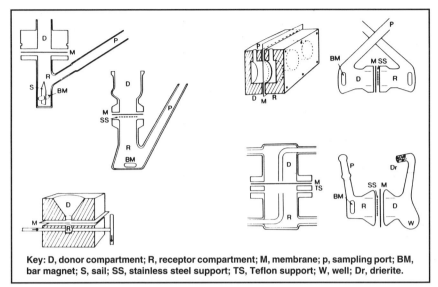

Key: D, donor compartment; R, receptor compartment; M, membrane; p, sampling port; BM, bar magnet; S, sail; SS, stainless steel support; TS, Teflon support; W, well; Dr, drierite.

Figure 3. Typical skin diffusion cells

On either side of the skin, for example, is a cell compartment that serves either as a donor or a receptor.

In a "wet-wet" setup, there is a liquid donor side and a liquid receptor side. The donor cell usually contains the drug either in suspension or solution. The receptor cell contains a liquid in which the drug can diffuse into for measurement. The receptor fluid can be water, normal saline, buffer, or some water with additional solvent to solubilize poorly soluble drugs. The simple membrane (or skin) is placed between the donor cell and the receptor cell compartments. As the drug migrates across the test membrane or skin, samples are removed from the receptor cell and tested for content at various sampling times. In a "dry-wet" cell set-up, a "dry" or "solid state" film (such as a polymeric matrix that contains dissolved or suspended drug or a transdermal system) is mounted at the opening of the donor side of the cell and receptor fluid is on the receptor or receiving side.

Some cells are designed to have a continuous circulating receptor solution. This allows for automated and continuous monitoring of concentration changes. In order to control temperature, some cells have water jackets surrounding the donor and receptor cell areas or the cells are placed directly in a water bath. Diffusion studies are typically performed at 37°C although some research groups prefer 32° to 35°C as a closer simulation of skin temperature. The data collected from these diffusion studies can be presented graphically in terms of release rate, J (mcg/cm^{2}h) or cumulative amount released, Q_t, (mcg/cm^2) at sampling time, t_n.

An awareness of how much drug is applied to the skin and the drug solubility in the test media has to be considered. The donor side may contain an "infinite" or a "finite"amount of drug. An "infinite"amount refers to the fact that there is more than enough drug present above its solubility on the donor side and far more

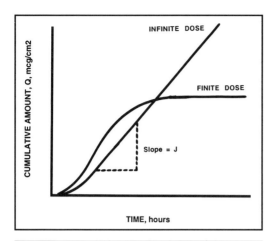

a. Cumulative amount of drug permeated versus time.

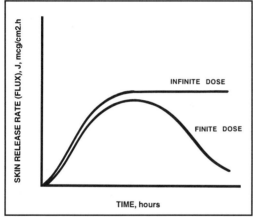

b. Skin flux of drug versus time.

Figure 4. Typical skin permeation data profile for finite and infinite dose.

available than will penetrate the skin during the lifetime of the experiment. For example, there may be a concentration of drug in excess of its solubility present in a transdermal system to maintain a steady state or zero order condition during the transit through the skin for long periods of time. In this case there is a constant amount of drug or an "infinite dose" available on the donor side to cross the membrane. Transdermal films or solutions can be placed on either vertical or horizontal cells with the drug diffusing in the direction of the receptor fluid only (e.g., a "dry-wet" or "wet-wet" cell setup). Figure 4a illustrates a typical curve that describes cumulative amount of drug that diffuses through a membrane or skin with either a finite or infinite dose. The graphical representation of the cumulative amount absorbed can also be interpreted in terms of rate of absorption or skin release rate (J), in the case where skin is used (figure 4b). Figure 4b shows typical skin flux profiles of drugs studied under either finite or infinite dose techniques.

In the case of the "finite dose" technique, a steady state flux of the drug is not necessarily reached. Only a small amount of drug, usually 5 to 10 µl of drug

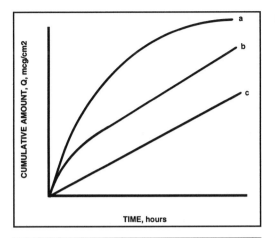

a. cumulative amount of drug released into water versus time.

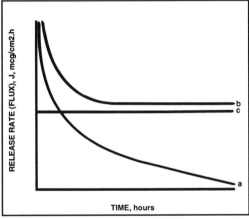

b. release rate of drug into water versus time.

Figure 5. Typical data profile of drug release into water from a transdermal for:
1. non-steady state (first order) delivery.
2. initial burst (non-steady state or first order) with continuous (zero order) delivery.
3. Continuous (zero order) delivery.

suspension or solution (2 to 5 mcg total drug content) is placed on a square centimeter skin sample that is mounted in the chamber. This type of test method is a better reflection of what occurs when a drug is delivered to skin with an ointment or lotion that is rubbed into the skin as a very thin film.

Figure 5 depicts typical release rate and cumulative amount profile curves found with transdermals releasing drug directly into water in the absence of skin. These curves are helpful in the characterization of transdermals and are discussed in the release rate testing section.

Skin toxicology. Skin irritation and sensitization are issues that must also be addressed in the early stages of system development. A skin reaction may be caused by the drug itself, any vehicles, enhancers, or polymers that may be present in the final formulation of the transdermal system.

Changing the formulation, particularly in the post-IND stage, can be costly. Adding a new component at this stage can completely change skin adhesion, or skin permeation of the drug, or even create new skin toxicological problems. Depending on the degree of change, the system design process may have to essentially start over, thus losing a year or two of hard work besides losing opportunity in the marketplace.

Animal screening for irritation and sensitization is used in the preclinical phase. Typically, 28-day cumulative irritation and 6-12 week sensitization studies are performed on humans with the final formulation in Phase II human clinicals (5,6).

Skin Properties. Properties of the skin vary as the result of interaction of one or any combination of the drug, vehicle and polymer with the skin. This includes the plasticization of the skin by vehicles, penetration enhancers, or even water passing up through the skin from beneath the skin. These interactions potentially have the capacity to change diffusional parameters within skin and the transdermal system, drug binding in skin, drug partitioning between phases of the skin and vehicle and the total amount of drug residing in the system. The skin releases lipids from the sebaceous glands and water continuously migrates from the tissues below and is intermittently expressed through the skin's sweat glands. These secretory dynamics can have an effect on adhesion and drug delivery.

Adhesion has to be managed no matter if one is considering short or long term wearing of a transdermal system. Properties that can affect the ability of the transdermal system to adhere to the skin are related to the skin's mechanical properties and to the environmental conditions as well. The stretchability, wrinkling and ability of the skin to change shape are factors of adhesion as is the continuous sloughing of the outer layers of the stratum corneum. Environmental factors such as excess water from swimming or showering, sweating from heat or exercise, and movements of the body have an impact on transdermal design. Since skin is a living organ, there are surface changes that take place over time that affect short (24 hours) and long (one week) term wearing. The transdermal system must be designed to accommodate these vagaries of skin properties.

Modulating the formula, such as part of the laminate structure, skin adhesive, a rate controlling membrane (if necessary), the release of the drug can be changed to achieve the required rate of drug release. The designer has to be cautious in selecting the materials to achieve the desired release rate profile and patch adhesiveness. There are few polymers and enhancers that have undergone the characterization and scrutiny necessary to be medically used on skin.

Transdermal Patch Design

Table II lists transdermal products that have reached the marketplace to date. There are various ways to view these products. Often, they are referred to as "membrane controlled," "reservoir," or "monolithic" types. These terms describe the drug release mechanism used and can be misleading when it comes to design and manufacturing considerations. There are many different types of transdermal systems under development today, and it is useful to attempt to classify them in order to differentiate them. How can one best classify the different types of transdermals? One way is to consider the design of the transdermal without regard to the drug release mechanism itself. This will give a visual perception of the total product and its components in addition to how it might be formulated and fabricated.

The designs of the four types of transdermals presently on the market (Figure 6) are:

- Type I–*Semi-solid amorphous ointment, cream lotion, or viscous dispersion applied directly to the skin:* Nitrobid (Marion Merrell Dow); Progestagel and Estragel (Besins-Iscovesco)
- Type II–*Liquid form, fill and seal laminate structure:* Transderm-Nitro and Estraderm (Ciba); Duragesic (Janssen)
- Type III–*Peripheral adhesive laminate structure:* Nitro TDS (Bolar); Nitro-Disc (Searle); Nitro-Dur I (Key); Prostep (Lederle)
- Type IV–*Solid-state laminate structure:* Transderm Scop V (Ciba); Transderm-Catapres (Boehringer-Ingelheim); Nitro-Dur II (Key); Deponit (Wyeth); Minitran (Riker); Nicotrol (Parke-Davis); Habitrol (Ciba); Nicoderm (Marion Merrell Dow)

In Table II, note the differences between the area of the total system and the active delivery area. For example, Key Pharmaceutical's first transdermal nitroglycerin product delivered 10 mg/day over a 20 cm^2 active delivery area (equal to 0.5 mg/cm^2-day).* This transdermal was actually a 90 cm^2 system because of the peripheral adhesive (Type III Design), and yet was still accepted by patients. This extra surface area is seen with other products found in this design type.** Key's second generation nitroglycerin system*** was a Type IV Design, where the active delivery area was identical to the size of the product. An examination of both systems clearly reveals that the first generation product was over three times as large as the second generation product, used more material, had a more complicated construction, and was more costly to fabricate.

The appearance and size of any transdermal system will always have an effect on its degree of patient acceptance. The optimum amount of drug to be delivered may be as high as 20 mg/day. However, esthetics aside, the size of the system will also be dependent on skin flux and the blood level needed to elicit the desired therapeutic results.

The four types of designs shown in Figure 6 (pg. 224) are not all inclusive since new approaches and combinations of each design are always possible. All of these systems, however, have the potential to deliver a drug to the skin surface so that the drug can migrate through the skin. By understanding these basic designs and their relative advantages and disadvantages, the system designer can better incorporate the most suitable drug release mechanism for the application required. Using the appropriate plasticizers or vehicles, polymers, films or membranes to match the diffusivity of the drug through the skin, the desired delivery rate and the optimum blood level can be effectively achieved. The selection of a specific system design, however, will affect and be affected by many of the desired attributes listed in the initial product profile.

Drug Release from the System

The correct drug release profile for a transdermal system can be built into any of the four system designs described here. There are two considerations, however,

---

* Nitro-Dur I
** Prostep and Nitro-Disc
*** Nitro-Dur

when evaluating release profiles for application in a transdermal system:
1) release into water or into an in vitro test media and
2) release through skin.

In most cases the skin will provide some or all of the resistance, so that the profile will be greatly influenced by the presence of skin. In essence, the skin becomes part of the system.

The drug can be released from a system or its structural components into the skin using any of a number of different diffusion mechanisms. Physical and chemical properties of both the drug and the system components can be optimized to achieve the desired drug release profile. The drug must leave the system in some manner (release) and enter the skin at some amount over time (rate) then reach the systemic circulation at a therapeutic level. The system therefore serves as a method or device to hold the drug in place (a reservoir) and provides a diffusive pathway to reach the surface of the skin (a bridge to the skin).

Diffusion Processes

There are special cases that describe mechanisms of how a drug leaves a matrix or passes through a membrane. Figure 7 (pg. 225) shows six simple drug release mechanisms (Cases I-VI) for transdermal systems that have been described elsewhere.[2] These mechanisms can provide some insight into the relationships between various parameters affecting the release of a drug molecule from a matrix or through a membrane. For example, a Type II transdermal design (liquid-filled/form-fill-seal type),* contains at least two drug releasing mechanisms (Cases I and V) within its construction, not to mention the additional influences of the skin (Case IV). The drug release profiles for Cases I, IV and V are related to parameters such as drug diffusion coefficient (D), drug loading and solubility (C_o and C_s) in the polymers and skin, the concentration gradient in the membrane (ΔC_m), and film/membrane or skin thickness. By keeping these parameters and how they may be modulated in mind, these illustrative cases can serve as a guide to designing and understanding the dynamics of a transdermal system.

Each of the diffusion mechanisms described is relatively simple, and assumes that the drug is diffusing in one direction from a matrix or through a membrane into an infinite sink that is well stirred. However, some caution should be used since all of the models are based on a particular set of boundary conditions. Some are even based on specific assumptions that are normally not well approximated in the complex mechanisms found in transdermal delivery systems. The release of a drug can be modulated by varying any of the parameters, such as the selection of a different polymer with inherently different drug solubility or diffusion, degree of crosslinking, vehicle/enhancer concentrations, and thickness.

These cases are not all inclusive but generally describe what may be occurring (Figure 7). There are other complex cases that describe how a drug leaves a matrix or passes through a membrane. There may be combinations of these mechanisms or transitions from one case to another as well as more elaborate models. It is beyond the scope of this chapter to describe each mathematical model. However, a knowledge of these models can give the transdermal designer a better understanding of the parameters involved in mass transport.

* such as the Transderm Nitro (Ciba)

Material Selection

Drugs, vehicles (solubilizers or enhancers), and polymers are the main components found in transdermal products. The various materials that have reached the U.S. marketplace include:

1) Drugs: scopolamine, nitroglycerin, clonidine, estradiol, fentanyl and nicotine
2) Vehicles: mineral oil, isopropyl myristate, glycerin, water, ethanol and silicone oil
3) Polymers:
   a. Skin pressure sensitive adhesives: acrylates, silicone, and rubber-based adhesives
   b. Release liners: silicone and fluorocarbon coatings on paper, polyester or polycarbonate films
   c. Backings/laminates: ethylene vinyl acetate, polypropylene, polyester, polyethylene, polyvinyl chloride and aluminum films
   d. Specialty films: foams, non-wovens, micro-porous films, vapor-deposited aluminum films

The candidate drug that is selected to be delivered transdermally has to be evaluated like the other constituents that are incorporated into the transdermal system regarding, purity stability, toxicology and processing constraints. Of course, it will be assumed in this chapter that a suitable permeation rate regarding skin to reach the therapeutic blood level and profile has been determined. Drugs have their own inherent diffusive characteristics within each polymer type and through skin as shown in Table I. These natural diffusive characteristics are often referred to as "passive transport." These molecules typically have low diffusivity in the rubber and acrylic polymers while silicone has a higher order of magnitude of diffusivity. Vehicle or enhancer consideration is the same as the drug. They not only affect drug diffusivity within the polymer, but also the adhesive property of the transdermal.

Basic Structural Layers: A Simple Type IV Design

Figure 8 illustrates the basic layers that are most often found in a Type IV designed transdermal delivery system. These layers can be found in other designs but Type IV is the simplest to describe. The backing material can be

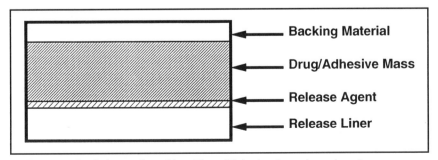

Figure 8. Basic layers found in a Type IV design transdermal system

occlusive (impermeable to gases and liquids) or non-occlusive (allowing gases and water vapor to diffuse through the structure). Typical of occlusive materials are barrier (dense) films made from polyvinyl, polyethylene, polyester or aluminized polymer films and composite films. This type of material allows the skin to be hydrated. Non-occlusive materials are usually films made from non-woven, woven, or foamed polymers, or occlusive films made porous by other techniques. Non-occlusive materials, which allow moisture to pass through, leave the skin less hydrated. The backing serves as a platform, or carrier, for the adhesive and is essential to provide film integrity for application to, and removal from, the skin. This backing layer characteristically has to have good tensile strength to perform its function properly.

The layer next to the backing is the "adhesive mass" layer (Figure 8). It is this layer that anchors subsequent layers and the entire transdermal delivery system to the skin site. This layer is often called the "skin contact adhesive." The adhesive mass has to be formulated to provide adhesion of the system to the skin, and yet be easily removed without removing any skin or leaving a residue. What is desirable is a material that will adhere very aggressively to the backing material, and to a lesser extent to skin, with the slightest pressure. The entire structure can then be removed from the skin or the release liner without leaving any residue. To provide instant anchoring to the skin, the adhesive must adhere aggressively and instantaneously with only very slight pressure. This quality is known as "tack." Pressure sensitive adhesives are viscoelastic materials, which, in solvent-free form, remain permanently "tacky."

The most common pressure sensitive adhesives having a history of skin use are based on rubber, acrylate, or silicone polymer chemistry. Materials that are used in pressure adhesive mass should have a history of being used on human skin (or on animals if the application is for animals). Again, the physical chemistry of these polymers plays an important role in the selection of the adhesive as an integral part of the transdermal system. Drugs will have their own inherent diffusive characteristics depending upon which polymer is selected. Drugs typically have low diffusivity in the rubber and acrylic polymers while silicone has a higher order of magnitude of diffusivity. The addition of plasticizers or vehicles not only has an affect on drug diffusivity, but also on the adhesive. To assess the effect of a change of adhesive properties on the skin, backing, or the protective liner, the system designer measures the degree of cohesive and adhesive failure, peel strength, tack, and creep with specific test methods.

The final layer, a protective or release liner, is important to protect the adhesive mass until the tape or transdermal patch is used. This protective liner is a film which is easily removed from the adhesive mass just prior to application on the skin. There should be greater adhesion of the backing to the adhesive mass than to the release liner, such that the backing layer serves as the carrier for the adhesive to make it possible to hold the entire system in one's hand for application to and removal from the release liner. A release agent, in the form of a thin coating, is applied to paper, polymer coated paper, or polymer film, which provides structure to the liner. This release agent is necessary to prevent the adhesive mass from sticking to its protective liner. Silicone- and fluorocarbon-coated release liners are commonly used in transdermal systems for this reason.

Physical, Chemical and Transport Properties of the Materials

In the design of a transdermal delivery system, the drug can be released from a system and into the skin in a number of different ways. Physical chemical properties of both the drug and the materials used in the system are essential to achieve a suitable design. The physicochemical properties of a polymer can affect the mechanical properties as well as the diffusional properties. Understanding the influence of the skin's properties, the transdermal patch may have to be flexible or be able to stretch with the skin. Stiffness of the transdermal system, thus selection of the polymer, may influence the wearing time and degree of irritation. The chemical properties of the polymer or adhesive can affect the ability of the patch to load an appropriate amount of drug, the mass transport properties as well as cutaneous toxicity.

The physical structure that contains the drug is often referred to as a matrix, drug reservoir, monolith or slab. For simplicity, the term matrix (or matrices) will be used in this chapter. The drug and other excipients are incorporated into the matrix. The matrix could be a (1) liquid, (2) semisolid, (3) non-flowing, three dimensionally stable material, or (4) any combination of these three forms. Liquid and semisolid systems have the ability to leak and flow away from the desired site and must be contained in place if a constant area is desirable. Containment of a liquid reservoir can be achieved by sealing the liquid between two films (Type II design). A matrix, usually a polymer, offers a structural means for incorporating a drug within a transdermal system. The solute or drug molecule diffuses through the matrix to its interface with the skin or with an interfacing rate controlling membrane. A rate controlling membrane can be thought of as a polymeric barrier that a solute or drug molecule must pass through but at a slower rate than diffusion within the matrix or skin.

Release rate testing: One way to understand the degree of release of the drug from the matrix model over time is to perform release rate tests. Releasing the drug directly into a receptor fluid that provides infinite sink condition, such as water, will provide the system designer with a drug release profile that can determine the maximal time course of the system and in which direction to modulate the formulation. The equations that describe the release of the drug can be put in terms of either:

1) M_t, the total amount of drug released per unit area at any time, t (mcg/cm^2)
2) M_t/M_∞, the fraction (or percent) released at any time, t (no unit)
3) or J or (dM/dt), the rate of drug release or flux (mcg/cm^{2}h).

When plotted against time or the square root of time, different shaped profiles will occur in each of these three type of plots. The profiles of these plots will vary in shape depending on the conditions of the diffusion mechanism. Figure 5 illustrates the release profile curves generated by transdermals that release drugs with different mechanisms of release. Figures 5a and b present three typical cumulative amount profiles and their respective curves in terms of release rate. In these cases the drug is released in

1) a non-steady state (first order) delivery
2) an initial burst (non-steady state or first order) followed with a continuous (zero order) delivery
3) continuous (zero order) only delivery.

These tests are also useful in characterizing and establishing specifications of the final product for quality control. A good estimate for skin permeation will be to release the drug from the system through human cadaver skin and test in vitro. The in vitro skin study will show to what degree the system controls the release of the drug through skin, the drug's availability and whether a rate controlling membrane is needed. The in vivo human study will validate the in vitro skin testing and give the blood level and profile.

Adhesive materials: Adhesion plays an important role in the efficacy of a transdermal delivery system. Adhesives are used to hold layers of film together, as well as anchor the entire transdermal system to skin.

Adhesion to the skin is one of the characteristics that contributes to the functionality of the transdermal system. It is desirable to apply the system to the application site as simply as possible, yet have it remain in place for a specific period of time with easy and painless removal. *Pressure sensitive adhesives* can be formulated to adhere aggressively to surfaces with a permanent bond, or form less than a permanent bond where the adhesive on one layer can be removed relatively easily from another layer. This type of adhesive lends itself to use in anchoring the transdermal delivery systems to the skin, or maintaining the integrity of various layers of the system itself. Structural adhesives are used to maintain a permanent bond where a specific type of surface property is needed, or holding laminate structures together within the system and not easily debonded.

Theory or phenomena of adhesion: An understanding of adhesion theory, adhesive physical and chemical properties and adhesive materials can provide some insight to the designer of transdermals. The theory of adhesion is still evolving; most of what has been developed has been done in the last 50 years or so.

Understanding the theoretical basis for adhesion is no trivial matter. It is a complex number of interacting sets of phenomena that science has attempted to bring from the empirical to a scientific basis. Again, one who formulates pressure sensitive adhesives in transdermals is confronted with a full set of problems that requires a working knowledge of chemistry, physics, dermatology, pharmaceutics and especially polymer and material sciences. The literature presents a number of contradictory proposals for the explanation of adhesion.[7,8] The theories have not necessarily simplified our understanding or encouraged agreement between the various phenomena. However, one can generalize adhesion theory in terms of four principal areas associated with mechanical, adsorption, electrostatic and diffusional phenomena.

Types of bonding: There are two types of adhesive bonding that are found in transdermal systems—permanent and semi-permanent adhesion. The permanent adhesion is required when laminate structures have to be bonded to adjacent layers and not become separated during storage or wearing. Pressure sensitive adhesives provide a semi-permanent adhesion. The semi-permanent bonding is where a laminate structure has to be removed so that the transdermal system can be functional. Pressure sensitive adhesives are used in transdermals so that the system can be temporarily anchored to the skin for a specific time and then be easily removed later. Both structural and pressure sensitive adhesives technology play an important role in transdermal product development.

Properties of pressure sensitive adhesives: Understanding the mechanical properties of polymers, especially pressure sensitive adhesives, can give direction to the system designer with regard to adhesive-cohesive properties. This proves also useful for stability and quality control of the polymer raw material and final transdermal product as well as validating the effect of the manufacturing process on the adhesive. A number of test methodologies and rheological measurements that describe properties of pressure sensitive adhesives that empirically incorporate our understanding of the four phenomena of adhesion under constant and variable stresses and strains. Because most polymers and pressure sensitive adhesives are non-Newtonian and shear rate dependent, one can use tools that follow simple linear viscoelastic properties (constant stress and strain) as well as dynamic mechanical analysis (sinusoidally varying stress and strain). To assess the effect of a change of adhesive properties on the skin, backing or release liner, one can measure the degree of cohesive and adhesive failure, peel strength, tack and creep with specific test methods.

Cohesive and adhesive properties: The ability of the adhesive mass to remain a coherent layer is a function of its cohesive properties. The stronger its cohesive forces (the ability of the adhesive mass to stick to itself), the more likely the layer will not split apart during removal from an adherend. The adhesive properties reflect the adhesive mass's ability to adhere to unlike materials. Figure 9 describes four cases of how an adhesive mass can separate from a substrate or from itself. Ideally, a pressure sensitive adhesive should perform as illustrated in Case 1 shown in Figure 9. Here, the adhesive mass leaves no residue on the adherend but adheres well enough to the backing during removal. The adherend could be a release liner or skin in the case of transdermal delivery systems.

However, there are other potential areas where the adhesive mass may debond. The other cases in Figure 9 depict these adhesive-cohesive failures. Case II shows the delamination of the backing layer when the adhesive mass has greater adhesion to the adherend. When the adhesive mass adheres too well to both the

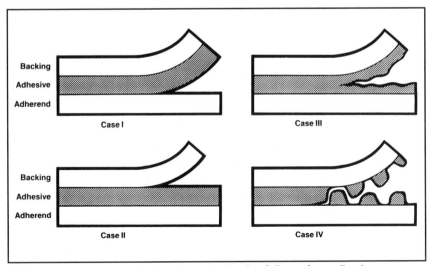

Figure 9. Four types of adhesive and cohesive failure of an adhesive mass

backing and the adherend, cohesive failure takes place as shown in Case III. Case III failure can arise by a low viscosity adhesive mass or poor cohesive strength. Case IV failure is a combination of cohesive and adhesive failure at the same time. Here, the adhesive mass does not know whether to adhere to the backing or the adherend or whether to cohere to itself. In effect, the energy of cohesion is of the same magnitude as the energy of adhesion. It is undesirable to undergo a Case III and IV failure with a transdermal delivery system because a sticky residue will be left behind when the system is removed.

Adhesive Strength: The adhesive strength is measured by the amount of force it takes to remove the adhesive from a surface. Adhesive strength is often referred to as adhesive force, peel adhesion, peel force or peel strength. Peel strength, Pø, is dependent on a number of parameters including those inherent in the adhesive mass, the backing, the bond width and the peel angle, ø. Kaeble has derived an equation that attempts to relate these parameters at a high angle peel (9,10)

$$P_\emptyset = waK^2\sigma_0^2/2Y \ (1 - \cos\emptyset)$$ Equation 4

where $$K = \beta m/(\beta m + \sin\emptyset)$$ Equation 5

and $$\beta = (Yw/4Ela)^{1/4}$$ Equation 6

and at a 180° angle peel, the peel force is:

$$P_{180°} = wa^2/2Y$$ Equation 7

where w = bond width; a = adhesive thickness; K = dimensionless parameter relating to cleavage stress, adhesive modulus, bond width, adhesive and backing thicknesses; β = cleavage stress concentration; Y = adhesive Young's modulus; m = momentum arm of peel force; El = bending modulus of the flexible strip (backing).

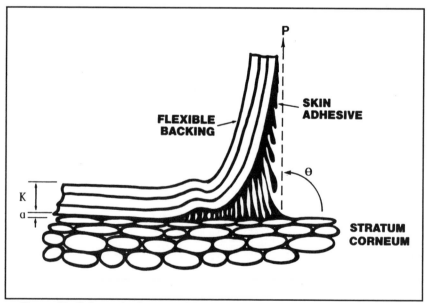

Figure 10. Schematic diagram of forces and parameters affecting adhesive strength in pressure sensitive adhesives (References 9,10)

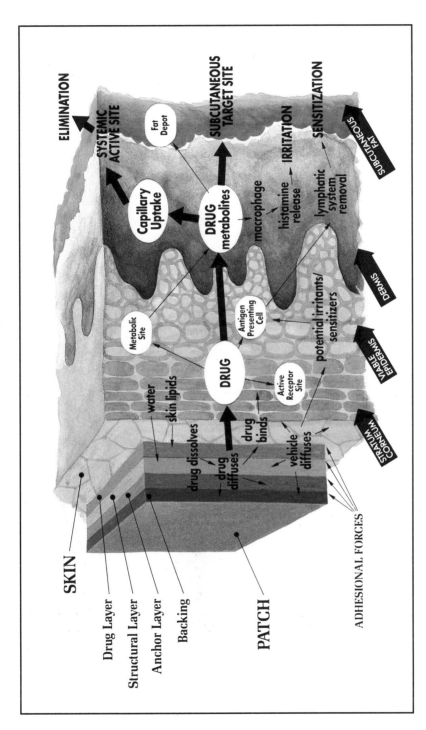

Figure 1. Factors in transdermal delivery.

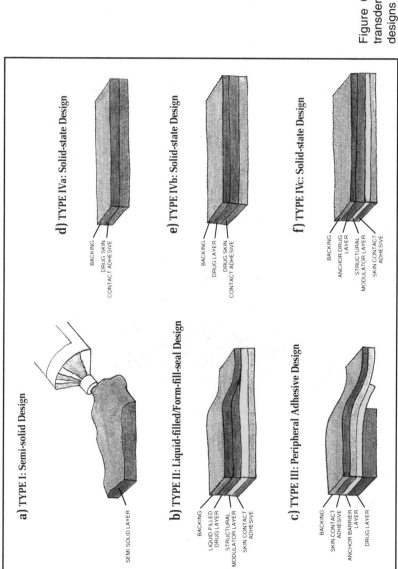

a) TYPE I: Semi-solid Design

SEMI-SOLID LAYER

b) TYPE II: Liquid-filled/Form-fill-seal Design

BACKING
LIQUID FILLED DRUG LAYER
STRUCTURAL MODULATOR LAYER
SKIN CONTACT ADHESIVE

c) TYPE III: Peripheral Adhesive Design

BACKING
SKIN CONTACT ADHESIVE
ANCHOR BARRIER LAYER
DRUG LAYER

d) TYPE IVa: Solid-state Design

BACKING
DRUG SKIN CONTACT ADHESIVE

e) TYPE IVb: Solid-state Design

BACKING
DRUG LAYER
DRUG SKIN CONTACT ADHESIVE

f) TYPE IVc: Solid-state Design

BACKING
ANCHOR DRUG LAYER
STRUCTURAL MODULATOR LAYER
SKIN CONTACT ADHESIVE

Figure 6. Four types of transdermal drug delivery designs

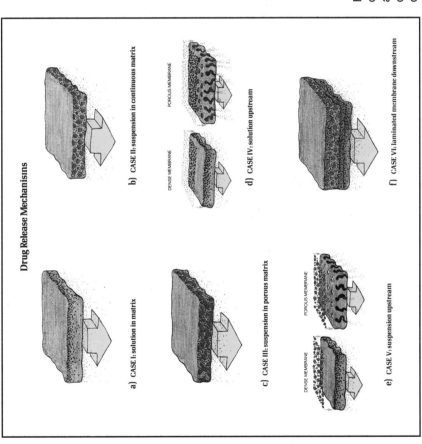

Drug Release Mechanisms

a) CASE I: solution in matrix

b) CASE II: suspension in continuous matrix

c) CASE III: suspension in porous matrix

d) CASE IV: solution upstream

e) CASE V: suspension upstream

f) CASE VI: laminated membrane: downstream

DENSE MEMBRANE   POROUS MEMBRANE

Figure 7. Six different cases of drug release mechanisms found in transdermal drug delivery designs (Reference 2)

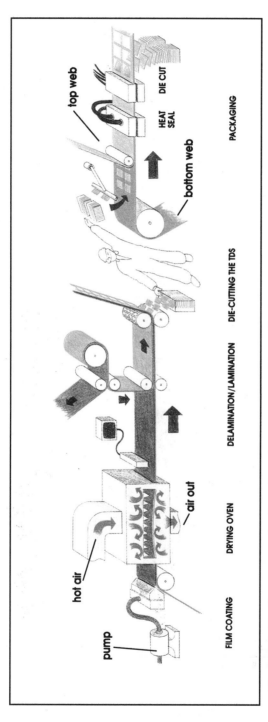

Figure 15. Coating process for transdermal pressure sensitive adhesive polymer

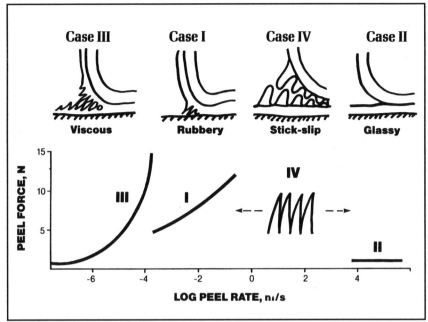

Figure 11. Effect of unwinding speed on adhesive and cohesive failure of pressure sensitive adhesives (Reference 11)

Figure 10 is a schematic diagram of some of the forces and parameters described in equations 4-7 that are present when peeling an adhesive tape. Cohesive failure can be caused by poor formulation or improper bonding to surfaces; it can also occur because of environmental factors. A change in temperature or peel speed can change the property of an adhesive mass from a desired adhesive failure to an unwanted cohesive failure. Figure 11 illustrates the effect of low and high speeds of unwinding of polyacrylic tapes with respect to the adhesive's viscosity (cohesiveness) and peel force (adhesiveness).[11] As the adhesive's property goes from a low viscosity to rubbery to a glassy condition, the adhesive force can be quite variable and cohesiveness causes different types of debonding failure.

Note that width, adhesive thickness and bending modulus of the backing are important parameters that relate to peel strength. These parameters must be kept in mind when selecting film material and the geometry of the system during its design phase.

Tack: Tack is an adhesive property that relates the immediacy of the bond formation of a system (such as a transdermal) with an adherend (such as skin). ASTM defines tack as the property of an adhesive that enables it to form a bond of measurable strength immediately after adhesive and adherend are brought into contact under low pressure.[12] Tack is related to viscosity of the adhesive, adhesive formulation, type of adhesive system and surface of the adherend. A thin layer of oil or moisture on the skin can modify the surface such that initial tack is decreased. Pressure sensitive adhesives are viscoelastic materials, which, in solvent-free form, remain permanently "tacky."

In the measurement of tack, both bonding and debonding processes take place. The bonding process is difficult to quantitate, since it is usually the debonding process that has been measured and analyzed. The rheological models used to describe mechanisms for debonding are controversial. It is not understood whether the process could be described in terms of linear viscoelasticity such as a shear (G) or tensile (E) process or a combination of both. It is not clear whether storage (G') or loss (G") components of the modulus or compliance (inverse modulus) are dominant in dynamic mechanical analysis. Either adhesive or cohesive failure may occur. It is the shear strength measurements that indicated the degree of cohesiveness of an adhesive mass.

Shear strength: In order for the adhesive to exhibit its pressure sensitive nature, it must be able to conform to surface textures and undergo relaxation in its stress-strain behavior. Its resistance to flow under stress, or more broadly, the stress-strain behavior of the elastic mass, is treated as the shear phenomenon ("creep" or "cold" flow). Creep is associated with tack and peel force. It is an example of flow between parallel plates and can be related to steady state viscosity, η, by:[13]

$$\eta = \frac{Fa}{A} \left(\frac{1}{dx/dt} \right) \qquad \text{Equation 8}$$

where F = load, a =- thickness, A = contact area, dx/dt = slope of displacement vs time curve.

A unique shear test that determines shear properties in a transdermal delivery system has been reported.[14]

Bright et al. studied the effect of temperature on cohesive/adhesive failure.[15] At a temperature of 15 to 40°C, adhesive mass underwent adhesive failure similar to that shown in Case I adhesive failure. When the temperature was increased to between 40 and 55°C, the adhesive underwent mixed failure (Case IV). With further increase to higher temperature regions, 55 to 75°C, the adhesive underwent cohesive failure (Case III) when peeled.

In designing transdermals, the formulator has to consider the temperatures at which the formula will change its peel strength and its cohesive integrity, the effect of plasticization of vehicles or enhancers, uptake of the skin's physiological fluids, the speed at which a patient will remove a patch or if high-speed delamination/lamination will be part of the manufacturing steps. In other words the designer has to be aware of many factors in adhesion properties that encompass from conceptualization of the product through development, manufacture and ultimately patient use.

Selection of pressure sensitive adhesives: In selecting a suitable polymer for a transdermal adhesive, one considers the adhesive properties needed, the diffusivity required, and any inherent problems found with the polymer in general. For skin adhesion, one considers peel strength, tack and shear strength. Each of the common polymers used in pressure-sensitive adhesive formulas, such as those based on rubbery, acrylates and silicone polymers has its own positive and negative attributes depending on the product profile that has been described for the transdermal designer. Drugs listed in Table I typically have low diffusivity in the rubber and acrylic polymers while silicone has a higher order of magnitude of diffusivity. Acrylics and silicone are inherently tacky and adhesive by themselves and do not need any additives to enhance adhesive properties. Rubber pressure-sensitive adhesives have to be compounded with tackifers, plasticizers, binders (optionally), and antioxidants which tend to complicate the formulation of the adhesive mass. Silicones have a tendency to stick well to a wide range of materials such that even removal from a release liner can be difficult. Rubber-based systems have the widest range of tack, while silicones have a marginal range of tack. Initial tack is important when applying adhesives to the skin since movement of the body may not allow the adhesive to bond well. The adhesive portion of system design is most complex since it involves both the formulation and the ability of that formulation to respond appropriately to the skin site application.

Adhesion and the Skin

There is very little information in the literature regarding behavior of pressure-sensitive adhesives on the skin.[16,17] There have been some studies using stainless steel plates, gelatin or collagen films to simulate adhesion to the human skin. Stainless steel plates are typically used as a standard test substrate, but only to observe any change of adhesiveness in stability or quality control testing. The use of other materials as skin substitute substrates has not been successful as models for skin adhesion.

One has to keep in mind that the structure of the skin is highly complex, and the skin's outer layers vary from person to person. The skin cells at the surface adhere loosely together while those deeper within the stratum corneum are more firmly anchored to one another.[18] Under occlusion, more cells are pulled off the skin than when non-occlusive tape is used.[19] Bothwell showed that the force to remove an occlusive tape was about half the value to remove a non-occlusive tape.[20] After a rapid build-up of initial peel strength, the occlusive tape then has a dramatic lowering of peel strength after four hours of wearing and large quantities of stratum corneum adhere to the adhesive when the tape is removed. The non-occlusive tape has a slower build-up of adhesive strength with smaller amounts of stratum corneum on the tape after removal. This suggests that the hydration of the skin by the occlusive layer loosens up the adhesive forces between the cells in the stratum corneum. Thus a premature or accidental removal of a patch from a skin site may be highly influenced by the cellular adhesion of the skin.

System Functionality

The function of a transdermal delivery system is to provide a systemic blood level that is therapeutically efficacious. Additionally, it must not only be nonirritating, nonsensitizing, and adhere to the skin for the delivery time but it must also be manufacturable.

Several transdermal products have achieved these criteria and have reached the marketplace. They deliver drugs through the skin effectively anywhere from one to seven days. Table III summarizes what transdermal technology has contributed to drug delivery and therapy in the last 10 years. The following discussion describes in more detail how this dosage form has performed:

Different blood level profiles from different dosage forms: A good example of how transdermals provide different types of blood level profiles is demon-

Table III. Transdermal contribution to drug delivery
1. Blood level profiles different than other dosage forms (e.g. eliminate large peak to trough differences 2. Same blood level profile with different transdermal designs 3. Same blood level profile with different drug release mechanism 4. Active surface area directly proportional to blood level 5. Different ratios of metabolites than from oral delivery 6. Used in several therapeutic areas 7. Drug delivery from 1/2 to 7 days 8. Handles difficult to formulate drugs 9. Better compliance potential 10. Avoids "first pass" effect

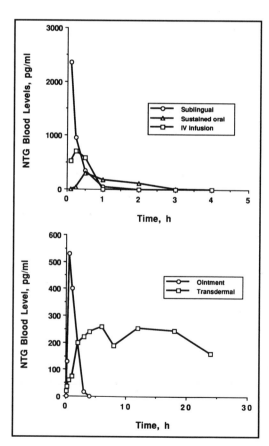

Figure 12. Nitroglycerin blood level profile from different dosage forms, (a) sublingual, sustained oral, IV infusion; (b) ointment, transdermal (References 21-23)

strated by comparisons of various nitroglycerin dosage forms. Figure 12 shows the blood levels produced by various nitroglycerin dosage forms: IV infusion, ointment, sublingual and sustained release tablets, and a transdermal system.[21-23] Note that the more traditional forms give shorter bursts of nitroglycerin and, sometimes, a lot higher concentration, as in the case of the sublingual tablet. The transdermal dosage form gives prolonged levels with less difference between peak and trough levels. Similar reduction in peak to trough values in plasma concentration have also been noted with other commercial transdermal drugs such as scopolamine, clonidine, and estradiol.

Different designs can achieve same blood levels: There are now several drug companies in the United States marketing nitroglycerin transdermal patches. They all provide similar blood levels and profiles, yet the patches have very different designs and built-in drug release mechanisms. Examples of each of the four designs presented in Table II are shown with their blood level profiles in Figure 13.[23-25] Note that they all provide for 24 hours of drug delivery in the same range of constant blood levels, except for the ointment that was shown in Figure 12. Because of a slight variance in flux rates per area (e.g. per cm² basis) through skin, the size of each system is slightly different.

Different mechanisms can achieve comparable blood levels: The release profiles of nitroglycerin into in vitro media (e.g. water) are dramatically different for differing transdermal devices, as shown in Figure 14.[26] These differences indicate the variety of drug release profiles obtainable from systems with different mechanisms. Figure 13 indicates plasma levels of the Ciba, Wyeth, Key and Searle patch at nearly the same levels, yet Figure 14 depicts different mechanisms of release. This also indicates that not all transdermals release nitroglycerin at the same rate per unit area. However, by increasing or decreasing the size of a particular system, comparable plasma levels can be reached even though different designs and different release mechanisms are used. Although these release profiles are often referred to as "reservoir," "matrix" or "rate controlling" systems, the barrier properties of the skin tend to normalize the amount of drug allowed through the skin despite the effectiveness of the specific system design and drug release mechanism selected.

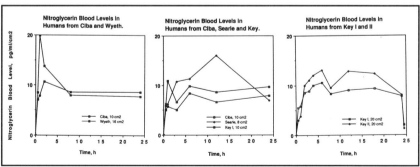

Figure 13. Nitroglycerin blood levels found in various commercial nitroglycerin transdermals, (a) Ciba, 10 cm² and Wyeth, 16 cm² (Reference 24); (b) Ciba, 10 cm², Searle, 8 cm², and Key I, 10 cm² (Reference 25); and (c) Key I, 20 cm² and Key II, 20 cm² (Reference 23)

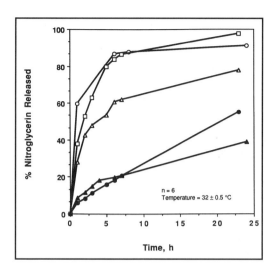

Figure 14. Percent nitroglycerin released into water from various commercial nitroglycerin transdermals (○ Ciba, ● Key, Δ Searle, □ Bolar, ■ Wyeth (Reference 26)

It is interesting to note that three commercial transdermal nitroglycerin patches have the same 24 hour nitroglycerin release rate in vivo, yet each system has a different surface area (16 to 30 cm^2). The values for in vivo release in 24 hours can also be determined by placing a patch on a subject, then assaying the remaining amount in the system after 24 hours of wear. Wolfe et al. found a linear relationship of the Deponit system surface area to the amount released in a 24-hour in vivo release of nitroglycerin.[24] Karim found slightly higher values for Nitrodisc and Transderm-Nitro of 6.2 and 5.4 mg/24 hr., respectively.[27]

Size is linearly related to blood levels: Once a formulation has been selected, the size (surface area) of a transdermal patch will dictate the total amount of drug delivered over time, and thus the amount found in the plasma. The direct linear relationship of a transdermal system area to blood levels of drug (e.g., clonidine, nitroglycerin, estradiol, nicotine and fentanyl) has been shown.[28-32]

Different ratios of metabolites and lipids: Comparing the effects of transdermal estradiol with those of oral preparations of estrogens, Powers et al. showed differences in the blood level of a metabolite, estrone, in postmenopausal women.[33] Transdermal systems with delivery rates of 0.025, 0.05 or 0.1 mg/day (5, 10, or 20 cm^2 respectively) were compared to the oral dosage forms of 2 mg 17b-estradiol or 1.25 mg conjugated equine estrogen. The transdermal estradiol system (0.05 mg/day) produced serum levels of about 40 pg/ml for both estradiol and estrone 1:1 ratio. Administration of the oral dosage forms gave similar blood levels for estradiol, between 40 and 60 pg/ml after the third dose, but the estrone levels were in the 200 to 400 pg/ml range 1:5 ratio. Since estrone does not appear to be effective at the pituitary-hypothalamic level and is not relative to the decrease in gonadotropins, it is evident that the oral estrogens are putting an increased amount of nonphysiological estrone into the plasma. The 1:1 estradiol/estrone ratio resulting from the administration of the transdermal delivery system is closer to the ratio normally found during a woman's reproductive years.[34]

Different therapeutic areas: The therapeutic areas of angina pectoris, hormone replacement, hypertension, motion sickness, smoking cessation and pain control currently have a transdermal product as part of their armamentarium. Patients and physicians have both accepted transdermals as a logical alternative to other dosage forms.

Different delivery and wearing time: Another advantage that transdermals offer a patient, which other dosage forms do not, is the convenience of the dosage regimen of the drug. Patients are now wearing a single transdermal patch for 1 day (nitroglycerin, nicotine), 3 or 3.5 days (scopolamine, estradiol fentanyl), or 7 days (clonidine), instead of administering single or multiple dosings per day with other dosage forms. Transdermals have therefore helped improve patient compliance.

Drugs with difficult to formulate properties: A very volatile enhancer or drug may preclude use of heat to drive off any solvents such as found with the process used to make the solid state laminate structure (Type IV Design). A form-fill-seal fabrication (Type II Design, such as Transderm-Nitro, Estraderm, Duragesic) solves the problem of losing volatile materials such as liquid nitroglycerin and ethanol during production by trapping the liquid in a pouch-like reservoir. Potential problems with the liquid system are: unintentional leakage of liquids that could compromise patient safety, and intentional diversion of a controlled drug. Recent advances in processing techniques now allow volatile drugs to be incorporated into the solid state laminate structure (Type IV Design).[35] These more volatile drugs would be more difficult to stabilize in other dosage forms.

These are just some of the problematic issues that must be addressed as project development reaches larger scale production. Many of these problems should be alleviated or avoided by considering the consequences of design choices early enough in the development process.

Other drugs: Drugs other than those listed in Table II have recently reached human clinical testing but have not been commercialized. Beta-blockers (timolol and bupranolol), antihistamines (triprolidine and azatadine), and a hormone replacement (testosterone) have all been shown to achieve potentially therapeutic blood levels.[36-40]

Manufacturing Processes and Costs

Once a prototype transdermal system has been identified as one that fits the desired product profile, then the method of manufacture can be conceptualized, the necessary regulatory documents can be readied and filed, and human clinical trials can begin. Since the manufacturing process and the equipment for fabricating transdermals are essentially new to the pharmaceutical industry, equipment may not be available to produce sufficient quantities for testing in early clinical studies.

In the early stages of development a transdermal system may be fabricated by hand or manufactured on bench or pilot equipment. Ultimately, however, final systems have to be made on equipment that is capable of producing commercial quantities for the marketplace. There isn't any off-the-shelf transdermal manufacturing equipment available today. Equipment has to be custom engineered to be able to fabricate a particular designed transdermal system.

Materials that have been selected to be part of a new transdermal system in the early stages of development, will help determine how the product will be manufactured and what processes will be necessary, thus how efficient and costly the equipment, the resultant product, and quality control will be.

A very volatile enhancer or drug may preclude the manufacturing process that may use heat to drive off any solvents. Putting a peripheral adhesive on the patch may involve intricate or repeated passes through a machine that can drive costs up. Using form, fill and seal of liquids in a system may compromise the safety of an individual using the transdermal product. The ultimate process may not be able to drive off enough residual solvent such that the coating process will take several passes through an oven or a more efficient oven may take up more room and be costlier. Another scenario that takes place is that the new prototype product design has to be the same as the first transdermal system because the company has made extremely large capital investment and cannot afford to buy totally new and different equipment. These are just some of the issues that become apparent as the project reaches larger scale production. Some of these issues can be avoided by considering the consequences early in the development of a transdermal system.

Processing steps: Once the decision has been made to proceed with a particular process, there is still a lot more work left to do to reach commercialization. Like other dosage forms, there is a "wet" end process, a fabrication function and a packaging step (Figure 15). The wet end portion consists of incorporating the drug into a polymer or polymer dispersion that may be initially a liquid and is ultimately surrounded by films or formed into a solid state film or matrix. The fabrication part of the process consists of bringing all the various components (films, laminate structures, adhesive layers, release liners, etc.) together and die cutting the system to size. Finally, the transdermal system is placed in a pouch as a unit dose in a fashion typically found in the pharmaceutical industry.

Several papers have described manufacturing processes for transdermals that have reached the marketplace in the United States.[41-43] The wet end portion of the manufacturing process usually involves a polymer that may be either in the liquid or "solid state." In all cases, viscous polymer solutions, slurries or melts are involved in the process. From this process the final drug reservoir may remain a viscous dispersion, cross-linked with or without heat. It is important in this stage of the operation to assure that the drug or other components do not degrade or volatilize during the heating processes, interact with the cross-linking materials, or interact with the other components. Finally, the formulation and the process must be adjusted and analyzed to assure that batches can be made reproducibly and within desired specification limits.

In the second stage of the fabrication process, films that consist of special laminate structures are brought together either encase a liquid drug reservoir, a molded polymer matrix, or laminate to other film structures, or a sliced piece of matrix. These films are in the form of rolls or webs that are interleaved on machines that are capable of either continuous or intermittent type of motion. Intermittant motion machines have the webs of film stop at a particular station where possibly a tray forming, filling operation, bonding operation, die cutting, or heat sealing takes place on the web of polymer film before moving on to the next station. A continuous motion machine does not stop at a particular station but the web of film moves through the machine in a continuous motion. Usually laminating, bonding, printing and die cutting operations can be done in a continuous manner.

The construction of an adhesive laminate structure as well as the nature of the backing (facestock) material, adhesive mass and release liner must be considered in fabrication. Depending on the materials, there are the impact of the materials on the wear of the dies used to cut the transdermal out of the web, the depth of the die and how far it will cut into the web, how well the dies withstand wear with each material, and the speed at which the web moves. If not properly formulated, the adhesive mass in roll form may have a tendency to flow causing a sticky mass to develop on the sides of the roll, making it difficult to process on the machine. If the adhesive mass builds up adhesive strength during storage, it may be impossible to unwind the roll. A good understanding of the peel strengths of the adhesive at the machine unwind speeds and the release values for the release liners will prevent the difficult unwind and processing problems on the machine.

The type of machinery used in fabricating the transdermal has to be considered depending on the design of the transdermal system. The complexity of the system design, the need for high output, and the need for specialized stations to perform a particular task are useful in selecting a continuous web or an intermittent web machine. The stations that perform a specialized task have to be placed in an optimal order for assembly. Consideration for cleanliness and potential contamination by the equipment parts will allow for the fabrication of clean transdermal systems. Web speeds that are too fast or slow may impact on how the rolls of web material will perform on the machine. For instance, registration of the material has to be within a tight range at the correct station within a limited tolerance. When laminating or delaminating a laminated material, angle of peel, build-up of static electricity, and surface contamination have to be considered as well in machine design.

Validation of process—By now it can be recognized that fabricating a transdermal delivery system utilizes equipment and the skilled know-how that is not found in the traditional pharmaceutical company. One still has to accomplish the same objectives in process development and manufacturing that are found in tabletting and other common dosage forms that include:

- establish process parameters and their effect on system functionality
- reproducibility from batch to batch
- documentation for regulatory filings
- process optimization with high economic output
- transfer to the production department and repeat the four objectives listed above

In the validation of equipment where experiments are performed to see the processing parameters and their effect on system functionality, the studies can be complex, labor intensive and costly. Take for instance the coating operation shown in Figure 15. Here the polymer being extruded may contain a drug and enhancer that is being coated onto another substrate. The processing engineer is now faced with determining the effect of machine variability on residual solvent content, drug and enhancer content uniformity and thickness of the film. The various stations along the coating line have to be considered:

Web handling: tension, registration, speed, thickness
Coating station: speed, temperature/humidity, viscosity, drug concentration, die opening, pump rate
Drying ovens: temperature, air volume, air velocity, solvent content
Lamination: pressure, gap, speed, material thicknesses, tension

The coating process described above relates only to the seemingly simple adhesive film laminate that may contain the drug and the enhancer. As the complexity of the transdermal system design increases the complexity in manufacturing takes place along with the unwieldy number of variables that can make validation of the equipment extremely difficult, long, tedious and costly. Again, the design of the product can greatly influence the cost of its manufacturing equipment, batch reproducibility and cost of goods.

Quality Control and Regulatory Approvals

Transdermal systems contain drugs, and therefore are considered drugs, and must undergo a government review process, which requires approval of an Investigative New Drug (IND) and a New Drug Application (NDA) by the FDA before reaching the market. Logically, federal regulators of new dosage forms are requesting clinical efficacy studies for those drugs given transdermally where there is no other clinically proven, officially approved product that delivers the same drug through the skin. Where there is a product on the market that has approval in the US for transdermal delivery, the FDA allows the new transdermal to reach the market by submitting an Abbreviated New Drug Application (ANDA), only if clinical trials demonstrate the same blood levels and profiles as the approved product. The Waxman-Hatch Act requires that after the innovative, or first, transdermal with a given drug reaches market approval, the subsequent transdermals having that same drug and desiring regulatory approval must also be subjected to efficacy studies as well as blood level studies. Otherwise, there is a three-year grace period before another transdermal can have market approval based solely only on blood levels, bioequivalence and skin toxicity studies.

Quality control testing: All raw materials and components undergo the scrutiny of strict standards and are tested by validated analytical test methods. Documentation similar to that of other drug dosage forms is also required for transdermal batch testing (e.g. batch records, reconciliation, weights, measurements, specifications and packaging). Two assays that are unique for testing transdermals are the total content per area assay and the release of drug into water assay. In the case of the total content assay, the drug often has to be extracted from undissolved polymer. This involves extraction procedures longer than those normally found with other dosage forms or when the adhesive or polymer cannot be dissolved.

As with other sustained release or long acting dosage forms, the transdermal release of the drug needs to be characterized by its release rate. Figure 14 shows the release of nitroglycerin from various commercial products. The differences in release profiles reflect different release mechanism, formulation or drug content. Changes in the drug release profile may be seen in stability testing or batch to batch processing. Although there are many ways to study the release of the drug, regulatory agencies and official compendia have suggested a couple of methods that relate release to the labelled drug content.[26]

In the final analysis, a system designer will find it very difficult to develop a transdermal product in the sequential fashion that we have become accustomed to using with the traditional dosage forms. First, there must be a product profile to serve as a road map for the system designer and the manufacturing group. Second, there has to be simultaneous conceptualizations of the system design, delivery mechanism, skin toxicology, adhesion, component constraints, and the commercial manufacturing process, all fed continuously to the development team if there is to be a timely and successful outcome. All of these aspects obviously affect the final cost of the transdermal system, which must often compete with less costly traditional dosage forms, higher retail profit margins and existing product acceptance by the patient.

The Future

The more advanced transdermal designs have been in the marketplace for about a decade now. These new dosage forms are complex to develop, and use technologies that are new to the pharmaceutical industry. Initially, transdermals have been developed for generic drugs and have reached a worldwide market niche of nearly $1 billion in 1991.

With all the new technologies that abound outside the pharmaceutical arena, there is more room to explore, in which transdermal technology may grow. Better understanding of skin immunology, new polymer materials and advanced transdermal fabrication techniques can be brought to bear to advance the state of the art. Genetically engineered polypeptides and microelectronics offer opportunity to non-invasively treat diseases in either continuous or pulsatile delivery. Pharmaceutical companies now have an alternative dosage form by which to market new chemical entities that are needed to meet stringent patient compliance, unique blood level profiles or that may not be marketable in the traditional dosage forms. The future is very bright for the transdermal approach as we enter the second decade of this specialized technology.

Iontophoresis

By Pramod P. Sarpotdar

Iontophoresis is a technique used to deliver compounds across the skin under the influence of an electrical current. It is analogous to electrophoresis in that it makes use of the mobilities of molecules in an electrical field. Iontophoresis is used clinically in the treatment of hyperhidrosis[1,2] where a typical treatment involves periodic tap water iontophoresis. Shen et al.[3] have recently suggested further improvement in the treatment by the inclusion of glycopyrrolate, an anticholinergic agent, and aluminum chloride during iontophoresis. It is also used diagnostically in the detection of cystic fibrosis.[4]

Iontophoresis has been extensively evaluated in dentistry for the delivery of local anesthetic,[5] tooth desensitization,[6] and lowering dentin sensitivity.[7] Its applications in ophthalmology have been evaluated by Hobden et al.[9] They compared the effectiveness of ciprofloxacin after iontophoretic treatment of rabbit cornea infected with P. aeruginosa to the topical treatment alone. They noticed that one iontophoretic treatment was equivalent to about 11 topical treatments of the drug.

Recently, Iomed introduced the first transdermal patch which uses iontophoresis to deliver lidocaine and dexamethasone. The improved version is called Phoresor II® and its usefulness is described by Glass et al.[9] Zeltzer et al.[10] evaluated the usefulness of lidocaine iontophoresis for local anesthesia during dialysis in children. A current of 3 mA for 10 minutes was judged as less painful compared to the subcutaneous (sc) injection. However, the overall effectiveness of a sc injection was considered to be better. The results are encouraging, since it appears that lidocaine iontophoresis may provide an alternative to needles, which could be traumatic, especially in children.

A large number of therapeutic agents under investigation as candidates for iontophoretic delivery are listed in an excellent review article by P. Tyle.[11] Readers are encouraged to examine reviews by Banga and Chien,[12] Sloan and Soltani,[13] Singh and Roberts,[14] and Parasrampuria,[15] all of which in combination provide a complete listing of previous publications.

Although the usefulness of iontophoresis was initially demonstrated almost 100 years ago, its application in the field of drug delivery has only been explored in the past decade. Three main factors have contributed to the renewed interest. The first is increased attention to the general field of transdermal therapy. There have also been vast advances in battery technology which now make possible a small, inconspicuous power source, at little expense. Finally, there is an increased understanding of the critical formulation and electrical factors of iontophoretic delivery. These elements have combined to make iontophoresis a potentially useful technique for the controlled delivery of therapeutic agents.

Advantages and Limitations

The potential advantages of iontophoresis include:

1. Increased capability of delivering larger amounts of therapeutic agents compared to passive delivery systems. For example, a reasonably-sized transdermal patch (25 to 50 cm^2 area) using passive technology would be capable of delivering a maximum of about 10 mg of a small molecular weight (< 1,000 Dalton) drug. An iontophoretic patch of similar dimensions would be capable of delivering at least 100 mg of the same compound under optimal conditions. Needless to say, the list of compounds which could be delivered transdermally at therapeutic concentrations now includes drugs with medium potency, reflecting this increased capability.

2. Ability to deliver significantly higher amounts of relatively large molecular weight compounds. The possibility of delivering peptides is particularly attractive since they are, as a class, highly potent agents used in illnesses which require chronic therapy. These agents are generally water-soluble compounds and unstable in the GI fluids, limiting their administration to injectable routes. However, most of them exist as charged species at physiological pH. They are fairly large molecules for delivery by passive transdermal techniques. There have been reports in the literature which suggest that insulin (MW~5,400) could be delivered at therapeutic levels by an iontophoretic patch.[16-18] Based on the transport studies with various molecular weight polyethylene glycols, Ruddy and Hadzija[19] estimated that the effective pore size for iontophoretic transport is approximately 36 Å. The authors predict that larger molecular weight compounds such as insulin could be transported through these channels.

3. Better control of the delivery profile, including nonzero-order profiles. Insulin is, again, an excellent example which could make use of this capability. As will be seen later, the rate of transport of the drug is directly related to the applied current. Thus, one can effectively turn on the delivery as needed and turn it off at other times. Gonadotropin releasing hormone (GnRH), a decapeptide, is yet another example where a continuous delivery would result in depressed sexual function while a pulsed release is attractive for the treatment of female infertility and hypogonadism.[20]

Potential disadvantages of iontophoresis include:

1. Complexity of the delivery system. Even though prototype iontophoresis patches which are identical in appearance to transdermal patches are available, they are significantly more complex in nature. There are at least three compartments inside an iontophoresis patch. One of these is for the power source and the remaining two are for the electrodes. Evaluation of these patches is also more complex since one must understand not just the contribution of chemical factors but those of electrical factors as well.

2. Chemical stability of the therapeutic agent. Generally, in a transdermal patch, a compound is stabilized in the vehicle in which it is contained. Its stability

during transport across the skin is then assessed. In an iontophoretic patch, one also has to consider the effects of applied current on the stability of the compound. In our laboratory, we have observed that a peptide may be stable in solution, in contact with skin tissue, and in an applied electric field alone. However, when a current is applied to facilitate transport across the skin, the peptide breaks down.

3. Relatively unknown toxicology of prolonged exposure to current. Historically, iontophoresis has been used for short-term treatments. For example, in the treatment of hyperhidrosis, a patient is exposed to a low-level current for <1 hour every 4-6 weeks.[1-3] Similarly, in the diagnosis of multiple sclerosis, a patient is exposed to a low-level current for 10-15 minutes.[4] The proposed uses of iontophoresis in drug delivery mandate exposure to low-level current for longer periods of time. The effects of chronic exposure to these low-level currents are unknown.

Monteiro-Reviere[21] studied the effect of lidocaine iontophoresis on the morphology of porcine skin in-vivo. Gross observation of pig skin showed that erythema was common under the active electrode while edema was typically noticed under the counter electrode. Small pinpoint petechiae were also noticed under the active electrode. The effects were reversible. The initial intensity and the duration of these effects were dependent upon the total applied current. Microscopic evaluations showed epidermal alterations which consisted of dark basophilic nuclei oriented parallel to the stratum corneum but located within the stratum spinosum and stratum granulosum layers. These changes were observed even in the absence of the gross observations mentioned above. They were also noticed in in-vitro studies run under similar conditions. This suggested that the changes were non-immune mediated and have minimal toxicological significance. Based on her unpublished work with other compounds the author also concluded that the observed effects were not entirely due to electrical factors, but were specific to lidocaine iontophoresis.

4. Cost. It is obvious that the costs of development and manufacture for the iontophoretic patch would be significantly higher than the passive transdermal patch. Thus, the commercialization of technology would be limited to those compounds which are orally inactive, used in chronic therapy and which could not be delivered by passive transdermal patches.

Theoretical Background

The schematic diagram of the skin in Chapter 5 of this book clearly demonstrates its complex nature. It is generally accepted that, under passive conditions, the transport of molecules across the skin is governed by Fick's first law of diffusion:

$$J = P * C$$

For electrical transport, one relies on Ohm's law:

$$I = 1/R * V$$

where I is the intensity of the applied current (amperes), R is the resistance (ohms) of the barrier and V is the potential difference (volts) across the barrier. The two equations appear analogous and, in fact, Dugard and Scheuplein[22] recognized the similarities between the two equations during their studies on the effect of ionic surfactants on the permeability of epidermis.

We now know that under iontophoretic conditions the flux is directly proportional to the intensity of the applied current.[23] This then also suggests that the rate of transport is independent of the membrane. However, Magerl et al.[24] observed differential effects of not only body region and gender, but also of season, when they studied the transport of histamine by laser doppler flowmetry. Bannon et al.[25] pointed out that for a univalent ion the passage of 96485 coulombs will result in the transport of the molecular weight of the compound. This is true only when the transport number is one, or in other words, when there are no other species competing for the charge. Thus, the maximum rate of transport could be expressed as follows:

$$J_{max} = MW * I/96485$$

where, J_{max} = maximum rate of transport and MW = molecular weight of the compound.

In reality, however, the transport number will be significantly lower than one due to the presence of other ionic species which compete for the charge. Efficiency,[26] is a more versatile term and is related to the transference number as follows:

$$T = Z*E$$

where T = transference number, Z = valence and E = efficiency of the drug delivery.

In designing a new drug delivery system it is then of utmost importance to optimize efficiency. This is further discussed under critical factors affecting iontophoretic transport.

It is commonly noticed that the passive flux of a species immediately after the withdrawal of iontophoretic treatment is significantly higher than the passive flux for the same species before iontophoretic treatment. This increase is reversible and is generally attributed to skin capacitance. Figure 1 is a schematic diagram depicting the flow of current through the skin.

The resistance of the skin to the transport is not linear and is altered by several factors. The nonlinearity is more apparent with a larger current and at lower frequencies.[27] Chien et al.[28] also noticed that the impedance of the skin is lowered after continuous application of the current. This could be due to the saturation of skin capacitance which results in the apparent lowering of voltage necessary to maintain the same level of current. Koizumi et al.[29] modified the simple model drawn above in studying the transport of diclofenac sodium. They concluded that the product of skin resistance and capacitance is independent of the applied voltage.

In humans, shunt pathways occupy <0.1% of the total surface area.[30] Passive transport through these pores is considered to be minimal for most drugs. However, these hydrophilic pores offer the least resistance to the passage of current. One can view them as several resistances in parallel. Thus the fraction of the total applied current passing through each pore is inversely proportional to the resistance of that pore pathway.

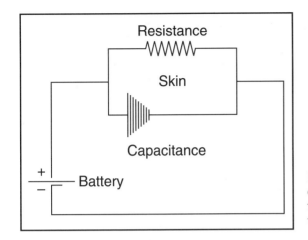

Figure 1. A schematic diagram depicting the flow of current through the skin

It is believed that the transport of drugs under iontophoretic conditions predominantly occurs through these pore pathways. Burnette and Ongpipattanakul[31] demonstrated this by studying the transport of methylene blue across excised human skin. They placed the dye in the receptor compartment in an in-vitro setup. At the end of the experiment, a dotted pattern on the skin surface suggested that the dye had traveled predominantly through the pores. This hypothesis was further confirmed by measuring voltage drop across the pores using microprobes. As expected, they noticed minimal voltage drop across the pores, suggesting that the pores are the path of least resistance Another interesting method of determining the barrier layer used the transport of ferric ions across pig skin in-vivo.[32] At the end of the experiment the skin tissue was removed and treated with potassium ferrocyanide and observed microscopically. Iontophoretic treatment showed deeper ferric ion penetration compared to the controls. Recently Pikal[33-35] has explained the contribution of electroosmotic flow on the enhancement of flux during iontophoretic transport. The author concludes that, while all the pores are negatively charged at physiological pH, there is a heterogeneity in the net negative charge and diameter of each pore.

Another interesting phenomenon relates to the isoelectric point of the skin (pH_{iso}), which is typically between pH 3 and 4. At physiological pH, these pores are negatively charged. When an electric field is applied, cations form bonds with the negatively-charged proteins on the skin surface. For a monovalent cation, the bonds are sufficiently weak to allow them to be broken, allowing the cation to be further advanced. This facilitates the transport of monovalent cations.[36] Burnette has termed this "permselectivity of the skin." These positively-charged ions also carry the solvent molecules in which they are dissolved, thus increasing the transport rate of solvent molecules. This, in turn, enhances the rate of transport of any solute that is dissolved in the solvent. This mass flow of solvent, electroosmosis, is responsible for the enhanced transport of neutral species under iontophoresis. Pikal demonstrated the transport of water by measuring volume changes in capillaries in a slightly modified diffusion cell

Table I. Structures and properties of TRH, dTGP and dTLP			
Name	Structure	Mol. Wt.	pKa
TRH	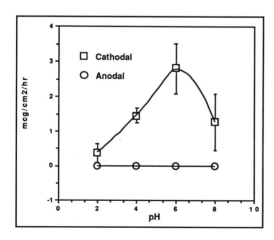	362	6.2
dTGP	X=CH2.CH2.COOH	401	~4.5
dTLP	X=(CH2)5.NH2	414	~10.5

design.[37] In general then, at pH above the pH_{iso} of skin, transport of cations is faster than for neutral species, which in turn travel faster than anions.

One would intuitively expect that anions may be preferentially transported across the skin if the pH of the solution is lowered below the isoelectric point of the skin. Miller et al.[20] showed this to be the case when they compared the transport of GnRH, GnRH agonist and GnRH antagonist. They found that the agonist, whch was cationic, had higher transport rates compared to the antagonist, which was anionic. The author's laboratory investigated transport of three tripeptides which were very similar (Table I). Figure 2 shows the transport of desamino tyrosyl glutamyl prolineamide (dTGP), an anion, at a wide range of pH values and at differing polarities. Figure 3 shows the effect of similar conditions on the transport of desamino tyrosyl lysyl prolineamide

Figure 2. The effect of pH of the formulation and polarity of the applied current on the penetration of dTGP across cadaver skin in-vitro

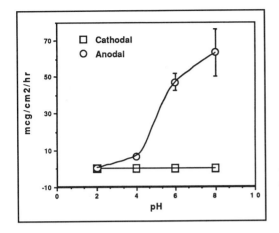

Figure 3. The effect of the formulation pH and polarity of the applied current on the penetration of dTLP across cadaver skin in-vitro

(dTLP), a cation. Note that no transport is detected in either case if the polarity of the applied current and the penetrating species is complimentary. Thus, for the anion dTGP, no transport is achieved when an anode is inserted in the donor compartment. Conversely, for dTLP, no transport is achieved when a cathode is inserted in the donor compartment. It is interesting to note that dTLP is charged at all the experimental pH values. Thus, the electrophoretic mobility of the compound is constant throughout the experiment. Therefore, the increase in the observed rates of transports is due to the increasing electroosmotic flow, which increases as the pH of the solutions is increased.

Another interesting observation is that the highest rate of transport for the anion dTGP is achieved at pH 6. One explanation for this is the fact that dTGP is neutral at pH 2. Thus, its electrophoretic mobility is almost zero at this pH. Also, even though the skin is now positively charged, it is very weakly charged; thus, electroosmotic transport at this pH is weak. At higher pHs, even though the electroosmotic flow is countering the electrophoretic transport of dTGP, the net gain is higher, up to pH 6. Since the pKa of the compound is 4.5, it is fully charged above pH 6.5. Thus, its electrophoretic mobility is constant beyond pH 6.5. As the pH is increased to 8, transport rates drop due to the stronger electroosmotic flow, countering the transport of dTGP. Finally, it is important to note that the highest rate of transport of dTLP is at least 25 times higher than the highest rate of transport of dTGP. This preferential transport of cations over anions has also been demonstrated by other workers.[38,39] Interestingly, the transport of divalent cations is significantly lower than the monovalent species.[36] This is perhaps due to tighter bonds between the divalent species and skin proteins which prevent gliding (as in the monovalent species). Finally, almost identical rates of penetration were obtained for TRH at pH 4 (where it is ionized) and at pH 8 (where it exists as a neutral species) by careful optimization of formulation factors.[40]

The primary factors affecting electroosmosis have been summarized by Srinivasan[41] as the net charge density of the membrane, the ionic strength and viscosity of the electrolyte, and the magnitude of the applied electric field. The dimensionless grouping characterizing convective mass flow is defined as the Peclet number:

$$P = v*1/D$$

where, P = Peclet number, v = velocity of the solvent, 1 = membrane thickness and D = diffusion coefficient of the compound.

It is important to note that Peclet number is inversely related to the diffusion coefficient of the compound. Thus for a larger molecular weight compound with smaller diffusion coefficient, the contribution of electroosmosis to the overall transport will be higher. Wearley et al.[42] confirmed this by studying four different amino acids, all of which had an identical pH_{iso} of 6.

Critical Factors Affecting Iontophoresis

In general, methods of evaluation are quite similar to those used for studying the transport of compounds under passive conditions. The in-vitro setup is typically modified by the insertion of electrodes in the donor and receptor compartments. Several versions of diffusion cells, incorporating minor variations, have been reported.[20, 38, 43-46] While each variation offers some advantages, the key is to be uniform in usage and treatment, and to use cross references whenever possible.

A comment about the positioning of electrodes is warranted here. In any in-vitro setup, the counter electrode is positioned under the skin. This situation is not desirable for medical use. However, it is generally accepted that positioning the counter electrode next to the active electrode is equally effective in transporting the drug across the skin. This holds true as long as the electrical circuit is completed through the skin. Use of proper insulating materials between the two electrodes is critical to prevent a short circuit.

Some of the critical factors that significantly affect iontophoretic transport are:

1. *Electrical considerations*: While a large number of electrode materials has been investigated, the most common materials appear to be platinum, carbon or silver/silver chloride. Transport of a cationic compound is enhanced by inserting the anode in the formulation and the cathode in the receptor. This configuration further results in an electroosmotic flow from donor to receptor, and is therefore preferred for the neutral compounds. Polarities are reversed to study the transport of an anionic compound. While the surface area of the electrode does not appear to be a major factor during iontophoresis, there are several other complications of which one must be aware. The electrolysis of water at the applied voltage results in the formation of gas, which gets trapped beneath the skin in an in-vitro setup. This problem appears to be more acute with platinum electrodes and with the vertical cell geometry. One alternative is to use cells with side-by-side geometry, thus preventing bubbles from contacting the skin. However, platinum electrodes are preferred during the transport of peptides since silver/silver chloride electrodes can cause precipitation of peptides.[28]

2. *pH*: In addition to bubble formation, the electrolysis of water also causes a significant shift in solution pH. It is important to note that this shift in pH occurs in opposing directions, meaning that the cathode becomes increasingly basic while the anode becomes increasingly acidic. This is an unacceptable situation

since, among other things, it could affect drug stability. In addition, the shift in pH could also affect the ionization of the drug in-situ which may severely alter transport of the drug. Therefore, it is absolutely critical to maintain the solution pH during iontophoresis. Maintaining the pH by use of typical buffer solutions gives rise to another problem: since buffers are made of small electrolytes they are, themselves, capable of carrying current. Therefore, in effect, they compete with the penetrating species for charge which results in decreased efficiency.

3. *Efficiency*: Efficiency of an iontophoretic system is defined as the fraction of charge (in %) carried by the penetrating molecule of interest. Higher efficiency will not only carry larger amounts of drug across the skin but will also require less current to deliver the desired quantities of drug. If one makes an assumption of linearity of relationship between the flux and applied current, the efficiency of transport for a given compound can be calculated from the slope of the curve which could be mathematically expressed as:[47]

$$E = S*F/MW$$

where, E = efficiency of iontophoretic transport, S = slope of the curve (flux vs. applied current), F = Farady's constant, MW = molecular weight of the species.

Lattin et al.[47] calculated the efficiencies for the two test compounds, pyridostigmine and hydromorphone using the above equation and reported them to be 24% and 11% respectively under the conditions selected. As the equation suggests, the difference in efficiencies of the two compounds could be simply due to the difference in molecular weights.

Incorporation of the highest possible concentration of the drug, while using minimal buffer concentration to maintain the pH, is one possible approach to increase efficiency of the iontophoretic transport. However, using high concentrations of the therapeutic agents may not be economically feasible. On the other hand, solubility of the therapeutic agent could be a rate-limiting factor. In our experience, addition of cosolvents sometimes alleviates this problem. However, to be conductive, the solvent must contain the equivalent of at least 40% normal saline solution.

Phipps and Untereker showed that the efficiency of transport could be significantly increased by use of silver/silver chloride electrodes, provided that chloride is present in solution as a counterion.[48] The usefulness of silver/silver chloride electrodes has also been demonstrated by Petelenz et al.[49] During iontophoresis, the silver chloride that is formed is insoluble in the aqueous solution, and no longer competes for the charge.

Sanderson et al.[50] used ion exchange resin in the donor compartment in an effort to increase the efficiency of transport. Essentially, in a two-compartment design, the ion exchange resin allows only the transport of the drug species, while removing the counterion from the solution. Nyambi et al.[46] carried this approach one step further by using ion exchange membranes in donor as well as receptor compartments. It is not clear if the increased efficiency observed in the in-vitro system under the above approach is applicable to in-vivo situations.

Finally, when Miller and Smith[51] compared the rates of transport of three anions (acetate, hexanoate, and dodecanoate) they noticed that the rates decreased as the anion became bulkier. Even though the authors did not evaluate the effect of anion size on the penetration of the common cation, it is possible that by using the bulkier counterion one may be able to deliver the cation of interest at higher rates.

Yet another approach is the use of polymeric buffers.[52] There are two potential advantages of using polymeric buffers. First, since these are large molecular weight compounds, they do not readily go across the skin. Second, they carry multiple charges on polymeric backbones and require a very small molar concentration to maintain the pH effectively. Tables II through V show the utility of these polymeric buffers in enhancing the transport of dTLP (Table II) and TRH (Table III) between pHs 4 and 8. The rates of both dTLP and TRH are increased two-fold at pH 8 when hydroxy polyethylimine (PEH) is used as a buffer instead of a McIlvaine buffer. Two concentrations of the polymeric buffer were evaluated in these experiments. The difference between the initial and the final formulation pH was minimal when 0.14 molar PEH is used. However, it is important to note that even at lower concentration of PEH (0.014M), the shift in pH during the experiment is comparable to the shift in pH when 0.2 M McIlvaine buffer is used.

A four- to six-fold increase in rate of penetration is observed for both compounds at pH 4 when 0.024 molar poly (methyl vinyl ether maleic anhydride) (PMVEMA) buffer is used instead of a 0.2 M McIlvaine buffer (Tables IV and V). It is important to note that the solution pH was adequately maintained during the experiment. Table V also shows that a combination of two polymeric compounds could be effective to obtain an intermediate pH (pH 6 in this case). It is important to note that, while dTLP is charged at all test pHs, TRH exists as a cation at pH 4 and as a neutral species at pH 8.

4. *Current*: So far the focus of discussion has been on the application of "DC" or direct current. It is believed that the skin acts as a capacitor. When an applied electric field is withdrawn, the current is maintained for some finite period, due to the discharging of the capacitor. The periodic application of electrical field was perceived to be helpful in reducing local toxicity. This was first shown by Okabe et al. when they studied the transport of metoprolol in human volunteers.[53] They claimed that the application of pulsed DC results not only in significant transport of metoprolol, but also in a significant reduction in the intensity of local irritation. Similar results have been reported for diclofenac sodium by Koizumi et al.[54] It is important to note that, just as with constant current application, a linear relationship between the applied current and flux is observed during pulsatile application. In the author's laboratory, the effects of applying DC vs. pulsed DC on the in-vitro transport of metoprolol were compared. Figure 4 shows that the metaprolol rates of transport obtained after applying pulsed DC above 50% duty cycle are comparable to the rates obtained after the application of DC. Below 50% duty cycle, the transport rates fall linearly. In yet another study[55] the plasma concentration of formeterol fumarate was found to be highest in guinea pigs after iontophoretic treatment at 30% duty cycle. Chien et al. have reported the effects of different wave shapes and duty cycles on the iontophoretic transport of insulin.[56]

5. *Chemical Enhancement*: Successful transport of peptides across human skin by iontophoresis has been reported several times. However, the total

Table II. The effect of the cationic polymeric buffer (PEH) on the penetration of dTLP at pH 8

Buffer	Rate	SEM	Initial pH	Final pH
McIlvaine 200mM	31.08	8.57	8.1	7.4
Poly-buffer 0.14mM	37.34	2.80	8.5	8.2
Poly-buffer 0.014mM	68.79	36.09	8.1	8.1

Table III. The effect of the cationic polymeric buffer (PEH) on the penetration of TRH at pH 8

Buffer	Rate	SEM	Initial pH	Final pH
McIlvaine 200mM	5.09	0.91	8.2	7.4
Poly-buffer 0.14mM	6.34	1.63	8.0	8.0
Poly-buffer 0.014mM	9.28	1.95	8.0	7.6

Table IV. The effect of the anionic polymeric buffer (PMVEMA) on the penetration of TRH at pH 4

Buffer	Rate	SEM	Initial pH	Final pH
McIlvaine 200mM	16.17	2.09	4.3	4.8
Poly-buffer 0.24mM	70.07	11.50	4.3	4.1
Poly-buffer 0.024mM	91.10	20.83	3.9	5.2

Table V. The effect of polymeric buffers in combination on the iontophoretic delivery of dTLP

pH	Rate(Polymeric Combination*)	pH (Polymeric buffers) Initial	Final	Rate (McIlvaine)
4	134.8 ± 15.9	3.7	5.2	18.2 ± 6.6
6	500.4 ± 60.2	5.7	6.9	NA
8	64.8 ± 11.4	7.9	8.2	31.1 ± 8.6

*PEH/PMVEMA
NOTE: All rates are expressed in $\mu g/cm^2 \bullet hr$
SEM=Standard error around mean

amounts of larger peptides transported are at subtherapeutic levels. Srinivasan et al.[57] observed that pretreating the hairless mouse skin with ethanol for two hours immediately prior to iontophoretic treatment resulted in significant increase in the transport rates of insulin compared to the iontophoretic

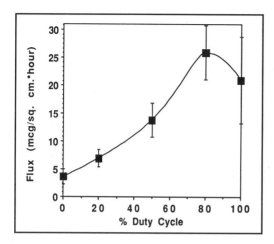

Figure 4. The effect of duty cycle on metoprolol penetration. Note: average current = 0.01 mA/cm.²

Table VI. Variables that influence iontophoretic transport of drugs	
VARIABLE	EFFECTS
ELECTRICAL:	
1. Electrode type	variable
2. Applied current intensity	+ transport rates
3. Duty cycle	equivalent to DC
PHYSICO-CHEMICAL:	
1. Buffer concentration	- transport rates
2. Drug concentration	+ transport rates
3. pH	drug dependant
4. Solvent effects	conductivity changes

treatment alone. It is important to note that the passive rate of transport of insulin is insignificant. Wearley and Chien[58] noticed similar synergy when they studied the transport of azidothymidine (AZT) across hairless rat skin. In this study the chemical enhancer (N-decylmethyl sulfoxide) was added as a part of the vehicle instead of being used to pretreat the skin as in the previous study.[57]

Conclusions

Table VI summarizes the effects of key formulation and electrical factors on the iontophoretic transport of drugs. Iontophoresis is an exciting technique which vastly increases the capability to deliver drugs across the skin. However, due to cost and unknown toxicity potential, this technique is limited at present to the drugs which require chronic therapy.

Physiological End Points: Instrumental Monitoring

By Jeffrey K. Mills, Joel L. Zatz, PhD and Richard S. Berger, MD

Penetration of topically-applied compounds appears to be dependent on several factors including skin thickness, age, disease, anatomical location, percent active concentration and vehicle. Efficacy of a given formulation is ultimately judged by clinical and/or symptomatic changes. However, approaches to aid in screening compounds and designing formulas are needed for the development of new products. This chapter addresses the application of various noninvasive instrumental approaches as they may help monitor and document the penetration of active compounds in vivo, as reflected by physiological end points.

Developments in bioinstrumental applications for the skin have increased greatly over the last two decades. As the body's most accessible organ, the skin lends itself to the application of noninvasive engineering principles and methods. Efforts have included development of instrumentation systems, interfacing data collection systems and analysis, and adaptation of computer technology. Some of the more traditional engineering areas which bioengineering uses are electronics, fluid mechanics, heat and mass transfer, materials, mathematics, mechanics, optics, radiation and thermodynamics. Our interest here is to describe instrumental interfaces with skin physiology and pharmacology.

One approach to measuring skin penetration of active compounds in vivo is to monitor physiologic or pharmacologic responses in the skin. For the purposes of this review, we will limit our survey to instrumental applications monitoring physiological end points. A physiological end point may be defined as the action of a drug when applied to healthy skin, as distinguished from its therapeutic action. As with any review, we shall describe some but not all of the published applications. We will, however, make some suggestions for additional applications based on the current literature.

Reflectance Spectrometry

Traditionally, irritation (erythema, redness) caused by various intrinsic and extrinsic factors has been evaluated by the trained eye. Skin color can now be instrumentally evaluated using reflectance techniques.[1-3] Various instruments which have been developed include the Minolta Chroma Meter and the Cortex DermaSpec-trometer.[4-9]

The Chroma Meter uses 0° view angle geometry to produce a reading that corresponds with skin color as seen under typical lighting. Using filtered photocells and a pulsed xenon arc lamp as its light source, it detects reflected light. The detected signals are fed to a microcomputer which uses the principle of tristimulus colorimetry to determine the values of the sample surface. There are different color systems for the data display. Several reports utilized the CIE (Commission Internationale de l'Eclairage) L*a*b* system as an expression of the skin color. The color is expressed in a three dimensional system with an a*-axis (green-red), a b*-axis (yellow-blue) and an L*-axis (levels of brightness between black and white). Each value increases as the color becomes more reddish, more yellowish, and brighter, respectively.

The Cortex DermaSpectrometer measures intensity of erythema and melanin-induced pigmentation. This instrument has two light emitting diodes (LEDs) with selected narrow bands of emitted wavelengths as light sources. The peaks of the two bands are centered in 568 nm (green) and 655 nm (red), the absorption spectra of hemoglobin and melanin. The two LEDs emit light onto the skin; the intensity of the reflected light is detected by a photodetector in sequence. Background light intensity is detected before and after measurements are made and the equipment is calibrated against black and white using a dual calibration standard. Data obtained is converted into digital form and compensation is made for temperature and ambient light influencing the sensor. An Erythema-index (E-index) and Melanin-index (M-index) are defined as:

$$\text{E-index} = 100 \ \log \frac{\text{intensity of reflected red light}}{\text{intensity of reflected green light}}$$

and

$$\text{M-index} = 100 \ \log \frac{1}{\text{intensity of reflected red light}}$$

Conner, Zanani, Nix et al. presented a poster exhibit at the American Society for Clinical Pharmacology and Therapeutics 1990 annual meeting describing the use of reflectance spectrometry as it might apply to the assay of McKenzie and Stoughton.[10] This assay uses blanching of the skin to assess the penetration and potency of corticosteroid formulations.[11] Conner and his coworkers used paired groups of active and placebo creams or ointments. One set was applied using a perforated guard; another set was applied to the opposite forearm and occluded with plastic wrap. The latter were kept in place for a shorter period of time. The ratings (0=no blanching, 3=maximum blanching) of two human trained observers were compared to the reflectance spectrophotometric technique results. The human observers and the reflectance spectrophotometric method correlated (p<0.001). Conner and colleagues concluded that reflectance spectrometry was a promising method showing potential for greater sensitivity in the skin blanching assay.

The Centre International de Recherches Dermatologiques group also presented data using reflectance spectrometry at the 8th International Symposium on Bioengineering and the Skin.[12] Drs. C. Queille-Roussel, M. Poncet and H. Schaefer used the Minolta tristimulus colorimeter CR 200 to quantify corticosteroid blanching. They looked at the influence of time on calorimetric parameters. On Day 1 they took measurements at six predetermined ventral forearm sites from six healthy volunteers at two-hour intervals over a 12-hour period. They found the colorimetric values to be site-related, with the two-hourly variations occurring with similar profiles for all sites. On the second day they applied four topical corticosteroid creams, each representative of its class of activity and vehicle bases, for two hours in a randomized double blind, without occlusion, on five of the six predetermined sites. They did a visual grading and colorimetric measurement every two hours over the following 12-hour diurnal period and repeated the same set of measurements on a third day. Dr. Schaefer's group reported that the colorimetric parameters L* (brightness) and a* (green-red), after subtraction of their baseline value, "gave an objective rank order identical to that of the clinical corticosteroid potency with superior discrimination compared with simple subjective visual grading." L* was a more precise parameter than a* for evaluating blanching.

Laser Doppler Velocimetry

Laser Doppler velocimetry has been widely used in medical studies. One reference guide lists over twenty organ-specific applications in addition to the skin.[13] Laser Doppler velocimetry uses a helium-neon laser to measure the blood flow of the superficial vasculature. The laser emits radiation through an optical fiber which penetrates 1-1.5 mm below the upper epidermis. This radiation is scattered, and its optical frequency is Doppler-shifted by passing blood cells, before reflected light is collected by a second fiber. The magnitude and frequency distribution of the Doppler shift are related to the numbers and velocities of blood cells. Measurements are, in principle, relative. Percutaneous penetration of methyl nicotinate (methyl 3-pyridincarbonylate) has been followed with both laser Doppler velocimetry and photopulse plethysmography.[14] Following topical application of this agent, correlation was observed between the recordings of both methods and the clinical observation of erythema. Lower drug concentrations were found to delay both the onset and the magnitude of microperfusion; they also reduced its period. In this study, noninvasive instrumental monitoring made it possible to follow the time course of drug action at the location where the application was made.

Wilkin et al. carried laser Doppler monitoring of topically applied methyl nicotinate further in an experiment designed to inhibit the response and, therefore, gain insight in the chemical's mechanism(s) of action.[15] Wilkin applied aqueous concentrations (0 to 100 ml) of methyl nicotinate in quadruplicate to the volar forearms of normal healthy volunteers following oral pretreatments with 25 mg doxepin hydrochloride, 600 mg ibuprofen, 50 mg indomethacin, 975 mg aspirin and a lactose placebo. Wilkin's group found indomethacin, ibuprofen and aspirin suppressed the nicotinate response. They pointed to inhibition of prostaglandin bioformation as the common denominator for these different chemical structures.

An interesting report by Dowd and his coworkers points to the potential value of instruments detecting physiological end-point changes without clinical change.[16] This group applied hexyl nicotinate in a lotion formulation to the skin and assessed the response by clinical evaluation of erythema and laser

Doppler velocimetry. Mean erythematous responses and increased blood flow were dose-related. However, several of the subjects showed an increase in blood flow but only a minimal erythematous response. Here laser Doppler velocimetry was detecting vasodilation with only slight clinical change.

Image Analysis

Digital imaging involves the mapping of an object in order to graphically represent it. Often just one measurable property of an object is utilized in creating the object's image. These images can then be stored, reproduced or analyzed at any time. Analysis of digital images is instantaneous, and the types of analysis possible have become virtually limitless with the computer programs now available. Various types of imaging include ultrasound, scanning electron microscopy and image analysis.[17]

The skin presents obvious opportunities to use image analysis for a variety of surface topography and histology evaluations.[18] Image analysis also has several interesting applications in the monitoring of active-agent effects on physiological end points. To do this, image analysis is used to evaluate other noninvasive sampling methods.

Image analysis has applications, for example, to follicular biopsy samples of the sebaceous follicle. The follicular biopsy technique allows for an assessment of the presence of sebaceous filaments or casts.[19,20]

A sample is taken by applying a thin layer of methyl cyanoacrylate adhesive to the surface of the skin and firmly holding in place a glass slide. The adhesive polymerizes in approximately one minute. The slide is then peeled off gently, removing some stratum corneum and follicular casts, if present. Recently, Groh et al. described image analysis of assay samples from a human comedogenic assay.[21] Groh used polarized illumination to achieve contrast for image analysis (Figures 1 and 2). This type of lighting consists of wavetrains running parallel in a given direction, achieved by using a polarizing filter over the light source and microscope lens. Groh used a digital image analysis system that captured the image through a light microscope with a high-resolution video camera. The captured video image was then digitized and analyzed. A computer program was developed to count the number, area and size distribution of horny impactions. The program decides, based on intensity range, which objects to evaluate. It then automatically edits, measures and records.

The assessment described by Groh evaluates extrinsically-caused hyperkeratinous impactions of the sebaceous follicle. This follicular biopsy image-analysis system would seem to have application in assessing the lytic activity of topically-applied compound on intrinsically-occurring follicular casts. The latter appear to occur in a large number of individuals who do not present with pathology. These casts are by histology a conglomeration of varying amounts of keratin, lipid, bacteria, water and hair(s). If applied compounds lyse these casts, the number of objects image analysis reports on slides should be reduced after a period of application.

Image analysis has also been combined with a silicone rubber impression technique to evaluate the activity of sweat glands.[22] Imprints of gland activity are made by applying a thin film of rubber silicone on the skin. This material

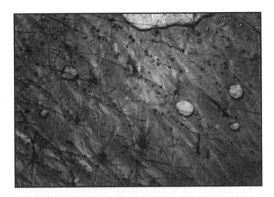

Figure 1. Follicular biopsy slide viewed through microscope with regular light.

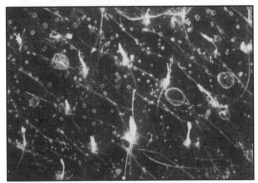

Figure 2. Sample biopsy slide using polarized light.

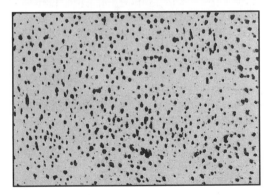

Figure 3. Sebum pore patterns resulting from Sebutape sampling.

cannot be mixed with water, thus sweat droplets create holes or impressions in the film as they reach the skin's surface. The film is then peeled away and scanned by image analysis. This technique has been used on the volar forearm where eccrine glands are concentrated. Application of the film is more difficult in the axilla, where apocrine glands are significant.

Another example of the interaction of image analysis and a noninvasive sampling method is the monitoring of the lipid from sebaceous glands as it reaches the skin surface.[23] This is done by using a sebum-sensitive adhesive tape.

Sebutape allows a measurement of sebum production and also records the output of sebum from individual follicles.[24] This adhesive film consists of a hydrophobic polymer film with small air spaces. The surface coat is a lipid-porous adhesive which allows the tape to be sealed to the skin during collection of sebum. As sebum reaches the skin's surface, it is absorbed into the tape, displacing the air. The now sebum-filled cavities become transparent to light. Each follicle, if active, leaves a well-defined spot whose size corresponds to the outline of the sebum droplet (Figure 3). This type of display lends itself well to image analysis. Topically-applied materials which safely reduce sebaceous gland output would be very valuable in dermatology.

Pulse Electrometry

Although local anesthetics produce a recognized physiological end point, which is the development of anesthesia, this end point has been hard to monitor because its demonstration relies on the absence of subjective response to some local stimulus. Testing methods have involved pin pricks which are difficult to quantitate or reproduce. Also, these probings pierce the skin, and that may affect the absorption process. Other test stimuli tried in this area have included thermal radiation and controlled electrical stimulation.

Pulse electrometry is a recently developed technique for in vivo measurement of the absorption of local anesthetics.[25] The instrument, the Vitality Scanner (Analytic Technology), is a handheld device developed for the measurement of tooth vitality. It delivers a current of 0.1 mA through a 2-mm diameter flat surface metal probe. Voltage slowly increases automatically from 15 V to approximately 300 V. Electrical stimulation is delivered as a burst of 10 pulses of negative polarity lasting about 150-200 microseconds, with a 3-15 millisecond pause between pulses. With each change in voltage, a digital counter on the instrument is advanced one digit. The range of the counter is from 0 to 80 units. When the subject feels the "tickle" of the voltage, he or she removes the probe from the skin; the digital reading is frozen and can be recorded as a measure of nerve ending sensitivity. There is no sign of skin damage, even at the highest voltage.

Validation of the instrument involved testing on different subjects at various body sites and measuring the response to an intradermal lidocaine injection. Instrument readings taken at each site were quite reproducible. A more thorough evaluation was conducted in several subjects, concentrating on the volar forearm. Both arms responded similarly and differences between evaluation sites were generally small. Some random fluctuations were noted but there was little drift in the readings taken over a period of time.

Further validation involved injection of lidocaine intradermally. Sodium chloride solution was used as the control. The results are shown in Figure 4. After injection of the control, a transient increase in instrument response was noted, and then readings returned to the baseline value. This was due to the influence of fluid within the skin (bleb) immediately after the injection. With the active preparations, instrument readings reached maximal value, 80, within a few minutes and remained there for some period of time before retreating. The duration of maximal response averaged 77 minutes following injection of a 1% lidocaine injection; mean time of maximal response was 128 minutes for a 2%

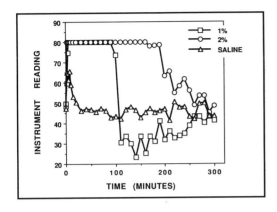

Figure 4. Typical Vitality Scanner instrument response following intradermal injection of lidocaine or saline control.

lidocaine solution.

Pulse electrometry was applied to the evaluation of anesthesia in 29 human subjects following application of several lidocaine formulations.[26] Hill Top Chambers containing the suspension vehicle (no lidocaine or surfactant) were applied to eight sites on the forearms for 30 minutes, after which the baseline reading (R_0) for each site was recorded. Hill Top Chambers containing test formulation or control were then applied to the sites in randomized pattern and left in place for three hours. Readings were taken at each site upon chamber removal (R_{180}) and one and two hours later (R_{240} and R_{300}, respectively). The effect, E, was taken as the mean instrument response corrected for baseline, as follows:

$$E = \frac{R_{180} + R_{240} + R_{300}}{3} - R_0 \qquad \text{Equation 1}$$

All of the formulations containing lidocaine gave significantly higher E values than the controls. Figure 5 shows data for 5% lidocaine formulations containing 20% propylene glycol and two alkyl trimethylammonium halides at a concentration of 81 mM. (The same figure contains data from an in vitro study using excised skin.) ER values represent enhancement ratios comparing formulations containing surfactants against a control.[27] Both pH values (7.9 and 10) produced essentially the same response in vivo as well as in vitro. The formulation containing myristoyl dimethylam-monium halide exhibited higher E and ER values than the formulation with the longer-chain surfactant.

None of the pulse electrometry subjects complained of pain or discomfort and there were no objective signs of skin damage. Based on the above studies, pulse electrometry appears to be a safe study technique capable of measuring anesthesia in skin. The technique responded differentially to lidocaine treatments that could have varied only in their degree of absorption, since all of them contained the same drug agent.

Limitations

The literature does have reports of noncor-respondence between bioinstrumental and clinical findings, such as the report of Dowd.[16] This type of report points to changes in the skin not detected by the clinical eye. This low

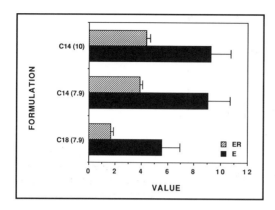

Figure 5. Response for formulations containing 5% lidocaine. Formulations are identified by surfactant chain length and pH (in parentheses). E represents instrument response in vivo calculated according to Eq.1; ER represents enhancement ratio for excised human skin in vitro. Bars indicate SEM.

level of activity could be very important given all the changes that can occur before we see results such as erythema or blanching. Formulations that could act at the subclinical level may be the most interesting ones of all and bioinstrumental monitoring should be very helpful here.

Also, there are reports concerning large scatter in bioinstrumental data. For example, Miller, Keller and Imlop found the reproducibility of resting blood flow over time to be poor and questioned the monitoring of pharmacological influences over a long-term, day-to-day situation.[28] They did feel from their work that laser Doppler velocimetry could be suitable for short-term investigation of drug effects on circulation.

Recognition of the limitations in applying bioinstrumentation to the skin has sometimes led to further engineering modifications specifically for the skin. For example, the laser Doppler monitors capillary flux in a small radius (1-1.5 mm). The flux can only be recorded at 1 or 2 points at a time depending on the number of channels. Recognizing this, Drs. Fauhtor, Selbam and Ziegerbagel reported on a computer-driven instrument which moves the probes of a laser Doppler flowmeter back and forth over the skin, stopping at preselected points to make measurements.[29]

Summary

Monitoring physiological end points with noninvasive bioinstrumentation represents another approach to gaining data on penetration of active compounds. This brief review has selected some noninvasive bioinstrumental approaches looking for reported measurements of physiological end points.

Bioinstrumental monitoring collects data at the local site where topical application occurs rather than collecting remote site information. These local changes should be relatively free of systemic effects as compared to blood or urine sampling. Also, results from traditional measurements of flux or skin concentration do not always relate to clinical responses. The suggestion to consider monitoring physiological end points is supported by some reports correlating clinical responses.[30-32]

Finally, applications of instrumental methods to the skin have been introduced relatively recently and, in some cases, there are insufficient data to affirm their utility. However, there appears to be sufficient information in the literature to suggest that bioinstrumental applications promise to expand our ability to measure drug absorption objectively.

References

Chapter 1

1:1. PW Wertz and DT Downing, Stratum corneum: biological and biochemical considerations, in *Transdermal Drug Delivery,* J Hadgraft and RH Guy, eds, New York: Dekker (1989) p 1

1:2. RJ Feldmann and HI Maibach, Regional variation in percutaneous penetration of ^{14}C cortisol in man, *J Invest Dermatol* **48** 181 (1967)

1:3. JA Parrish, *Dermatology and Skin Care,* New York: McGraw-Hill (1975)

1:4. RJ Scheuplein and IH Blank, Permeability of the skin, *Phys Rev* **51** 702 (1971)

1:5. B Illel, H Schaefer, J Wepierre and O Doucet, Follicles play an important role in percutaneous absorption, *J Pharm Sci* **80** 424 (1991)

1:6. GL Flynn, Mechanism of percutaneous absorption from physicochemical evidence, *Percutaneous Absorption,* 2nd Ed, R Bronaugh and H Maibach, eds, New York: Dekker (1989) p 27

1:7. RH Guy and J Hadgraft, Physicochemical aspects of percutaneous penetration and its enhancement, *Pharm Res* **5** 753 (1988)

1:8. ER Cooper, Increased skin permeability for lipophilic molecules, *J Pharm Sci* **73** 1153 (1984)

1:9. GP Kushla and JL Zatz, Correlation of Water and Lidocaine Flux Enhancement by Cationic Surfactants In Vitro, *J Pharm Sci* (in press)

1:10. AH Ghanem, H Mahmoud, WI Higuchi, UD Rohr, S Borsadia, P Liu, JL Fox and WR Good, The effects of ethanol on transport of b-estradiol and other permeants in hairless mouse skin, *J Control Rel* **7** 75 (1987)

1:11. H Schaefer, A Zesch and G Stuttgen, *Skin Permeability,* New York: Springer-Verlag (1982)

1:12. CFH Vickers, Existence of reservoir in stratum corneum, *Arch Dermatol* **88** 20 (1963)

1:13. RD Carr and RG Wieland, Corticosteroid reservoir in the stratum corneum, *Arch Dermatol* **94** 81 (1966)

1:14. A Rougier, D Dupuis, C Lotte and HI Maibach, Stripping method for measuring percutaneous absorption in vivo, *Percutaneous Absorption,* 2nd Ed, R Bronaugh and H Maibach, eds, New York: Dekker (1989) p 415

1:15. WG Riefenrath, GS Hawkins and MS Kurtz, Percutaneous penetration and skin retention of topically applied compounds: an in vitro/in vivo study, *J Pharm Sci* **80** 526 (1991)

1:16. JE Riviere, B Sage and NA Monteiro-Riviere, Transdermal lidocaine iontophoresis in isolated perfused porcine skin, *Cutan Ocular Toxicol* **8** 493 (1989-1990)

1:17. LK Pershing and GG Krueger, Human skin sandwich flap model for percutaneous absorption, in *Percutaneous Absorption,* RL Bronaugh and HI Maibach, eds, New York: Dekker (1989) p 397

1:18. J Kao, FK Patterson and J Hall, Skin penetration and metabolism of topically applied chemicals in six mammalian species, including man: an in vitro study with benzo[a]pyrene and testosterone, *Toxicol Appl Pharmacol* **81** 502 (1985)

1:19. EW Smith and JM Haigh, In vitro systems for assessment of drug release from topical formulations and transmembrane permeation, *Percutaneous Absorption,* 2nd ed, R Bronaugh and H Maibach, eds, New York: Dekker (1989) p 465

1:20. JL Zatz, Influence of depletion on percutaneous absorption characteristics, *J Soc Cosm Chem* **36** 237 (1985)

1:21. GP Kushla and JL Zatz, Lidocaine penetration through human and hairless mouse skin in vitro, *J Soc Cosm Chem* **40** 41 (1989)

262

1:22. K Sato, K Sugibayashi and Y Morimoto, Species differences in percutaneous absorption of nicorandil, *J Pharm Sci* **80** 104 (1991)

1:23. AD Pozzo, G Donzelli, E Liggeri and L Rodriguez, Percutaneous absorption of nicotinic acid derivatives in vitro, *J Pharm Sci* **80** 54 (1991)

1:24. BD Anderson and PV Raykar, Solute structure-permeability relationships in human stratum corneum, *J Invest Dermatol* **93** 280 (1989)

1:25. GP Kushla and JL Zatz, Influence of pH on lidocaine penetration through human and hairless mouse skin in vitro, *Int J Pharm* **71** 167 (1991)

1:26. JL Zatz, Simulation studies of skin permeation, *J Soc Cosm Chem* **43** 37 (1992)

Chapter 2

2:1. PV Raykar, MC Fung and BD Anderson, The role of protein and lipid domains in the uptake of solutes by human stratum corneum, *Pharm Res* **5** 140-150 (1988)

2:2. RC Wester and HI Maibach, Cutaneous Pharmocokinetics; 10 steps to percutaneous absorption, *Drug Metab Rev* **14** 169-205 (1983)

2:3. RS Scheuplein and IH Blank, Permeability of the skin, *Physiological Review* **51** (IV) 702-747 (1971)

2:4. PM Elias, Lipids and the epidermal permeability barrier, *Arch Dermatol Res* **270** 95-117 (1981)

2:5. G Grubauer, KR Feingold, RM Harris and PM Elias, Lipid content and lipid type as determinants of the epidermal permeability barrier, *J Lip Res* **30** 89-96 (1989)

2:6. WP Smith, MS Christensen, S Nacht and EH Gans, Effects of lipids on the aggregation and permeability of human stratum corneum, *J Invest Dermatol* **78** 7-11 (1982)

2:7. MM Rieger, Skin lipids and their importance to cosmetic science.*Cosm & Toil* **102** (7) 366-50 (1987)

2:8. S Rothman, The mechanism of percutaneous penetration and absorption. *J Soc Cosm Chem* **6** 193-200 (1955)

2:9. RJ Scheuplein, Mechanism of percutaneous absorption. I. Route of penetration and the influence of solubility, *J Invest Dermatol* **45** 334-346 (1965)

2:10. M Suzuki, K Asaba, H. Komatsu and M Mochizuka, Autoradiographic study on percutaneous absorption of oils useful in cosmetics, *J Soc Cosm Chem* **29** 265-282 (1978)

2:11. H Loth, Vehicular influence on transdermal drug penetration, *Int J Pharm* **68** 1-10 (1991)

2:12. GL Flynn, SH Yalkowsky and TJ Roseman, Mass transport phenomena and models: Theoretical concepts, *J Pharm Sci* **63** 479-510 (1974)

2:13. T Higuchi, Physical chemical analysis of percutaneous absorption process from creams and ointments, *J Soc Cosm Chem* **11** (11) 85-97 (1960)

2:14. RJ Scheuplein, Mechanism of percutaneous absorption. I. Routes of penetration and the influence of solubility, *J Invest Dermatol* **45** 334-346 (1965)

2:15. PH Dugard, Skin permeability theory in relation to measurements of percutaneous absorption in toxicology, Ch 22 in *Dermatotoxicology and Pharmacology,* FN Marzulli and HI Maibach, eds, New York: John Wiley & Sons (1977)

2:16. RH Guy and J Hadgraft, Mathematical models of percutaneous absorption, Ch 1 in *Percutaneous Absorption,* RL Bronaugh and HI Maibach, eds, New York: Marcel Dekker (1985)

2:17. C Surber, K-P Wilhelm, M Hori, HI Maibach and RH Guy, Optimization of topical therapy, partitioning of drugs into stratum corneum, *Pharm Res* **7** 1320-1324 (1990)

2:18. R Warner, MC Myer and DA Taylor, Electron probe analysis of human skin; Determination of the water concentration profile, *J Invest Dermatol* **90** 218-224 (1988)

2:19. D Bommannan, RO Potts and RH Guy, Examination of stratum corneum barrier function

263

in vivo by infrared spectroscopy, *J Invest Dermatol* **95** 403-408 (1990)

2:20. J Hadgraft, The epidermal reservoir: A theoretical approach, *Int J Pharm* **2** 265-274 (1979)

2:21. GS Hawkins and WG Reifenrath, Influence of skin source, penetration cell fluid and partition coefficient on in vitro skin penetration, *J Pharm Sci* **75** 378-381 (1986)

2:22. RL Bronaugh and RF Stewart, Methods for in vitro percutaneous absorption studies, IV: The flow-through diffusion cell, *J Pharm Sci* **74** 64-67 (1985); RL Bronaugh and RF Stewart, Methods for in vitro percutaneous absorption studies, VI: Preparation of the barrier layer, *J Pharm Sci* **75** 487-491 (1986); RL Bronaugh and RF Stewart, Methods for in vitro percutaneous absorption studies. III: Hydrophobic compounds, *J Pharm Sci* **73** 1255-1258 (1984)

2:23. RL Bronaugh, RF Stewart, RC Wester, D Bucks, HI Maibach and J Anderson, Comparison of percutaneous absorption of fragrances by humans and monkey, *Fd Chem Toxicol* **23** 111-114 (1985)

2:24. DB Guzek, AH Kennedy, SC McNeill, E Wakshull and RO Potts, Transdermal drug transport and metabolism, I: Comparison of in vitro and in vivo results, *Pharm Res* **6** 33-36 (1989); see also J Kao, The influence of metabolism on percutaneous absorption, Ch 17 in *Percutaneous Absorption*, 2nd Ed, RL Bronaugh and HI Maibach, eds, New York: Marcel Dekker (1989)

2:25. T Higuchi, Analysis of data on the medicament release from ointments, *J Pharm Sci* **51** 802-804 (1962); see also Reference 12.

2:26. RJ Scheuplein and LW Ross, Mechanism of percutaneous absorption. V. Percutaneous absorption of solvent deposited solids. *J Invest Dermatol* **62** 353-360 (1974)

2:27. K Wolter, H Schaefer, K-H Fromming and G. Stüttgen, Particle size and permeation, *Am Cosm Perf* **87** (III) 45-47 (1972); see also H Schaefer, A Zesch and G Stüttgen, *Skin Permeability*, Berlin: Springer (1982) p 758

2:28. W Schalla, JC Jamoulle and H Schaefer, Localization of compounds in different skin layers and its use as an indicator of percutaneous absorption, Ch 18 in *Percutaneous Absorption*, 2nd Ed, RL Bronaugh and HI Maibach, eds, New York: Marcel Dekker (1989)

2:29. J-C Tsai, M Cappel, N Weiner, G Flynn and J Ferry, Solvent effects on the harvesting of stratum corneum from hairless mouse skin through adhesive tape stripping in vitro, *Intern J Pharm* **68** 127-133 (1991)

2:30. H Schaefer, A Zesch and G Stüttgen, *Skin Permeability*, Berlin: Springer Verlag (1982)

2:31. BD Anderson, WI Higuchi and PV Raykar, Heterogeneity effects on permeability-partition coefficient relationships in human stratum corneum, *Pharm Res* **5** 566-573 (1988); see also BD Anderson and PV Raykar, Solute structure-permeability relationships in human stratum corneum, *J Invest Dermatol* **93** 280-286 (1989)

2:32. WJ Lambert, WI Higuchi, K Knutson and SL Krill, Effects of long-term hydration leading to the development of polar channels in hairless mouse stratum corneum, *J Pharm Sci* **78** 925-928 (1989)

2:33. UG Dalvi and JL Zatz, Effect of skin binding on percutaneous transport of benzocaine from aqueous suspensions and solutions, *J Invest Dermatol* **62**, 217-223 (1974)

2:34. K Adachi, Receptor proteins for androgen in hamster sebaceous glands, *J Invest Dermatol* **62**, 217-223 (1974)

2:35. RJ Feldman and HI Maibach, Penetration of ^{14}C-hydrocortisone through normal skin, *J Invest Dermatol* **91** 661-666 (1965)

2:36. E Menczel and HI Maibach, In vitro human percutaneous penetration of benzyl alcohol and testosterone: epidermal retention, *J Invest Dermatol* **54** 368-394 (1970); see also *Acta Dermatovenereol (Stockh)* **52** 38-42 (1972)

2:37. DE Wurster and KH Yang, Water vapor sorption and desorption by human callus, I: Anomalous diffusion, *J Pharm Sci* **71** 1235-1238 (1982)

2:38. IH Blank, J Moloney, AG Emslie, I Simon and C Apt, The diffusion of water across the

264

stratum corneum as a function of its water content, *J Invest Dermatol* **82** 188-194 (1984)

2:39. RS Scheuplein and LJ Morgan, Bound water in keratin membranes measured by a microbalance technique, *Nature* **214** 456 (1967)

2:40. CR Robbins and KM Fermee, Some observations on the swelling of human epidermal membrane, *J Soc Cosm Chem* **34** 21-34 (1983)

2:41. JR Bond and BW Barry, Limitations of hairless mouse skin as a model for in vitro permeation studies for human skin: Hydration damage, *J Invest Dermatol* **90** 486-489 (1988)

2:42. RS Hinz, CD Hodson, CR Lorence and RH Guy, In vitro percutaneous penetration: Evaluation of the utility of hairless mouse skin, *J Invest Dermatol* **93** 87-91 (1989)

2:43. KV Roskos and RH Guy, Assessment of skin barrier function using transepidermal water loss: Effect of age, *Pharm Res* **6** 949-953 (1989)

2:44. RO Potts, Stratum corneum hydration: Experimental techniques and interpretation of results, *J Soc Cosm Chem* **37** 9-33 (1986)

2:45. RC Winter and HI Maibach, Influence of hydration on percutaneous absorption, Ch 18 in *Percutaneous Absorption*, RL Bronaugh and HI Maibach, eds, New York: Marcel Dekker (1985)

2:46. MM Breuer, The interaction between surfactants and keratinous tissues, *J Soc Cosm Chem* **30**, 41-64 (1979)

2:47. EJ Singer and EP Pittz, Interaction of surfactants with epidermal tissues: biochemical and toxicological aspects, Ch 6 in *Surfactants in Cosmetics*, MM Rieger, ed, New York: Marcel Dekker (1985)

2:48. IH Blank and E Gould, Penetration of anionic surfactants (surface active agents) into skin. I. Penetration of sodium laurate and sodium dodecyl sulfate into excised human skin, *J Invest Dermatol* **33** 327-336 (1959)

2:49. D Howes, The percutaneous absorption of some anionic surfactants, *J Soc Cosm Chem* **26** 47-63 (1975)

2:50. JA Faucher and ED Goddard, Interaction of keratinous substrates with sodium lauryl sulfate: I. Sorption, *J Soc Cosm Chem* **29** 323-337 (1978)

2:51. JA Faucher and ED Goddard, Interaction of keratinous substrates with sodium lauryl sulfate. II. Permeation through stratum corneum, *J Soc Cosm Chem* **29** 339-352 (1978)

2:52. LD Rhein, CR Robbins, K Fermee and R Cantore, Surfactant-structure effects on swelling of isolated human stratum corneum, *J Soc Cosm Chem* **37** 125-139 (1986)

2:53. U Zeidler, Der Einfluss des pH-Werts von Körperreinigungsmitteln auf die Hautquellung, Poster, 15th IFSCC Congress, London, 26-29 Sept (1988)

2:54. C Tondre, Interaction of poly(ethylene oxide) with sodium dodecyl sulfate micelles: a fast kinetic study by temperature jump, *J Phys Chem* **89** 5101-5106 (1985)

2:55. RB Kundsin and CW Walter, Investigation on adsorption of benzalkonium chloride USP by skin, gloves, and sponges, *Arch Surg Chicago* **75** 1036-1042 (1957)

2:56. JA Faucher and ED Goddard, Sorption of a cationic polymer by stratum corneum, *J Soc Cosm Chem* **27** 543-553 (1976)

2:57. GV Scott, CR Robbins, and JD Barnhurst, Sorption of quaternary ammonium surfactants by human hair, *J Soc Cosm Chem* **20** 135-152 (1969)

2:58. PP Sarpotdar and JL Zatz, Percutaneous absorption enhancement by nonionic surfactants, *Drug Develop Ind Pharm* **12** 1625-1647 (1986)

2:59. R Salzman, JE Manson, GT Griffing, R Kimmerle, N Ruderman, A McCall, El Stoltz, C Mullin, D Small, J Armstrong and JC Melby, Intranasal aerosolized insulin, mixed-meal studies and long-term use in type I diabetes, *New England J Med* **312** 1078-1084 (1985)

2:60. BW Barry, Mode of action of penetration enhancers in human skin, *J Contr Release* **6** 85-97 (1987)

2:61. GH Golden, JE McKie and RO Potts, Role of stratum corneum lipid fluidity in transdermal drug flux, *J Pharm Sci* **76** 25-28 (1987)

265

2:62. PK Wotton, B Mollgaard, J Hadgraft and A Hoelgaard, Vehicle effect on topical drug delivery. III. Effect of Azone on the cutaneous permeation of metronidazol and propylene glycol, *Int J Pharm* **2** 19-26 (1985)

2:63. KS Ryatt, JM Stevenson, HI Maibach and RH Guy, Pharmacodynamic measurements of percutaneous penetration enhancement in vivo, *J Pharm Sci* **75** 374-377 (1986)

2:64. VHW Mak, RO Potts and RH Guy, Percutaneous penetration enhancement in vivo measured by attenuated total reflectance infrared spectroscopy, *Pharm Res* **7** 835-841 (1990)

2:65. M Goodman and BW Barry, Lipid-Protein-Partitioning (LPP) theory of skin enhancer activity: Finite dose technique, *Int J Pharm* **57** 29-40 (1989)

2:66. H Sasaki, M Kojima, Y Mori, J Nakamura and J Shibasaki, Enhancing effect of pyrrolidone derivatives on transdermal penetration of 5-fluorouracil, triamcinolone acetonide, indomethacin and flurbiprofen, *J Pharm Sci* **80** 533-538 (1991)

2:67. B Berner, R-H Juang and GC Mazzenga, Ethanol and water sorption into stratum corneum and model systems, *J Pharm Sci* **78** 472-476 (1989); see also *J Pharm Sci* **78** 402-407 (1989)

2:68. SK Chandrasekaran, PS Campbell and AS Michaels, Effect of dimethylsulfoxide on drug permeation through human skin, *A I Ch E* **23** 810-816 (1977)

2:69. SG Elfbaum and K Laden, The effect of dimethylsulfoxide on percutaneous absorption: a mechanistic study. Part II, *J Soc Cosm Chem* **19** 841-847 (1968)

2:70. IH Blank and DJ McAuliffe, Penetration of benzene through human skin, *J Invest Dermatol* **85** 522-526 (1985)

2:71. SR Miselnicky, JL Lichtin, A Sakr and RL Bronaugh, The influence of solubility, protein binding, and percutaneous absorption on reservoir formation in skin, *J Soc Cosm Chem* **39** 169-177 (1988)

2:72. CFH Vickers, The role of the epidermis as a reservoir for topically applied agents, in *Progress in the Biological Sciences in Relation to Dermatology*, 2nd Ed, E Rook and RH Champion, eds, Cambridge: Cambridge University Press (1964)

2:73. AW McKenzie and RB Stoughton, Method of comparing percutaneous absorption of steroids, *Arch Dermatol* **86** 608-610 (1962)

2:74. CFH Vickers, Reservoir effect of human skin: Pharmacological speculation, in *Percutaneous Absorption of Steroids*, P. Mauvais-Jarvis, CFH Vickers and J Wepier, eds, New York: Academic Press (1980)

2:75. M Artuc, C Reinhold, G Stüttgen and J Gazith, A rapid method for measuring drug enrichment in epidermis, *Arch Dermatol Res* **268** 129-140 (1980)

2:76. A Zesch and H Schaefer, Penetration kinetics of four drugs in human skin, *Acta Dermatovenereol (Stockh)* **54** 91-98 (1974)

2:77. MI Foreman, I Clanachan and JP Kelly, The diffusion of nandrolone through occluded and non-occluded human skin, *J Pharm Pharmacol* **30** 152-157 (1978); see also *idem* *Brit J Dermatol* **108** 549-553 (1983)

2:78. MI Foreman and I Clanachan, Steroid diffusion and binding in human stratum corneum, *J Chem Soc, Farad Trans, I* **80** 3439-3444 (1984)

2:79. WS Watson and AY Finlay, The effect of vehicle formulation on the stratum corneum penetration characteristics of clobetasol 17-propionate in vivo, *Brit J Dermatol* **118** 523-530 (1988)

2:80. A Rougier, D Dupuis, C Lotte, R Roguet and H Schaefer, In vivo correlation between stratum corneum reservoir function and percutaneous absorption, *J Invest Dermatol* **81** 275-278 (1983)

2:81. D Dupuis, A Rougier, R Roguet, C Lotte and G Kalopissis, In vivo relationship between horny layer reservoir effect and percutaneous absorption in human and rat, *J Invest Dermatol* **82** 353-356 (1984)

2:82. A Rougier, D Dupuis, C Lotte and R Roguet, The measurement of the stratum corneum

266

reservoir. A predictive method for in vivo percutaneous absorption studies: Influence of application time, *J Invest Dermatol* **84** 66-68 (1985)

2:83. D Dupuis, A Rougier, R Roguet and C Lotte, The measurement of the stratum corneum reservoir: A simple method to predict the influence of vehicles on in vivo percutaneous absorption, *Brit J Dermatol* **115** 233-238 (1986)

2:84. A Rougier, C Lotte and HI Maibach, In vivo percutaneous penetration of some organic compounds related to anatomic site in humans: Predictive assessment by the stripping method, *J Pharm Sci* **76** 451-454 (1987); see also The hairless rat: A relevant animal model to predict in vivo percutaneous absorption in humans, *J Invest Dermatol* **88** 551-581 (1987)

2:85. A Rougier, C Lotte and D Dupuis, An original predictive method for in vivo percutaneous absorption studies, *J Soc Cosm Chem* **38** 397-417 (1987)

2:86. E Menczel, DAW Bucks, RC Wester and HI Maibach, Skin binding during percutaneous penetration, Ch 3 in *Percutaneous Absorption*, RL Bronaugh and HI Maibach, eds, New York: Marcel Dekker (1985)

2:87. SA Akhter and BW Barry, Absorption through human skin of ibuprofen and flurbiprofen; effect of dose variation, deposited drug film, occlusion and the penetration enhancer N-methyl-2-pyrrolidone, *J Pharm Pharmacol* **37** 27-37 (1985)

2:88. J Wepierre, M Corroller, D Dupuis, A Rougier and C Berrebi, In vivo cutaneous distribution of linoleic acid following topical application in the hairless rat *J Soc Cosm Chem* **37** 191-198 (1986)

2:89. RH Guy and HI Maibach, Drug delivery to local subcutaneous structures following topical administration, *J Pharm Sci* **72** 1375-1380 (1983)

2:90. DM Oakley and J Swarbrick, Effects of ionization on the percutaneous absorption of drugs: Partitioning of nicotine into organic liquids and hydrated stratum corneum, *J Pharm Sci* **76** 866-871 (1987)

2:91. RH Guy and J Hadgraft, Physicochemical aspects of percutaneous penetration and its enhancement, *Pharm Res* **5** 753-758 (1988)

2:92. Y Iwata, Y Moriya, and T Kobayashi, Percutaneous absorption of aliphatic compounds, *Cosm & Toil* **102** (11), 53-68 (1987)

2:93. HM Klimisch and G Chandra, Use of Fourier transform infrared spectroscopy with attenuated total reflectance for in vivo quantitation of polydimethylsiloxanes on human skin, *J Soc Cosm Chem* **37** 73-87 (1986)

2:94. LJ Murphy, Sorption of acyl lactylates by hair and skin as documented by radio tracer studies, *Cosm & Toil* **94** (3) 43-47 (1979)

2:95. RV Petersen, MS Kislalioglu, WQ Liang, SM Fang, M Emam and S Dickman, The athymic nude mouse grafted with human skin as a model for evaluating the safety and effectiveness of radiolabelled cosmetic ingredients, *J Soc Cosm Chem* **37** 249-265 (1986); see also LK Pershing and GG Krueger, Human skin sandwich flap model for predicting absorption, Ch 24 in *Percutaneous Absorption*, 2nd Edition, RL Bronaugh and HI Maibach, eds, New York: Marcel Dekker (1989)

2:96. F Wingen, C Gloxhuber and W Holtmann, Screening-Untersuchung zur Frage der Hautresorption von Kosmetikfarbstoffen: Parts I and II, *J Soc Cosm Chem* **34** 47-72 (1983)

2:97. U Hoppe and G Sauermann, Modern cosmetic agents: Evidence of their function, *H&G Z Hautkrankh* **65** (II), 123-131 (1990)

2:98. F Yackovich, NK Poulsen and JE Heinze, Validation of the agar patch test using soap bars which deposit different amounts of triclocarban, *J Soc Cosm Chem* **37** 99-104 (1986); see also *J Soc Cosm Chem* **36** 231-236 (1985)

2:99. E Eigen, A Legenyei and W Weiss, An in vivo method for the detection of residual antimicrobial activity on human skin *J Soc Cosm Chem* **26** 411-425 (1975)

2:100. T Rutherford and JG Black, The use of autoradiography to study the localization of germicides in skin, *Brit J Dermatol* **81**, Suppl 4, 74-86 (1969)

2:101. AF Kaul and JF Jewett, Agents and techniques for disinfection of the skin, *Surg Gynecol Obstet* **152** 677-685 (1981)

2:102. H North-Root, N Corbin and JL Demtrulias, Skin deposition and penetration of triclocarban, Ch 11 in *Percutaneous Absorption*, RL Bronaugh and HI Maibach, eds, New York: Marcel Dekker (1985)

2:103. H Schaefer and G Stüttgen, Absolute concentrations of an antimycotic agent, econazole, in the human skin after local application, *Arzneim-Forsch* **26** 429-435 (1976)

2:104. LH Jansen, T Hojyo, and AM Kligman, Improved fluoresence staining technique for estimating turnover of the human stratum corneum, *Brit J Dermatol* **90** 9-12 (1974)

2:105. M Takahashi, Y Machida and R Marks, Measurement of turnover times of stratum corneum using dansyl chloride fluorescence, *J Soc Cosm Chem* **38** 321-331 (1987)

2:106. S Nakagawa, H Ueki and K Tanioku, The distribution of 2,4-dinitrophenyl groups in guinea pig skin following surface application of 2,4-dinitrochlorobenzene: an immunofluorescent study, *J Invest Dermatol* **57** 269-277 (1971)

2:107. MH Samitz and SA Katz, Nickel-epidermal interactions: Diffusion and binding, *Environm Res* **11** 34-39 (1976)

2:108. A Fullerton, JR Andersen and A Hoelgaard, Permeation of nickel through human skin in vitro-effect of vehicles *Brit J Dermatol* **118** 509-516 (1988)

2:109. H Elling, Transkutane Penetration eines Mucopolysaccharidpolyschwefelsäureesters beim Menschen, *Arzneim-Forsch* **37** 212-213 (1987)

2:110. RD Griesemer, Biological factors affecting percutaneous absorption, *J Soc Cosm Chem* **11** 79-85 (1960)

2:111. IH Blank and RJ Scheuplein, The epidermal barrier in *Progress in the Biological Sciences in Relation to Dermatology*, A Rook and RH Champion, eds, 2nd ed, Cambridge: University Press (1964) p 245

2:112. B Idson, Biophysical factors in skin penetration, *J Soc Cosm Chem* **22** 615-634 (1971)

2:113. B Idson, Percutaneous absorption, *J Pharm Sci* **64** 901-924 (1975)

2:114. J Zatz, Percutaneous absorption, Chapter 4 in *Controlled Drug Availability*, v3, VR Smolen and WA Ball, eds, New York: John Wiley and Sons (1985)

2:115. JRJ Baker, RA Christian, P Simpson and AM White, The binding of topically applied glucocorticoids to rat skin, *Brit J Dermatol* **96** 171-178 (1977)

2:116. RC Wester and HI Maibach, Dermal decontamination and percutaneous absorption, Ch 20 in *Percutaneous Absorption*, 2nd ed, RL Bronaugh and HI Maibach, eds, New York: Marcel Dekker (1989)

Chapter 3

3:1. FD Malkinson and EH Ferguson, Percutaneous absorption of hydrocortisone-4-^{14}C in two subjects, *J Invest Dermatol* **25** 281 (1955)

3:2. FD Malkinson, EH Ferguson and MC Wang, Percutaneous absorption of cortisone-4-^{14}C through normal human skin, *J Invest Dermatol* **28** 211 (1957)

3:3. FD Malkinson, Studies on the percutaneous absorption of ^{14}C labelled steroids by use of the gas-flow cell, *J Invest Dermatol* **31** 19 (1958)

3:4. FD Malkinson and MB Kirschenbaum, Percutaneous absorption of C14-labelled triamcinolone acetonide, *Arch Dermatol* **88** 427 (1963)

3:5. RJ Feldmann and HI Maibach, Penetration of ^{14}C hydrocortisone through normal skin: The effect of stripping and occlusion, *Arch Dermatol* **91** 661 (1965)

3:6. RJ Feldmann and HI Maibach, Regional variation in percutaneous penetration of ^{14}C cortisol in man, *J Invest Dermatol* **48** 181 (1967)

3:7. RJ Feldmann and HI Maibach, Percutaneous penetration of steroids in man, *J Invest*

268

Dermatol **54** 399 (1969)

3:8. RJ Feldmann and HI Maibach, Absorption of some organic compounds through the skin in man, *J Invest Dermatol* **54** 399 (1969)

3:9. J Kao, FK Patterson and J Hall, Skin penetration and metabolism of topically applied chemicals in six mammalian species including man: An in-vitro study with benzo[a]pyrene and testosterone, *Toxicol Appl Pharmacol* **81** 502 (1985)

3:10. RO Potts, SC McNeill, CR Desbennet and E Wakshull, Transdermal drug transport and metabolism. II. The role of competing kinetic events, *Pharm Res* **6** 119 (1989)

3:11. RL Bronaugh, RF Stewart and JE Storm, Extent of cutaneous metabolism during percutaneous absorption of xenobiotics, *Toxicol Appl Pharmacol* **99** 534 (1989)

3:12. A Rougier and C Lotte, Correlation between horny layer concentration and percutaneous absorption, in *Pharmacology and the Skin, Skin Pharmacokinetics*, v 1, B Shroot and H Schaefer, eds, Basel, Switzerland: S Karger (1987) pp 81-102

3:13. HI Maibach, RJ Feldmann, TH Milby and WF Serat, Regional variation in percutaneous penetration in man, *Arch Environ Health* **23** 208 (1971)

3:14. RH Guy and HI Maibach, Calculations of body exposure from percutaneous absorption data, in *Percutaneous Absorption*, R Bronaugh and H Maibach, eds, New York: Marcel Dekker (1985) pp 461-466

3:15. TJ Franz, Percutaneous absorption of minoxidil in man, *Arch Dermatol* **121** 203 (1985)

3:16. DAW Bucks, HI Maibach and RH Guy, Percutaneous absorption of steroids: Effect of repeated application, *J Pharm Sci* **74** 1337 (1985)

3:17. CA Schlagel, EC Sanborn, The weights of topical preparations required for total and partial body inunction, *J Invest Dermatol* **42** 253 (1964)

3:18. TJ Franz, Kinetics of cutaneous drug penetration, *Int J Dermatol* **22** 499 (1983)

3:19. TJ Franz and PA Lehman, Systemic absorption of retinoic acid, *J Cut & Ocular Toxicol* **8** 517 (1989)

3:20. TJ Franz and PA Lehman, Percutaneous absorption of sulconazole nitrate in man, *J Pharm Sci* **77** 489 (1988)

3:21. TJ Franz, The finite dose technique as a valid in-vitro model for the study of percutaneous absorption in man, in *Skin: Drug Application and Evaluation of Environmental Hazards, Current Problems in Dermatology*, v7, G Simon, Z Paster, M Klingberg and M Kaye, eds, Basel, Switzerland: S Karger (1978) pp 58-68

3:22. MJ Bartek and JA LaBudde, Percutaneous absorption, in-vivo, in *Animal Models in Dermatology*, HI Maibach, ed, New York: Churchill-Livingstone (1975) pp 102-120

3:23. BK Jensen, BA McGann, V Kachevsky and TJ Franz, The negligible systemic availability of retinoids with multiple and excessive topical application of isotretinoin 0.05% (Isotrex) in acne, *J Amer Acad Dermatol* **24** 425 (1991)

3:24. T Chiang, Gas chromatographic-mass spectrometric assay for low levels of retinoic acid in human blood, *J Chromatog* **182** 335 (1980)

3:25. A Mizuchi, Y Miyachi, K Tamaki and A Kukita, Percutaneous absorption of betamethasone 17-benzoate measured by radioimmunoassay, *J Invest Dermatol* **67** 279 (1976)

3:26. DP West, JM Halket, DR Harvey, J Hadgraft, LM Solomon and JI Harper, Percutaneous absorption in preterm infants, *Ped Dermatol* **4** 234 (1987)

3:27. DAW Bucks, JR McMaster, HI Maibach and RH Guy, Bioavailability of topically administered steroids: A mass balance technique, *J Invest Dermatol* **91** 29 (1988)

3:28. W Schalla, JJ Jamoulle and H Schaefer, Localization of compounds in different skin layers and its use as an indicator of percutaneous absorption, in *Percutaneous Absorption, Mechanisms-Methodology-Drug Delivery*, 2nd Ed, RL Bronaugh, HI Maibach, Eds, New York: Marcel Dekker, Inc, (1989) pp283-312; Klingberg and M Kaye, eds, Basel, Switzerland: S Karger (1978) pp 80-94

3:29. US Nuclear Regulatory Commission, Title 10, Code of Federal Regulations, Part 20 (May 21, 1991)

3:30. International Commission on Radiological Protection, *Report of the Task Group on Reference Man*. Oxford: Pergamon Press, ICRP Publication 23 (1975)

3:31. National Council on Radiation Protection and Measurements. Recommendations on limits of exposure to "hot particle" on the skin. NCRP Scientific Committee 80-1, Draft, Rev 3 (June 1988)

3:32. International Commission on Radiological Protection, Recommendations of the ICRP, Oxford: Pergamon Press; ICRP Publication 26; *Ann ICRP* **1** 3 (1977)

3:33. E Konishi and Y Yoshizawa, Estimation of depth of basal layer of skin for radiation protection, *Rad Prot Dos* **11** 29 (1985)

3:34. Microshield, Ver 2.0, Washington Grove, MD: Grove Engineering Inc. (1985)

3:35. RJ Traub, WD Reece, RI Scherpelz and LA Sigalla, Dose calculation for contamination of the skin using the computer code VARSKIN, Springfield, VA: National Technical Information Service, NUREG/CR-44118 (PNL-5610) (1987)

3:36. EL McGuire and GV Dalrymple, Beta and electron dose calculations to skin due to contamination by common nuclear medicine radionuclides, *Health Physics* **58**:399 (1990)

3:37. R Loevinger and MA Berman, A schema for absorbed dose calculations for biologically distributed radionuclides, MIRD Pamphlet No 1, *J Nucl Med* (Supp 1) S48 (1989)

Chapter 4

4:1. TY Fan, U Goff, L Song, DH Fine, GP Arsenalt and K Biemann, N-Nitrosodiethanolamine in cosmetics, lotions and shampoos, *Fd Cosmet Toxicol* **15** 423 (1977)

4:2. RJ Scheuplein, Mechanism of percutaneous absorption I. Routes of penetration and the influence of solubility, *J Invest Dermatol* **45** 334 (1965)

4:3. TJ Franz, On the relevance of in vitro data, *J Invest Dermatol* **64** 190 (1975)

4:4. RL Bronaugh and RF Stewart, Methods for in vitro percutaneous absorption studies IV: the flow-through diffusion cell, *J Pharm Sci* **74** 64 (1985)

4:5. RL Bronaugh and HI Maibach, Percutaneous absorption of nitroaromatic compounds: In vivo and in vitro studies in the human and monkey, *J Invest Dermatol* **84** 180 (1985)

4:6. RL Bronaugh, RF Stewart, RC Wester, D Bucks, HI Maibach and J Anderson, Comparison of percutaneous absorption of fragrances by humans and monkeys, *Fd Chem Toxicol* **23** 111 (1985)

4:7. TS Spencer, JA Hill, RJ Feldmann and HI Maibach, Evaporation of diethyltoluamide from human skin in vivo and in vitro, *J Invest Dermatol* **72** 317 (1979)

4:8. WG Reifenrath and PB Robinson, In vitro skin evaporation and penetration characteristics of mosquito repellents, *J Pharm Sci* **71** 1014 (1982)

4:9. RL Bronaugh, ER Congdon and RJ Scheuplein, The effect of cosmetic vehicles on the penetration of N-nitrosodiethanolamine through excised human skin, *J Invest Dermatol* **76** 94 (1981)

4:10. Z Felsher, Studies on the adherence of the epidermis to the corium, *J Invest Dermatol* **8** 35 (1947)

4:11. RL Bronaugh and RF Stewart, Methods for in vitro percutaneous absorption studies III: Hydrophobic compounds, *J Pharm Sci* **73** 1255 (1984)

4:12. NF Wolejska and VR Usdin, Comparison of guinea pig and fetal hog skin, *J Soc Cosmet Chem* **30** 375 (1979)

4:13. HY Ando, A Escobar, RL Schnaare and ET Sugita, Skin potential changes in the guinea pig due to depilation and the repeated application of polyethylene glycol and retinoic acid, *J Soc Cosmet Chem* **34** 159 (1983)

4:14. J Kao, J Hall, LR Shugart and JM Holland, An in vitro approach to studying cutaneous metabolism and disposition of topically applied xenobiotics, *Tox Appl Pharmacol* **75** 289 (1984)

270

4:15. SW Collier, NM Sheikh, A Sakr, JL Lichtin, RF Stewart and RL Bronaugh, Maintenance of skin viability during in vitro percutaneous absorption/metabolism studies, Tox Appl Pharmacol 99 522 (1989)

4:16. RL Bronaugh, RF Stewart and JE Storm, Extent of cutaneous metabolism during percutaneous absorption of xenobiotics, Tox Appl Pharmacol 99 534 (1989)

4:17. RL Bronaugh, SW Collier, and RF Stewart, In vitro percutaneous absorption of a hydrophobic compound through viable hairless guinea pig skin, Toxicologist 9 61 (1989)

4:18. IH Blank, Penetration of low molecular weight alcohols I. Effect of concentration of alcohol and type of vehicle, J Invest Dermatol 43 415 (1964)

4:19. H Durrheim, GL Flynn, WI Higuchi and CR Behl, Permeation of hairless mouse skin I: Experimental methods and comparison with human epidermal permeation of alkanols, J Pharm Sci 69 781 (1980)

4:20. M Leider and CM Bunce, Physical dimensions of the skin: Determination of the specific gravity of skin, hair and nail, Arch Dermatol 69 563 (1954)

4:21. PR Bergstresser and JR Taylor, Epidermal 'turnover time'—a new examination, Br J Dermatol 96 503 (1977)

4:22. A Pannatier, P Jenner, B Testa and JC Etter, The skin as a drug-metabolizing organ, Drug Metab Rev 8 319 (1978)

4:23. PK Noonan and RC Wester, Cutaneous metabolism of xenobiotics, in PercutaneousAbsorption, RL Bronaugh and HI Maibach, eds, New York: Marcel Dekker (1978) p 65

4:24. AP Alvares, A Kappas, W Levin and AH Conney, Inducibility of benzo[a]pyrene in human skin by polycyclic hydrocarbons, Clin Pharmacol Therapeutics 14 30 (1978)

4:25. P Andersson, S Edsbäcker, Å Ryrfeldt and C Von Bahr, In vitro biotransformation of glucocorticoids in liver and skin homogenate fraction from man, rat and hairless mouse, J Steroid Biochem 16 787 (1982)

4:26. YW Cheung, A Li Wan Po and WJ Irwin, Cutaneous biotransformation as a parameter in the modulation of the activity of topical corticosteroids, Int J Pharmaceutics 26 175 (1985)

4:27. AP Kulkarni, JL Nelson and LL Radulovic, Partial purification and some biochemical properties of neonatal rat cutaneous glutathione S-transferases, Comp Biochem Physiol 87B 1005 (1987)

4:28. MW Coomes, AH Norling, RJ Pohl, D Müller and JR Fouts, Foreign compound metabolism by isolated skin cells from the hairless mouse, J Exp Pharmacol Therapeutics 225 770 (1983)

4:29. RR Warner, MC Myers and DA Taylor, Electron probe analysis of human skin: Element concentration profiles, J Invest Dermatol 90 78 (1988)

4:30. RR Warner, MC Myers and DA Taylor, Electron probe analysis of human skin: Determination of the water concentration profile, J Invest Dermatol 90 218 (1988)

4:31. RD Cohen and RA Iles, Intracellular pH: Measurement, control and metabolic interrelationships, CRC Crit Rev Clin Lab Sci 6 101 (1975)

4:32. J Kao, J Hall and JM Holland, Quantitation of cutaneous toxicity: An in vitro approach using skin organ culture, Toxicol Appl Pharmacol 68 206 (1983)

4:33. J Kao, FK Patterson and J Hall, Skin penetration and metabolism of topically applied chemicals in six mammalian species, including man: An in vitro study with benzo[a]pyrene and testosterone, Toxicol Appl Pharmacol 81 502 (1985)

4:34. J Paul, in Cell and Tissue Culture, Baltimore: Williams and Wilkins, Baltimore, (1961) p 1

4:35. H Blank, S Sagami, C Boyd and FJ Roth Jr, The pathogenesis of superficial fungus infections in cultured human skin, Arch Derm 79 524 (1959)

4:36. EP Reaven and AJ Cox, Organ culture and human skin, I Invest Dermatol 44 151 (1965)

4:37. RG Ham, Survival and growth requirements of nontransformed cells, in Handbook of Experimental Pharmacology; Tissue Growth Factors, v57, R Baserga, ed, New York: Springer-Verlag (1981) p 14

4:38. HE Swim, Nutrition of cells in culture–a review, in *Lipid Metabolism in Tissue Culture Cells*, GH Rothblat and D Kritchevsky, eds, Philadelphia: The Wistar Institute (1967) p 1

4:39. K Higuchi, Cultivation of animal cells in chemically defined media, a review, *Adv Appl Microbiol* **16** 111 (1973)

4:40. A Rizzino, H Rizzino and G Sato, Defined media and the determination of nutritional and hormonal requirements of mammalian cells in culture, *Nutr Rev* **37** 369 (1979)

4:41. D Barnes and G Sato, Serum-free cell culture: a unifying approach, *Cell* **22** 649 (1981)

4:42. R Dulbecco and G Freeman, Plaque production by the polyoma virus, *Virology* **8** 396 (1959)

4:43. JH Hanks and RD Wallace, Relation of oxygen and temperature in the preservation of tissues by refrigeration, *Proc Soc Exp Biol Med* **71** 196 (1949)

4:44. CW Boone, A surveillance procedure applied to sera, in *Tissue Culture: Methods and Applications*, P Kruze and M Patterson, eds, New York: Academic Press (1973) p 677

4:45. CD Yu, JL Fox, HFH Ho and WI Higuchi, Physical model evaluation of topical prodrug delivery—Simultaneous transport and bioconversion of vidarabine-5'-valerate II: Parameter determinations, *J Pharm Sci* **69** 1347 (1979)

4:46. H Bundgaard, A Hoelgaard and B Moligaard, Leaching of hydrolytic enzymes from human skin in cutaneous permeation studies as determined with metronidazole and 5-fluorouracil prodrugs, *Int J Pharm* **15** 285 (1983)

4:47. JE Storm, SW Collier, RF Stewart and RL Bronaugh, Metabolism of xenobiotics during percutaneous penetration: Role of absorption rate and cutaneous enzyme activity, *Fundam Appl Toxicol* **15** 132-141 (1990)

4:48. SW Collier, JE Storm, A Sakr, JL Lichtin and RL Bronaugh, The percutaneous absorption of azo colors, presented at the Society of Cosmetic Chemists Annual Scientific Meeting, New York, NY (December 1, 1988)

4:49. GE Burch and T Winsor, Rate of insensible perspiration locally through living and through dead skin, *Arch Intern Med* **74** 437 (1944)

4:50. TJ Franz, The finite dose technique as a valid in vitro model for the study of percutaneous absorption, *Curr Probl Dermatol* **7** 58 (1978)

4:51. RJ Feldmann and HI Maibach, Absorption of some organic compounds through the skin in man, *J Invest Dermatol* **54** 399 (1970)

4:52. DM Anjo, RJ Feldmann and HI Maibach, Methods for predicting percutaneous absorption in man, in *Percutaneous Absorption of Steroids,* P Mauvais-Jarvis, ed, London: Academic Press (1980) p 31

4:53. W Crutcher and HI Maibach, The effect of perfusion rate on in vitro percutaneous penetration, *J Invest Dermatol* **53** 264 (1969)

4:54. RL Bronaugh and TJ Franz, Vehicle effects on percutaneous absorption: In vivo and in vitro comparisons with human skin, *Br J Dermatol* **115** 1 (1986)

4:55. RL Bronaugh, RF Stewart and M Simon, Methods for in vitro percutaneous absorption studies VII: Use of excised human skin, *J Pharm Sci* **75** 1094 (1986)

4:56. H Tsuruta, Percutaneous absorption of organic solvents II. A method for measuring the penetration rate of chlorinated solvents through excised rat skin, *Ind Health* **15** 131 (1977)

4:57. RL Bronaugh, RF Stewart, ER Congdon and AL Giles Jr, Methods for in vitro percutaneous absorption studies I. Comparison with in vivo results, *Toxicol Appl Pharmacol* **62** 474 (1982)

4:58. M Ainsworth, Methods for measuring percutaneous absorption, *J Soc Cosmet Chem* **11** 69 (1960)

4:59. D Sekura and J Scala, The percutaneous absorption of alkylmethyl sulfoxides, in *Pharmacology and the Skin,* W Montagna, E VanScott and R Stoughton, eds, New York: Appleton-Century-Crofts (1972) p 257

4:60. NH Creasey, J Battensby and JA Fletcher, Factors affecting the permeability of skin,

272

Curr Probl Dermatol **7** 95 (1978)

4:61. RT Tregear, Molecular movement, the permeability of skin, *Physical Functions of Skin*, New York: Academic Press (1966) p 1

4:62. WG Reifenrath, EM Chellquist, EA Shipwash, WW Jederberg and GG Krueger, Percutaneous penetration in the hairless dog, weanling pig and grafted athymic nude mouse: evaluation of models for predicting skin penetration in man, *Br J Dermatol* (Supp 3) **27** 123 (1984)

4:63. RC Wester and HI Maibach, Percutaneous absorption in the Rhesus monkey compared to man, *Toxicol Appl Pharmacol* **32** 394 (1975)

4:64. RB Stoughton, Animal models for in vitro percutaneous absorption, in *Animal Models in Dermatology*, HI Maibach, ed, Edinburgh: Churchill Livingston (1975) p 121

4:65. RL Bronaugh, RF Stewart and ER Congdon, Methods for in vitro percutaneous absorption studies II. Animal models for human skin, *Toxicol Appl Pharmacol* **62** 481 (1982)

4:66. M Walker, PH Dugard and RC Scott, In vitro percutaneous absorption studies: A comparison of human and laboratory species, *Human Toxicol* **2** 561 (1983)

4:67. CR Behl, GL Flynn, EE Linn and WM Smith, Percutaneous absorption of corticosteroids: age, site and skin-sectioning influences on rate of permeation of hairless mouse skin by hydrocortisone, *J Pharm Sci* **13** 1287 (1984)

4:68. MI Foreman, I Clanachan and IP Kelly, Diffusion barriers in skin–a new method of comparison, *Br J Dermatol* **108** 549 (1983)

4:69. C Van Hooidonk, BI Ceulen, H Kienhuis and J Bock, Rate of skin penetration of organophosphates measured in diffusion cells, in *Mechanisms of Toxicity and Hazard Evaluation*, B Holmstedt, R Lauwerys, M Mercier and M Roberfroid, eds, Amsterdam: Elsevier/North Holland BiochemicalPress (1980) p 643

4:70. RL Bronaugh, RF Stewart and ER Congdon, Differences in permeability of rat skin related to sex and body site, *J Soc Cosmet Chem* **34** 127 (1983)

4:71. JB Knaak, K Yee, CR Ackennan, G Zwieg, DM Fry and BW Wilson, Percutaneous absorption and dermal dose-cholinesterase response studies with parathion and carbaryl in the rat, *Toxicol Appl Pharmacol* **76** 252 (1984)

4:72. RC Wester, PK Noonan and HI Maibach, Variations in percutaneous absorption of testosterone in the Rhesus monkey due to anatomic site of application and frequency of application, *Arch Dermatol Res* **267** 229 (1980)

4:73. RJ Feldmann and HI Maibach, Regional variation in percutaneous penetration of C_{14}-cortisol in man, *J Invest Dermatol* **48** 181 (1967)

4:74. CR Behl, GL Flynn, T Kurihara, N Harper, W Smith, WI Higuchi, NFH Ho and CL Pierson, Hydration and percutaneous absorption I. Influence of hydration on alkanol permeation through hairless mouse skin, *J Invest Dermatol* **75** 346 (1980)

4:75. HI Maibach, RJ Feldmann, TH Milby and WF Serat, Regional variation in percutaneous penetration in man: pesticides, *Arch Environ Health* **23** 208 (1971)

4:76. IH Blank, Further observations on factors which influence the water content of the stratum corneum, *J Invest Dermatol* **21** 259 (1953)

4:77. GL Flynn, H Durrheim and WI Higuchi, Permeation of hairless mouse skin II. Membrane sectioning techniques and influence on alkanol permeation, *J Pharm Sci* **70** 52 (1981)

4:78. Z Felsher and S Rothman, The insensible perspiration of the skin in hyperkeratotic conditions, *J Invest Dermatol* **6** 271 (1945)

4:79. MR Moore, PA Meredith, WS Watson, DJ Sumner, MK Taylor and A Goldberg, The percutaneous absorption of lead-203 in humans from cosmetic preparations containing lead acetate, as assessed by whole-body counting and other techniques, *Fd Cosmet Toxicol* **18** 399 (1980)

4:80. RL Bronaugh and RF Stewart, Methods for in vitro percutaneous absorption studies V. Permeation through damaged skin, *J Pharm Sci* **74** 1062 (1985)

4:81. ZT Chowan and R Pritchard, Effect of surfactants on percutaneous absorption of naproxin I. Comparisons of rabbit, rat and human excised skin, *J Pharm Sci* **67** 1272 (1978)

Chapter 5

5:1. NA Monteiro-Riviere, Comparative anatomy, physiology and biochemistry of mammalian skin, in *Dermal and Ocular Toxicology: Fundamentals and Methods*, DW Hobson, ed, Boca Raton, FL: CRC Press (1991) p 3

5:2. RJ Feldman and HI Maibach, Penetration of ^{14}C hydrocortisone through normal skin. The effect of stripping and occlusion, *Arch Dermatol* **91** 661 (1965)

5:3. RJ Scheuplein, Mechanism of percutaneous absorption. I. Routes of penetration and the influence of solubility, *J Invest Dermatol* **45** 334 (1965)

5:4. RJ Scheuplein, Mechanism of percutaneous absorption. II. Transient diffusion and the relative importance of various routes of skin permeation, *J Invest Dermatol* **48** 79 (1967)

5:5. GL Flynn, Mechanism of percutaneous absorption from physiochemical evidence, in *Percutaneous Absorption*, RL Bronaugh and HI Maibach, eds, New York: Marcel Dekker, Inc (1985) p 17

5:6. RC Scott, PH Dugard and AW Doss, Permeability of abnormal rat skin, *J Invest Derm* **86** 201 (1986)

5:7. KC Moon, RC Wester and HI Maibach, Diseased skin models in the hairless guinea pig: In vivo percutaneous absorption, *Dermatologica* **180** 8 (1990)

5:8. P Brisson, Percutaneous absorption, *CMA Journal* **110** 1182 (1974)

5:9. P Klemp and J Bojsen, Local variation in cutaneous and subcutaneous blood flow measured by CdTe(Cl) mini-detectors in normal and psoriatic skin, *J Invest Dermatol* **86** 109 (1986)

5:10. G Stuttgen, Drug absorption through intact and damaged skin, in *Dermal and Transdermal Absorption*, R Brandau and H Lippold, eds, Stuttgart: Wissenschaftliche Verlagsgesellschaft (1982) p 27

5:11. A Harpin and N Rutter, Barrier properties of the newborn infant's skin, *J Pediatr* **102** 419 (1983)

5:12. NJ Evans, N Rutter and J Hadgraft, Percutaneous administration of theophylline in the pre-term infant, *J Pediatr* **107** 307 (1985)

5:13. TJ Ryan, Cutaneous circulation, in *Biochemistry and Physiology of Skin*, vol 2, LA Goldsmith, ed, New York: Oxford University Press (1983) p 817

5:14. IM Braverman and A Keh-Yen, Ultrastructural abnormalities of the microvasculature and elastic fibers in the skin of juvenile diabetics, *J Invest Dermatol* **82** 1 (1984)

5:15. A Bollinger, J Frey, K Jager, J Furrer, J Seglias and W Siegenthaler, Patterns of diffusion through skin capillaries in patients with long-term diabetes, *New Engl J Med* **307** 1305 (1982)

5:16. MJ Bartek, JA LaBudde and HI Maibach, Skin permeability in vivo: Comparison in rat, rabbit, pig and man, *J Invest Dermatol* **58** 119 (1972)

5:17. RC Wester and HI Maibach, Animal models for percutaneous absorption, in *Models in Dermatology*, HI Maibach and NJ Lowe, eds, Basel: Karger (1985), p 159

5:18. WG Reifenrath, EM Chellquist, EA Shipwash, WW Jederberg and GG Kreuger, Percutaneous penetration in the hairless dog, weanling pig and grafted athymic nude mouse: Evaluation of models for predicting skin penetration in man, *Brit J Dermatol* **111** (Suppl 27), 123 (1984)

5:19. NA Monteiro-Riviere, DG Bristol, TO Manning, RA Rogers and JE Riviere, Interspecies and interregional analysis of the comparative histological thickness and laser Doppler blood flow measurements at five cutaneous sites in nine species, *J Invest Dermatol* **95** 582 (1990)

274

5:20. DE Wurtser and SF Kramer, Investigation of some factors influencing percutaneous absorption, *J Pharm Sci* **50** 288 (1961)

5:21. CR Behl, GL Flynn, T Kurihara, N Harper, H Smith, WI Higuchi, NFH Ho and C Pierson, Hydration and percutaneous absorption: I. Influence of hydration on alkanol permeation through hairless mouse skin, *J Invest Dermatol* **75** 346 (1980)

5:22. IH Blank, The effect of hydration on the permeability of skin, in *Percutaneous Absorption*, RL Bronaugh and HI Maibach, eds, New York: Marcel Dekker (1985) p 97

5:23. SK Chang and JE Riviere, Percutaneous absorption of parathion in vitro in porcine skin: Effects of dose, temperature, humidity, and perfusate composition on absorptive flux, *Fund Appl Toxicol* **17** 494 (1991)

5:24. A Danon, S Ben-Shimon and Z Ben-Zvi, Effect of exercise and heat exposure on percutaneous absorption of methylsalicylate, *Eur J Clin Pharmacol* **31** 49 (1986)

5:25. O Siddiqui, MS Roberts and AE Polack, Topical absorption of methotrexate: Role of dermal transport, *Int J Pharm* **27** 193 (1985)

5:26. LK Pershing, RL Conkling and GG Kreuger, Effects of reduced body temperature on blood flow and percutaneous absorption of ^{14}C benzoic acid across grafted nude rat skin, *Clin Res* **34** 418A (1986)

5:27. ZJ Wojciechowski, SA Burton, TJ Petelenze and GG Kreuger, Role of microcirculation in percutaneous absorption, *Clin Res* **33** 696A (1985)

5:28. JE Riviere, KJ Bowman, NA Monteiro-Riviere, MP Carver and LP Dix, The isolated perfused porcine skin flap (IPPSF) I. A novel in vitro model for percutaneous absorption and cutaneous toxicology studies, *Fund Appl Toxicol* **7** 444 (1986)

5:29. KF Bowman, NA Monteiro-Riviere and JE Riviere, Development of surgical techniques for preparation of in vitro isolated perfused porcine skin flaps for percutaneous absorption studies, *Am J Vet Res* **52** 75 (1991)

5:30. MP Carver, PL Williams and JE Riviere, The isolated perfused porcine skin flap. III. Percutaneous absorption pharmacokinetics of organophosphates, steroids, benzoic acid and caffeine, *Toxicol Appl Pharmacol* **97** 324 (1989)

5:31. PL Williams, MP Carver and JE Riviere, A physiologically relevant pharmacokinetic model of xenobiotic percutaneous absorption utilizing the isolated perfused porcine skin flap (IPPSF), *J Pharm Sci* **79** 305 (1990)

5:32. JE Riviere, B Sage and NA Monteiro-Riviere, Transdermal lidocaine iontophoresis in isolated perfused porcine skin, *Cutan Ocular Toxicol* **8** 493 (1989-90)

5:33. JE Riviere, B Sage and PL Williams, Effects of vasoactive drugs on transdermal lidocaine iontophoresis, *J Pharm Sci* **80** 615 (1991)

5:34. RB Stoughton and K Wullich, Relation of application time to bioactivity of a potent topical glucorticoid formulation, *J Am Acad Dermatol* **22** 1038 (1990)

5:35. KS Ryatt, JM Stevenson, HI Maibach and RH Guy, Pharmacodynamic measurement of percutaneous penetration enhancement in vivo, *J Pharm Sci* **75** 374 (1986)

5:36. PM Elias, Epidermal lipids, barrier functions and desquamation, *J Invest Dermatol* **80** 44 (1983)

5:37. RO Potts and ML Francoeur, The influence of stratum corneum morphology on water permeability, *J Invest Dermatol* **96** 495 (1991)

5:38. GM Golden, DB Guzek, RR Harris, JE McKie and RO Potts, Lipid thermotropic transitions in human stratum corneum, *J Invest Dermatol* **86** 255 (1986)

5:39. ML Williams and PM Elias, The extracellular matrix of stratum corneum: Role of lipids in normal and pathological function, *Crit Rev Ther Drug Carrier Syst* **3** 94 (1987)

5:40. C Prottey, Essential fatty acids and the skin, *Brit J Dermatol* **94** 579 (1976)

5:41. DR Bickers, H Mukhtar and SK Yang, Cutaneous metabolism of benzo(a)pyrene: Comparative studies in C57BL/GN and DBA/GN mice and neonatal Sprague-Dawley rats, *Chem Biol Interact* **43** 263 (1983)

5:42. J Kao, J Hall, LR Shugart and JM Holland, An in-vitro approach to studying cutaneous metabolism and disposition of topically-applied xenobiotics, *Toxicol Appl Pharmacol* **75** 289 (1984)

5:43. J Kao and J Hall, Skin absorption and cutaneous first-pass metabolism of topical steroids: In vitro studies with mouse skin in organ culture, *J Pharmacol Exp Therap* **241** 482 (1987)

5:44. RL Bronaugh, RF Stewart and JE Storm, Extent of cutaneous metabolism during percutaneous absorption of xenobiotics, *Toxicol Appl Pharmacol* **99** 534 (1989)

5:45. RO Potts, SC McNeill, CR Desbonnet and E Wakskull, Transdermal drug transport and metabolism II. The role of competing kinetic events, *Pharm Res* **6** 119 (1989)

5:46. MP Carver, P Levi and JE Riviere, Parathion metabolism during percutaneous absorption in perfused porcine skin, *Pesticide Biochem Physiol* **38** 245 (1990)

5:47. MP Carver, JE Riviere, Percutaneous absorption and excretion of xenobiotics after topical and intravenous administration to pigs, *Fund Appl Toxicol* **13** 714 (1989)

Chapter 6

6:1. L Gershenfeld and RE Miller, Ointment bases for bactericidal agents, *Amer J Pharm* **105** 194 (1933)

6:2. R Kadir, D Stempler, Z Liron and S Cohen, Delivery of theophylline into excised human skin from alkanoic acid solutions: a "push-pull" mechanism, *J Pharm Sci* **76** 774 (1987)

6:3. JL Zatz, Contact angles on human skin, *J Pharm Sci* **64** 1080 (1975)

6:4. ME Ginn, CM Noyes and E Jungermann, The contact angle of water on viable human skin, *J Colloid Interface Sci* **26** 146 (1968)

6:5. MM Rieger, Skin, water and moisturization, *Cosm & Toil* **104**(12) 41 (1989)

6:6. HLGM Tiemessen, HE Boddé and HE Junginger, A silicone membrane sandwich method to measure drug transport through isolated human stratum having a fixed water content, *Int J Pharm* **56** 87 (1989)

6:7. H Tsutsumi, T Utsugi and S Hayashi, Study on the occlusivity of oil films, *J Soc Cosm Chem* **30** 345 (1979)

6:8. T Higuchi, Physical chemical analysis of percutaneous absorption process from creams and ointments, *J Soc Cosm Chem* **11** 85 (1960)

6:9. JN Twist and JL Zatz, Influence of solvents on paraben permeation through idealized skin model membranes, *J Soc Cosm Chem* **37** 429 (1986)

6:10. BW Barry, O Fyrand, R Woodford, K Ulshagen and G Hogstad, Control of the bioavailability of a topical steroid; comparison of desonide creams 0.05% and 0.1% by vasoconstrictor studies and clinical trials, *Clin Exp Dermatol* **12** 406 (1987)

6:11. KB Sloan, The use of solubility parameters of drug and vehicle to describe skin transport, in *Topical Drug Delivery Formuations*, DW Osborne and AH Amann, eds, New York: Dekker (1990) p 245

6:12. JN Twist and JL Zatz, Membrane-solvent-solute interaction in a model permeation system, *J Pharm Sci* **77** 536 (1988)

6:13. JN Twist and JL Zatz, A model for alcohol-enhanced permeation through polydimethylsiloxane membranes, *J Pharm Sci* **79** 28 (1990)

6:14. JN Twist and JL Zatz, Interaction of vehicles with model skin membranes in the permeation process, *Percutaneous Absorption*, 2nd ed, R Bronaugh and H Maibach, eds, New York: Marcel Dekker (1989) p 147

6:15. JN Twist and JL Zatz, The effect of solvents on solute penetration through fuzzy rat skin, *J Soc Cosm Chem* **40** 231 (1989)

6:16. JL Zatz and UG Dalvi, Evaluation of solvent-skin interactions in percutaneous absorption, *J Soc Cosm Chem* **34** 327 (1983)

6:17. M Goodman and BW Barry, Action of penetration enhancers on human skin as assessed

276

by the permeation of model drugs 5-fluorouracil and estradiol. I. Infinite dose technique, *J Invest Dermatol* **91** 323 (1988)

6:18. JJ Windheuser, JL Haslam, L Caldwell and RD Shaffer, The use of N,N-dimethyl-m-toluamide to enhance dermal and transdermal delivery of drugs, *J Pharm Sci* **71** 1211 (1982)

6:19. MS Roberts and RA Anderson, The percutaneious absorption of phenolic compounds: the effect of vehicles on the penetration of phenol, *J Pharm Pharmacol* **27** 599 (1975)

6:20. MR Rahman and JL Zatz, to be published

6:21. B Mollgaard and A Hoelgaard, Permeation of estradiol through the skin effect of vehicles, *Int J Pharm* **15** 185 (1983)

6:22. B Mollgaard and A Hoelgaard, Vehicle effect on topical drug delivery. II. Concurrent skin transport of drugs and vehicle components, *Acta Pharm Suec* **20** 443 (1983)

6:23. MF Coldman, BJ Poulsen and T Higuchi, Enhancement of percutaneous absorption by the use of volatile/nonvolatile systems as vehicles, *J Pharm Sci* **58** 1098 (1969)

6:24. T Kurihara-Bergstrom, GL Flynn and WI Higuchi, Physicochemical study of percutaneousabsorption enhancement by dimethyl sulfoxide: Kinetic and thermodynamic determinants of dimethyl sulfoxide mediated mass transfer of alkanols, *J Pharm Sci* **75** 479 (1986)

6:25. BW Barry, Action of skin penetration enhancers—the lipid protein partitioning theory, *Int J Cosmet Sci* **10** 281 (1988)

6:26. HH Sharate and RR Burnette, Effect of dipolar aprotic permeability enhancers on the basal stratum corneum, *J Pharm Sci* **77** 27 (1988)

6:27. HE Bodde, MAM Kruithof, J Brussee and HK Koerten, Visualization of normal and enhanced $HgCl_2$ transport through human skin in vitro, *Int J Pharm* **53** 13 (1989)

6:28. T Kai, VHW Mak, RO Potts and RH Guy, Mechanism of percutaneous penetration enhancement: effect of n-alkanols on the permeability barrier of hairless mouse skin, *J Controlled Release* **12** 103 (1990)

6:29. LK Pershing, LD Lambert and K Knutson, Mechanism of ethanol-enhanced estradiol permeation across human skin in vivo, *Pharm Res* **7** 170 (1990)

6:30. T Kurihara-Bergstrom, K Knutson, LJ DeNoble and CY Goates, Percutaneous absorption enhancement of an ionic molecule by ethanol-water systems in human skin, *Pharm Res* **7** 762 (1990)

6:31. P Liu, WI Higuchi, W Song, T Kurihara-Bergstrom and WR Good, Quantitative evaluation of ethanol effects on diffusion and metabolism of β-estradiol in hairless mouse skin, *Pharm Res* **8** 865 (1991)

6:32. P Liu, T Kurihara-Bergstrom and WR Good, Cotransport of estradiol and ethanol through human skin in vitro: understanding the permeant/enhancer flux relationship, *Pharm Res* **8** 938 (1991)

6:33. J Rojas, F Falson, G Couarraze, A Francis and F Puisieux, Optimization of binary and ternary solvent systems in the percutaneous absorption of morphine base, *STP Pharma Sci* **1** 70 (1991)

6:34. PP Sarpotdar and JL Zatz, Evaluation of penetration enhancement of lidocaine by nonionic surfactants through hairless mouse skin in vitro, *J Pharm Sci* **75** 176 (1986)

6:35. H Okamato, K Muta, M Hashida and H Sezaki, Percutaneous penetration of acyclovir through excised hairless mouse and rat skin: effect of vehicle and percutaneous penetration enhancer, *Pharm Res* **7** 64 (1990)

6:36. BJ Aungst, JA Blake, NJ Rogers and MA Hussain, Transdermal oxymorphone formulation development and methods for evaluating flux and lag times for two skin permeation-enhancing vehicles, *J Pharm Sci* **79** 1072 (1990) 5

6:37. ML Francoer, GM Golden and RO Potts, Oleic acid: its effects on stratum corneum in relation to (trans)dermal drug delivery, *Pharm Res* **7** 621 (1990)

Chapter 7

7:1. JL Zatz, Modification of skin permeation by solvents, *Cosm & Toil* **106**(2) 91 (1991)

7:2. KA Walters, Penetration enhancers and their use in transdermal therapeutic systems, *Transdermal Drug Delivery* J Hadgraft and RH Guy, eds, New York: Dekker (1989) p 197

7:3. T Nishiyama, Y Iwata, K Nakajima and T Mitsui, In vivo percutaneous absorption of polyoxyethylene lauryl ether surfactants in hairless mice *J Soc Cosmet Chem* **34** 263 (1983)

7:4. UG Dalvi and JL Zatz, Effect of nonionic surfactants on penetration of dissolved benzocaine through hairless mouse skin, *J Soc Cosmet Chem* **32** 87 (1981)

7:5. UG Dalvi and JL Zatz, Effect of skin binding on percutaneous transport of benzocaine from aqueous suspensions and solutions *J Pharm Sci* **71** 824 (1982)

7:6. PP Sarpotdar and JL Zatz, Evaluation of penetration enhancement of lidocaine by nonionic surfactants through hairless mouse skin in vitro *J Pharm Sci* **75** 176 (1986)

7:7. PP Sarpotdar and JL Zatz, Percutaneous absorption enhancement by nonionic surfactants *Drug Dev Ind Pharm* **12** 1625 (1986)

7:8. R Kadir, D Stempler, Z Liron and S Cohen, Penetration of theophylline and adenosine into excised human skin from binary and ternary vehicle: effect of a nonionic surfactant *J Pharm Sci* **78** 149 (1989)

7:9. ER Cooper, Increased skin permeability for lipophilic molecules *J Pharm Sci* **73** 1153 (1984)

7:10. RO Potts, GM Golden, ML Francoeur, VHW Mak and R Guy, Mechanism and enhancement of solute transport across the stratum corneum *J Controlled Rel* **15** 249 (1991)

7:11. G M Golden, J E McKie and R O Potts, Role of stratum corneum lipid fluidity in transdermal drug flux, *J Pharm Sci* **76**(25) 149 (1987)

7:12. B Ongpipattanakul, RR Burnette, RO Potts and ML Francoeur, Evidence that oleic acid exists in a separate phase within stratum corneum lipids *Pharm Res* **8** 350 (1991)

7:13. BJ Aungst, JA Blake and MA Hussain, Contributions of drug solubilization, partitioning, barrier disruption and solvent permeation to the enhancement of skin permeation of various compounds with fatty acids and amines *Pharm Res* **7** 712 (1990)

7:14. H Okamato, K Muta, M Hashida and H Sezaki, Percutaneous penetration of acyclovir through excised hairless mouse and rat skin: effect of vehicle and percutaneous penetration enhancer *Pharm Res* **7** 64 (1990)

7:15. H Okamoto, M Hashida and H Sezaki, Effect of 1-alkyl- or 1-alkenylazacycloalkanone derivatives on the penetration of drugs with different lipophilicities through guinea pig skin *J Pharm Sci* **80** 39 (1991)

7:16. J A Bouwstra, LJC Peschier, J Brussee and HE Boddé, Effect of N-alkyl-azacycloheptan-2-ones including Azone on the thermal behavior of human stratum corneum *Int J Pharm* **52** 47 (1989)

7:17. HE Boddé, HLGM Tiemessen, H Mollee, FHN de Haan and HE Junginger, Modeling percutaneous drug transport in vitro: the interplay between water, flux enhancers and skin lipids, *Prediction of Percutaneous Penetration*, RC Scott, RH Guy and J Hadgraft, eds, London: IBC Technical Services (1990) p 93

7:18. E Touitou, Skin permeation enhancement by N-decyl methyl sulfoxide: effect of solvent systems and insights on mechanism of action *Int J Pharm* **43** 1 (1988)

7:19. BW Barry and SL Bennett, Effect of penetration enhancers on the permeation of mannitol, hydrocortisone and progesterone through human skin *J Pharm Pharmacol* **39** 535 (1987)

7:20. DD-S Tang-Liu, J Neff, H Zolezio and R Sandri, Percutaneous and systemic disposition of hexamethylene lauramide and its penetration enhancement effect on hydrocortisone in a rat sandwich skin-flap model *Pharm Res* **5** 477 (1988)

7:21. D Quan, K Takayama, T Mitsuzono, K Isowa and T Nagai, Influence of novel percutaneous absorption enhancers, cyclohexanone and piperidone derivatives, on histopathology of rat skin *Int J Pharm* **68** 239 (1991)

7:22. G Ridout, RS Hinz, JJ Hostynek, AK Reddy, RJ Wiersema, CD Hodson, CR Lorence and RH Guy, The effects of zwitterionic surfactants on skin barrier function *Fund Appl Toxicol* **16** 41 (1991)

7:23. M Takahashi, M Aizawa, K Miyazawa and Y Machida, "Effects of surface active agents on stratum corneum cell cohesion," *J Soc Cosmet Chem* **38** 21 (1987)

7:24. JG Black and D Howes, Absorption, metabolism and excretion of anionic surfactants *Anionic Surfactants. Biochemistry, Toxicology, Dermatology* C Gloxhumber, ed, New York: Dekker (1980) p 51

7:25. FR Bettley, "The irritant effect of soap in relation to epidermal permeability," *Brit J Dermatol* **75** 113 (1963)

7:26. PH Dugard and RJ Scheuplein, "Effects of ionic surfactants on the permeability of human epidermis: an electrometric study," *J Invest Dermatol* **60** 263 (1973)

7:27. ZT Chowhan and R Pritchard, "Effect of surfactants on percutaneous absorption of naproxen. I. Comparisons of rabbit, rat and human excised skin," *J Pharm Sci* **67** 1272 (1978)

7:28. RJ Scheuplein and L Ross, Effects of surfactants and solvents on the permeability of epidermis, *J Soc Cosmet Chem* **21** 853 (1970)

7:29. LD Rhein, CR Robbins, K Fernee and R Cantore, Surfactant structure effects on swelling of isolated human stratum corneum *J Soc Cosmet Chem* **37** 125 (1986)

7:30. M Lodén, The simultaneous penetration of water and sodium lauryl sulfate through isolated human skin *J Soc Cosmet Chem* **41** 227 (1990)

7:31. J Hirvonen, JH Rytting, P Paronen and A Urtti, Dodecyl N,N-dimethylamino acetate and Azone enhance drug penetration across human, snake and rabbit skin *Pharm Res* **8** 933 (1991)

7:32. GP Kushla and JL Zatz, "Correlation of Water and Lidocaine Flux Enhancement by Cationic Surfactants In Vitro *J Pharm Sci* **80** 1079 (1991)

Chapter 8

8:1. *Webster's New World Dictionary* of The American Language by William Collins Publishers, Inc., 1979

8:2. *Physician's Desk Reference*, 39th Edition, Medical Economics, Oradell, NJ, p. 403-446, 1985

8:3. H Gray, *Anatomy of The Human Body*, 28th edition, CM Goss, ed, Philadelphia: Lea & Febiger (1970) p. 1105

8:4. IH Blank and RJ Scheuplein, Transport Into and Within the Skin, *Br J Dermatol* **81** 4 (1969)

8:5. CR Behl, GL Glynn, T Kurihara, WM Smith, NH Bellantone, O Gatmaitan, WI Higuchi, NH Ho and CL Pierson, Age and Anatomical Site Influences on Alkanol Permeation of Skin of the Male Hairless Mouse, *J Soc Cosmet Chem* **35** 237 (1984)

8:6. DS Greene, Preformulation in *Modern Pharmaceutics,* GS Banker and CT Rhodes, eds, Marcel Dekker, NY p. 211 (1979)

8:7. T Higuchi, Physical-Chemical Analysis of the Percutaneous Absorption Process From Creams and Ointments, *J Soc Cosmet Chem* **11** 85 (1960)

8:8. CS Chandrasekaran, AS Michaels, PS Campbell and JE Shaw, Scopolamine Permeation Through Human Skin In Vitro, *AIChE Journal* **22** 828 (1976)

8:9. BJ Poulsen, Design of Topical Drug Products: Biopharmaceutics, in *Drug Design* vol 4, EJ Ariens, ed, New York and London: Academic Press pp 149-192 (1973)

8:10. MF Coldman, BJ Poulsen and T Higuchi, Enhancement of percutaneous absorption by the use of volatile/nonvolatile systems as vehicles, *J Pharm Sci* **58** 1098 (1969)

8:11. TJ Franz, Percutaneous absorption: On the relevance of in vitro data, *J Invest Dermatol* **64** 190 (1975)

8:12. ER Cooper and D Patel in *Skin Permeation,* J Zatz, ed, New York, Marcel Dekker (1986)

8:13. JL Zatz, Factors in percutaneous absorption, *CTFA Cos J* **15** 6 (1983)

8:14. BW Barry, Basic principles of diffusion through membranes in *Dermatological Formulations,* Marcel Dekker, Basel and New York, pp 49-233 (1983)

8:15. J Hadgraft, JW Hadgraft and I Sarkany, The effect of thermodynamic activity on the percutaneous absorption of methyl nicotinate from water/glycerol mixtures, *J Pharm Pharmacol* **25** 122 (1973)

8:16. WI Higuchi, Analysis of data on medicament release from ointments, *J Pharm Sci* **52** 802 (1962)

8:17. JW Ayers and PA Laskar, Diffusion of benzocaine from ointment bases, *J Pharm Sci* **63** 1402 (1974)

8:18. NF Billups and NK Patel, Experiments in physical pharmacy. V. In vitro release of medicament from ointment bases, *Am J Pharm Educ* **34** 190 (1970)

8:19. BJ Poulsen, E Young, V Coquilla and M Katz, Effect of topical vehicle composition on the in vitro release of fluocinolone acetonide and its acetate ester, *J Pharm Sci* **57** 928 (1968)

8:20. J Ostrenga, J Halesblian, BJ Poulsen, B Ferrel, N Mueller and S Shastri, Vehicle design for a new topical steroid, fluocinonide, *J Inv Dermatol* **56** 392 (1971)

8:21. J Ostrenga, C Steinmetz and BJ Poulsen, Significance of vehicle composition I: Relationship between topical vehicle composition, skin penetrability, and clinical efficacy, *J Pharm Sci* **60** 1175 (1971)

8:22. BW Barry and AR Brace, Permeation of aestrone, aestradiol, aestriol and dexamethasone across cellulose acetate membrane, *J Pharm Pharmacol* **29** 397 (1977)

8:23. M Tanaka, H Fukuda and T Naai, Permeation of drugs through a model membrane consisting of millipoore filter with oil, *Chem Pharm Bull,* **26** 9 (1978)

8:24. ZT Chowhan, R Pritchard WH Rooks II and A tomolonis, Effect of surfactants on the percutaneous absorption of naproxen II: In vivo and In vitro correlation in rats, *J Pharm Sci* **67** 1645 (1978)

8:25. AJ Aguiar and MA Weiner, Percutaneous absorption studies of chloramphenicol solutions, *J Pharm Sci* **58** 210 (1969)

8:26. AS Michaels, SK Chandrasekaran, JE Shaw, Drug permeation through human skin: theory and in vitro experimental measurement, *AIChE Journal* **21** 985 (1975)

8:27. R Bronaugh in *Skin Permeation,* J Zatz, ed, Marcel Dekker, New York (1986)

8:28. EM Chellquist, WG Reifeurath, EA Shipwash and WW Jederberg, Animal models for determining percutaneous absorption of chemicals, *Abstracts of the 35th Annual Meeting Acad Pharm Sci,* Miami Beach, Florida (November, 1983)

8:29. U Rohr, Z Wojciechowski, S Burton, WI Higuchi, JL Fox and GG Krueger, Comparison of in vivo and in vitro diffusion and metabolism of vidarabine using a unique isolation skin flap model, *Abstracts of the 37th National Meeting Acad Pharm Sci,* Philadelphia, Pennsylvania (November, 1984)

8:30. G Tonelli, L Thibault, I Ringer, A bio-assay for the comcomitant assessment of the antiphlogistic and thymolytic activities of topically applied corticoids, *Endocrinology* **77** 625 (1965)

8:31. E Drouhet, D Dompmartin, A Parachriston-Moraiti, Experimental dermatitis from pityrosporum-ovalae and/or pityrosporum-orbiculare in guinea pigs, *Bull de la société Française de Mycologie Med* **6** 167 (1977)

8:32. CJE Niemegeers, FJ Verbruggen and PAJ Janssen, Effect of various drugs on

280

carageenin-induced edema in the rat hind paw, *J Pharm Pharmacol* **16** 810 (1964)

8:33. A Robert and JE Nezamis, The granuloma pouch as a routine assay for antiphlogistic compounds, *Acta Endocrinol* **25** 105 (1957)

8:34. C Biachi and A Daird, Analgesic properties of 4-ethoxycarbonyl-1-(2-hydroxy-3-phenoxypropyl) 4-phenylpiperidine (BDH 200) and some related compounds, *J Pharm Pharmacol* **12** 449 (1960)

8:35. OH Mills, Jr. and AM Kligman, Assay of comedolytic agents in the rabbit ear, *Animal Models in Dermatology*, H Maibach, ed, New York and Edinburgh, London: Churchill Livingstone p 177 (1975)

8:36. PE Pochi, Sebaceous gland assay, *Animal Models in Dermatology*, H Maibach, ed, New York and Edinburgh, London: Churchill Livingstone p 184 (1975)

8:37. JA Mezick, MC Bhatia, LM Shea, EG Thorne and RJ Capetola, Anti-acne activity of retinoids in the rhino mouse, *Models in Dermatology 2*, H Maibach and NJ Lowe, eds, Basel: Karger p 59 (1985)

8:38. D Lobenberg, R Parmegiani, B Antonacci, T Yarosh-Tomaine, D Raue, JJ Wright and GH Miller, Sch 31153 a novel broad-spectrum antifungal agent, *Abstracts of the Twenty-Second Interscience Conference on Antimicrobial Agents and Chemotherapy No. 474* p 149 (1982)

8:39. H Schaefer, A Zesch and G Stuttgen, Penetration, permeation, and absorption of triamcinolone acetonide in normal and psoriatic skin, *Arch Dermatol* **258** 241 (1977)

8:40. AW McKenzie and RB Stoughton, Method for comparing percutaneous absorption of steroids, *Arch Dermatol* **86** 608 (1962)

8:41. RBP Burns and MV Shelanski, Histamine wheal and flare inhibition by clemastine fumarate, *Ann Allergy* **38** 339 (1977)

8:42. OH Mills and AM Kligman, A human model for assaying comedolytic substances, *Br J Dermatol* **107** 543 (1982)

8:43. RC Cornell and RB Stoughton, The use of topical steroids in psoriasis, *Dermatol Clin 2*, 397 (1984)

8:44. RC Cornell and RB Stoughton, Correlation of the vasoconstrictor assay and clinical in psoriasis, *Arch Dermatol* **121** 63 (1985)

8:45. L Lachman, HA Lieberman and JL Kanig, Kinetic principle and stability testing, *The Theory and Practice of Industrial Pharmacy*, 2nd ed, Lea & Febiger, Philadelphia, P 32-77 (1976)

8:46. AJ Woolfe and HEC Worthington, The determination of product expiry dates from short term storage at room temperature, *Drug Develop Comm*, **1** 185 (1974-75).

8:47. *Animal Models in Dermatology, Relevance to Human Dermatopharmacology and Dermatotoxicology,* H Maibach, ed, Edinburgh, London and New York, Churchill Livingstone, (1975)

8:48. *Models in Dermatology, Part I, Dermatology and Part II, Dermatopharmacology and Toxicology,* H Maibach and NJ Lowe, eds, Basel, Karger (1985)

8:49. S Nacht, J Close, D Yeung and EH Gans, Skin friction coefficient: changes induced by skin hydration and emollient application and correlation with perceived skin feel, *J Soc Cosmet Chem* **32** 55 (1981)

8:50. BW Barry and MC Meyer, Sensory assessment of spreadability of hydrophilic topical preparations, *J Pharm Sci* **62** 1349 (1973)

8:51. BW Barry, Continuous shear viscoelastic and spreading properties of a new topical vehicle, FAPG Base, *J Pharm Pharmacol* **25** 131 (1973)

Chapter 9

9:1. EM Jackson, Percutaneous absorption: scientific basis for new products or concern for safety, presented at the 38th International CIDESCO Conference, New York, NY (August 20, 1984)

9:2. FD Malkinson and L Gehlman, Factors affecting percutaneous absorption, in *Cutaneous Toxicity*, VA Drill and P Lazar, eds, New York: Academic Press (1977)

9:3. AH McCreesh, Percutaneous toxicity, *Toxicol Appl Pharmacol Suppl* **2** 20, 1965

9:4. RT Tregar, *Physical Functions of Skin*, New York: Academic Press (1966)

9:5. FN Marzulli, DWC Brown, et al, Techniques for studying skin penetration, *Toxicol Appl Pharmacol Suppl* **3** 76, 1969

9:6. DR Bickers, The skin as a site of drug and chemical metabolism, in *Cutaneous Toxicity*, VA Drill and P Lazar, eds, New York: Academic Press (1980)

9:7. BW Barry, Structure, Function, Diseases and Topical Treatment of Human Skin, Ch 1 in *Dermatological Formulations: Percutaneous Absorption*, New York: Marcel Dekker, Inc (1983)

9:8. RJ Scheuplein and RL Bronaugh, Percutaneous absorption, Ch 58 in *Biochemistry and Physiology of the Skin*, LA Goldsmith, ed, New York: Oxford University Press (1983)

9:9. C Benezra and G Dupuis, The concept of carrier in ACD, Ch 4 in *Allergic Contact Dermatitis to Simple Chemicals: A Molecular Approach*, New York: Marcel Dekker, Inc (1982)

9:10. EM Jackson, The cellular and molecular events of inflammation, *J Toxicol Cut & Ocular Tox* **3**(4) 347 (1984)

9:11. CR Robbins and KM Fernee, Some observations on the swelling of human epidermal membrane, *J Soc Cos Chem* **34** 21 (1983)

9:12. E Cronin and RB Stoughton, Percutaneous absorption, regional variations and the effect of hydration and epidermal stripping, *Br J Dermatol* **74** 265 (1962)

9:13. FD Malkinson, Permeating of the stratum corneum, Ch XXI in *Epidermis*, W Montagna and WC Lobitz, Jr, eds, New York: Academic Press (1964)

9:14. WC Fritsch and RB Stoughton, The effect of temperature and humidity on the penetration of C^{14} acetylsalicylic acid in excised human skin, *J Invest Dermatol* **41** 307 (1963)

9:15. RB Stoughton and WC Fritsch, Influence of dimethyl sulfoxide (DMSO) on human percutaneous absorption, *Arch Dermatol* **90** 512 (1964)

9:16. R. Bronaugh, RF Stewart et al, Comparison of percutaneous absorptions of fragrances by humans and monkeys, *Fd Chem Toxic* **23**(1) 111 (1985)

9:17. External analgesic drug products or over-the-counter human use; Establishment of a monograph and notice of proposed rule making, *Fed Reg* **44** (234) 69768, December 4, 1979

9:18. DA Wiegrand, C Haygood et al, *Racial Variations in the Cutaneous Barrier, in Cutaneous Toxicity*, VA Drill and P Lazar, eds, New York: Academic Press (1980)

9:19. JG Black and D Howes, In penetration of chemically related detergents, *J Soc Cos Chem* **30** 157 (1979)

9:20. BW Barry, Formulation of dermatological vehicles, Ch 6 in *Dermatological Formulations: Percutaneous Absorption*, New York: Marcel Dekker, Inc (1983)

9:21. *Code of Federal Regulations* **21** 720.1(c), Cosmetic product categories

9:22. EM Jackson, Industrial safety testing practices, Ch 5 in *Alternative Methods in Toxicology: Product Safety Evaluation*, AM Goldberg, ed, New York: Mary Ann Leibert, Inc (1983)

9:23. EJ Franz, Percutaneous absorption of minoxidil in man, *Arch Dermatol* **121**(2) 203 (1985)

9:24. EP Pittz, Skin barrier function and use of cosmetics, *Cos & Toil* **99**(12) 30 (1984)

9:25. EM Jackson, Percutaneous absorption: Safety considerations, presented at the Annual Scientific Conference of the Cosmetic, Toiletry and Fragrance Association (CTFA) Washington DC (October 25, 1983)

9:26. RB Stoughton and WO McClure, Azone™ enhances percutaneous absorption, presented at the 41st Meeting of the American Academy of Dermatology, New Orleans, LA (December 4-9, 1982)

282

9:27. BW Barry, Properties that influence percutaneous absorption, Ch 4 in *Dermatological Formulations: Percutaneous Absorption*, New York: Marcel Dekker, Inc (1983)

9:28. S Athanaselis, S Qammaz et al, Percutaneous paraquat intoxication, *J Toxicol Cut & Ocular Toxicol* **2**(1) 3 (1983)

9:29. TB Hart, On percutaneous paraquat intoxication, *J Toxicol Cut & Ocular Toxicol* **3**(3) 239 (1984)

9:30. T Shibamato and S Mihara, Photochemistry of fragrance materials I. unsaturated compounds, *J Toxicol Cut & Ocular Toxicol* **2**(2&3) 153 (1983)

9:31. T Shibamato, Photochemistry of fragrance materials II. Aeromatic compounds and phototoxicity, *J Toxicol Cut & Ocular Toxicol* **2**(4&5) 267 (1983)

9:32. PS Spencer, AB Sterman et al, Neurotoxic changes in rats exposed to the fragrance compound acetyl ethyl tetramethyl tetralin, *Neurotoxicology* **1** 221 (1979)

9:33. PS Spencer, AB Sterman et al, Neurotoxic fragrance produces ceroid and myelin disease, *Science* **204**(204) 633 (1979)

9:34. KH Kaidbey and AM Kligman, Photocontact allergy to 6-methylcoumarin, *Contact Derm* **4** 277 (1978)

9:35. DLJ Opdyke, The structure activity relationships of some substituted coumarins with respect to skin reactions, *Dragoco Report* **2** 43 (1981)

9:36. IE Kochevar, GL Zalar et al, Assay of contact photosensitivity to musk ambrette in guinea pigs, *J Invest Dermatol* **73** 144 (1979)

9:37. VJ Giovinnazo, LC Harber et al, Photoallergic contact dermatitis to musk ambrette, *J Am Acad Derm* **3**(4) 384 (1984)

9:38. E Cronin, Photosensitivity to musk ambrette, *Contact Derm* **11** 88 (1984)

9:39. R Suskind and V Majeti, Occupational and environmental allergic problems of the skin, *J Dermatol* **3** 3 (1976)

9:40. DLJ Opdyke, Inhibition of sensitization reactions induced by certain aldehydes, *Fd Chem Toxicol* **14** 197 (1976)

9:41. RL Goldemberg, Quenching sensitization potential, *Skin Allergy News*, **7**(9) 1976

9:42. RL Goldemberg, Perfume sensitization, *Drug Cosm Ind* **119** 28 (1976)

9:43. AA Fischer and A Dooms-Goosens, The effect of perfume aging on the allergy of individual perfume ingredients, *Contact Derm* **2** 155 (1976)

9:44. RL Goldemberg, Use of anti-irritants in cosmetic formulating, *J Soc Cos Chem* **16** 317 (1965)

9:45. RL Goldemberg and L Safrin, Reduction of topical irritation, *J Soc Cos Chem* **28** 667 (1977)

9:46. RL Goldemberg, Anti-irritants, *J Soc Cos Chem* **30** 415 (1979)

9:47. RD Kinsborough, Review of toxicity of hexachlorophene, including its neurotoxicity, *J Clin Pharmacol* **13** 439 (1973)

9:48. RN Sherman, RW Leech et al, Neuropathology in newborn infants bathed in hexachlorophene, *Morb & Mort* **22** 93 (1973)

9:49. D&C Green No. 6: Listing as a color additive in externally applied drugs and cosmetics, *Fed Reg* **47** (64) 14138 (April 2, 1982)

9:50. TY Fan, U Goff et al, N-nitrosodiethanolamine in cosmetics, lotion and shampoos, *Fd Cosm Toxicol* **15** 423 (1977)

9:51. GS Edwards, M Pang et al, Detection of N-nitrosodiethanolamine in human urine following application of a contaminated cosmetic, *Toxicol Lett* **4** 217 (1979)

9:52. TJ Franz, Percutaneous absorption of D&C orange no. 17 through human skin in vitro, A study conducted for the Cosmetic, Toiletry and Fragrance Association at the University of Washington School of Medicine, Seattle, Washington (March 25, 1983)

9:53. TJ Franz, Percutaneous absorption of D&C red no. 9 through human skin in vitro, A study conducted for the Cosmetic, Toiletry and Fragrance Association at the University of Washington School of Medicine, Seattle, Washington (August 8, 1983)

9:54. TJ Franz, Percutaneous absorption of D&C red no. 19 through human skin in vitro, A study conducted for the Cosmetic, Toiletry and Fragrance Association at the University of Washington School of Medicine, Seattle, Washington (February 16, 1983)

9:55. TJ Franz, Percutaneous absorption of FD&C red no. 3 through human skin in vitro, A study conducted for the Cosmetic, Toiletry and Fragrance Association at the University of Washington School of Medicine, Seattle, Washington (March 19, 1984)

9:56. A Schaefer, A Zesch et al, *General Rules for Percutaneous Absorption in Skin Permeability*, New York: Springer-Verlag (1982)

Supplementary Bibliography

9:57. Symposium on Pharmacokinetics and Topically Applied Cosmetics, *Scientific Monograph Series No. 2*, JM McNerney, ed, Washington, DC: The Cosmetic, Toiletry and Fragrance Association (May 9, 1983)

Chapter 10

10:1. AD Bangham, MM Standish and JC Watkins, The action of steroids and streptolysin S on the permeability of phospholipid structures to cations, *J Mol Biol* **13** 138 (1965)

10:2. G Gregoriadis, The carrier potential of liposomes in biology and medicine, *New Engl J Med* **295** 704 (1976)

10:3. JH Fendler and A Romero, Liposomes as drug carriers, *Life Sci* **20** 1109 (1977)

10:4. MC Finkelstein and NG Wessman, The introduction of enzymes into cells by means of liposomes, *J Lipid Res* **19** 289 (1978)

10:5. MB Yatvin and PI Lelkes, Clinical prospects for liposomes, *Medical Physics* **9** 149 (1982)

10:6. G Gregoriadis, CP Swain, EJ Wills and AS Travill, Drug-carrier potential of liposomes in cancer chemotherapy, *Lancet* **1** 1313 (1974)

10:7. M Mezei and V Gulasekharam, Liposomes - A selective drug delivery system for the topical route of administration, I. lotion dosage form, *Life Sci* **26** 1473 (1980)

10:8. M Mezei and V Gulasekharam, Liposomes - A selective drug delivery system for the topical route of administration: gel dosage form, *J Pharm Pharmacol* **34** 473 (1982)

10:9. A J Vermorken, M W Hukkelhoven, A M Vermeesch, C M Goos and P Wirtz, The use of liposomes in the topical application of steroids, *J Pharm Pharmacol* **36** 334 (1983)

10:10. MG Ganesan, ND Weiner, GL Flynn and NFH Ho, Influence of liposomal drug entrapment on percutaneous absorption, *Int J Pharm* **20** 139 (1984)

10:11. TC Rowe, M Mezei and J Hilchie, Treatment of hirsutism with liposomal progesterone, *The Prostate* **5** 346 (1984)

10:12. U K Pat GB2 143 433A, Dermatological ointment, HM Patel (1984)

10:13. MM Rieger, Skin lipids and their importance to cosmetic science, *Cosm & Toil* **102** 36 (1987)

10:14. C Prottey, PJ Hartop and M Press, Correction of the cutaneous manifestations of essential fatty acid deficiency in man by application of sunflower-seed oil to the skin, *J Invest Dermatol* **64** 228 (1975)

10:15. H Lautenschlager, J Roding and M Ghyczy, The use of liposomes from soya phospholipids in cosmetics, *SOFW* **14** 531 (1988)

10:16. H Lautenschlager, Comments concerning the legal framework for the use of liposomes in cosmetics preparations, *SOFW* **18** 761 (1988)

10:17. G Imokawa, S Akasaki, Y Minematsu and M Kawai, Importance of intercellular lipids in water-retention properties of the stratum corneum, *Arch Dermatol Res* **281** 45-51 (1989)

10:18. C Artman, J Röding, M Ghyczy and G Pratzel, Influence of various liposome preparations on skin humidity, *Parf Kosm* **5** 326 (1990)

10:19. US Pat 3,957,971, WS Oleniacz (1976)

10:20. M Tagawa, K Shinozaki, Y Kurata, K Matsumoto and Y Tabata, Application of hydrogenated lecithin for cosmetics, *14th IFSCC* **1** 335 (1986)

10:21. F Szoka, Papahadjopoulos, Procedure for preparation of liposomes with large internal aqueous space and high capture by reverse-phase evaporation, *Biochemistry* **75** 4194 (1978)

10:22. CJ Kirby and G Gregoriadis, A simple procedure for preparing liposomes capable of high encapsulation efficiency under mild conditions, in *Liposome Technology*, v1, G Gregoriadis, ed, Boca Raton, FL: CRC Press (1984) pp19-28

10:23. AM Downes, AG Matoltsy and TM Sweeny, Rate of turnover of the stratum corneum in hairless mice, *J Invest Dermatol* **49** 400 (1967)

10:24. K Egbaria, C Ramachandran, D Kittayanod and N Weiner, Topical delivery of liposomal INF, *Antimicrob Agents Chemother* **34** 107 (1990)

10:25. K Egbaria, C Ramachandran and N Weiner, Liposomes as a topical drug delivery system, *Advanced Drug Delivery Review* **5** 287 (1990)

10:26. K Egbaria, C Ramachandran and N Weiner, Topical delivery of ciclosporin: evaluation of various formulations using in-vitro diffusion studies in hairless mouse skin, *Skin Pharmacol* **3** 21 (1990)

10:27. A Rougier, D Dupuis, C Lotte, R Roguet and H Schafer, In-vivo correlation between stratum corneum reservoir function and percutaneous absorption, *J Invest Dermatol* **81** 275 (1983)

10:28. S Grayson and PM Elias, Isolation and lipid biochemical characterization of stratum corneum membrane complexes: Implication for the cutaneous permeability barrier, *J Invest Dermatol* **78** 128-135 (1982)

10:29. H Schafer, G Stuttgen, A Zesch, W Schalla and J Gazith, Quantitative determination of percutaneous absorption of radiolabeled drug, in-vitro and in-vivo by human skin, *Curr Probl Derm* **7** 80-94 (1979)

10:30. K Egbaria and N Weiner, Topical application of liposomal preparations, *Cosm & Toil* **106** 79 (1991)

10:31. PM Elias, Structure and function of stratum corneum permeability barrier, *Drug Development Res* **13** 97 (1988)

10:32. PM Elias, Epidermal lipids, barrier function and desquamation, *J Invest Dermatol* **80** (1983)

10:33. PM Elias, ER Cooper, A Kore and BE Brown, Percutaneous transport in relation to stratum corneum structure and lipid composition, *J Invest Dermatol* **76** 297 (1981)

10:34. S Grayson and PM Elias, Isolation and lipid biochemical characterization of stratum corneum cell membrane complexes: Implication for cutaneous permeability barrier, *J Invest Dermatol* **78** 128 (1982)

10:35. K Egbaria, C Ramachandran and N Weiner, Topical application of liposomally entrapped ciclosporin evaluated by in-vitro diffusion studies with human skin, *Skin Pharmacol* **4** 21 (1991)

10:36. N Weiner, N Williams, G Birch, C Ramachandran, Shipman Jr. and G Flynn, Topical delivery of liposomally encapsulated interferon evaluated in a cutaneous herpes guinea pig model, *Antimicrob Agents Chemother* **33** 1217 (1989)

10:37. A William, PW Wertz, L Landmann and DT Downing, Preparation of liposomes from stratum corneum lipids, *J Invest Dermatol* **87** 582 (1988)

Chapter 11

11:1. GL Flynn and BS Stewart, Percutaneous drug penetration: choosing candidates for transdermal development, *Drug Development Research* **13** 169 (1988)

11:2. GW Cleary, Transdermal controlled release systems, in *Medical Applications of Controlled Release* V 1, RS Langer and DL Wise, eds, Boca Raton: CRC Press (1984) p 203

285

11:3. DR Stanski and CC Hug, Jr., Alfentanil—a kinetically predictable narcotic analgesic, *J Anesthesiol* **57** 435 (1982)

11:4. AS Michaels, SK Chandrasekaran and JE Shaw, Drug permeation through human skin: theory and in vitro experimental measurement, *AIChE Journal* **21** 985 (1975)

11:5. JE Shaw, ME Prevo and AA Amkraut, Testing of controlled release transdermal dosage forms *Arch Dermatol* **123** 1548 (1987)

11:6. JJ Leyden and GL Grove, Transdermal delivery systems cutaneous toxicology, *Transdermal Delivery of Drugs* Vol 2, eds, AF Kydonieus and B Berner, CRC Press, Boca Raton, 1987, p 99

11:7. DH Kaeble, Physical Chemistry of Adhesion, John Wiley & Sons, New York, 1971

11:8. KW Allen, Theories of adhesion surveyed, in Aspects of Adhesion (DJ Alner, ed) vol 5, University of London Press, 1969, p 11

11:9. Y Inoue and Y Kobatake, *Appl Sci Res* **A8** 321 (1959)

11:10. DH Kaelble, *Trans Soc Rheol* **4** 45 (1960)

11:11. DW Aubrey and S Ginosatis, Peel adhesion behavior of carboxylic elastomers, *J Adhesion* **12** 189 (1981)

11:12. ASTM Designation: D907-74, Standard Definitions of Terms Relating to Adhesives, American Society for Testing and Materials, Philadelphia (1974)

11:13. MA Krenceski, JF Johnson and SC Temin, Chemical and physical factors affecting performance of pressure sensitive adhesives, *J Macromolec Sci—Rev Macromol Chem Phys* **C26** 143 (1986)

11:14. HL Leeper and D Enscore, Creep test developed for adhesive-backed skin patch used to deliver drugs, *Adhes Age* **25** 16 (1982)

11:15. WM Bright, The adhesion of elastomeric pressure sensitive adhesives: rate process, in Adhesion and Adhesives, Fundamentals and Practice, (F Clark, JE Rutzler and RL Savage, eds) John Wiley & Sons, New York, p 130 (1954)

11:16. DH Kaelble and FA Hamm, Adhesion properties of a new surgical tape. II. Rheology and creep resistance, *Adhes Age* **11** 28 (1968)

11:17. JF Komerska and N Moffett, *Collagen films as test surfaces for skin-contact pressure sensitive adhesives*, Norwood Medical Products Brochure (1985)

11:18. RT Tregear and P Dirnhuber, The mass of keratin removed from the stratum corneum by stripping with adhesive tape, *J Invest Derm* **38** 375 (1962)

11:19. N Orentreich, RA Berger and R Auerbach, Anhydrotic effects of adhesive tapes and occlusive film, *Arch Dermatol* **94** 709 (1966)

11:20. JW Bothwell, Adhesion to skin: effects of surgical tapes on skin, in *Adhesion in Biological Systems*, R Manly, ed, New York: Academic Press (1970) p 215

11:21. EF McNiff, A Yacobi, FM Young-Chang, LH Golden, A Goldfarb and HL Fung, Nitroglycerin pharmacokinetics after intravenous infusion in normal subjects, *J Pharm Sci* **70** 1054 (1981)

11:22. VH Maier-Lenz, Ringevelski and A Windorfer, Pharmacokinetics and relative bioavailability of nitroglycerin ointment formulation, *Arzneim-Forsch* **30** 320 (1980)

11:23. PK Noonan, MA Gonzalez, D Ruggirello, J Tomlinson, E Babcock-Atkinson, M Ray, A Golub and A Cohen, Relative bioavailability of a new transdermal nitroglycerin delivery system, *J Pharm Sci* **75** 688 (1986)

11:24. M Wolff, G Cordes and V Luckow, In vitro and in vivo release of nitroglycerin from a new transdermal therapeutic system, *Pharm Res* **1** 23 (1985)

11:25. JE Shaw, Pharmacokinetics of nitroglycerin and clonidine delivered by the transdermal route, *J Am Heart* **108** 217 (1984)

11:26. VP Shah, NW Tymes and JP Skelly, Comparative in vitro release profiles of marketed nitroglycerin patches by different dissolution methods, *J Controlled Release* **7** 79 (1988)

11:27. A Karim, Transdermal absorption of nitroglycerin from microseal drug delivery (MDD) system, *J Vascular Diseases* **34** 11 (1983)

11:28. TR MacGregor, KM Matzek, JJ Keirns, RGA van Wagjen and A van den Ende, Pharmacokinetics of transdermally delivered clonidine, *Clin Pharmacol and Therap* **38** 278 (1985)

11:29. WR Good, Transder-nitro controlled delivery of nitroglycerin via the transdermal route, *Drug Develop & Ind Pharm* **9** 647 (1983)

11:30. MS Powers, P Campbell and L Schenkel, A new transdermal delivery system for estradiol, *J Controlled Release* **2** 89 (1985)

11:31. JP Dubois, A Sioufi, P Muller, D Mauli and PR Imhof, Pharmacokinetics and bioavailability of nicotine in healthy volunteers following single and repeated administration of different doses of transdermal nicotine systems, *Meth Find* **II** 187 (1989)

11:32. CH McLeskey, Transdermal opioids, *Amer Soc Anesthes, Annual Meeting Abstract*, New Orleans, (October 1989)

11:33. MS Powers, et al, Pharmacokinetics and pharmacodynamics of transdermal dosage forms of 17b-estradiol: Comparison with conventional oral estrogens used for hormone replacement, *Am J Obst Gynecol* **152** 1099 (1985)

11:34. LR Laufer, JL DeFazio, JK Lu, DR Meldrum, P Eggena, MP Sambhi, JM Hershman and HL Judd, Estrogen replacement therapy by transdermal estradiol administration, *Am J Obst Gynecol* **146** 533 (1983)

11:35. J Miranda and GW Cleary, US Patent 4,915,950, Printed transdermal drug delivery device, (April 10, 1990)

11:36. JB McCrea, PH Vlasses, TJ Franz and L Zeoli, Transdermal Timolol: β blockade and plasma concentrations after application for 48 hours and 7 days, *Pharmacotherapy* **10** 289 (1990)

11:37. A Wellstein, H Kuppers, HF Pitschner and D Palm, Transdermal delivery of bupranolol: pharmacodynamics and beta-adrenoceptor occupancy, *Eur J Clin Pharmacol* **31** 419 (1986)

11:38. MV Miles, R Balasubramanian, A Wayne Pittman, SH Grossman, KA Pappa, MF Smith, WA Wargin, JWA Findlay, RI Poust and MF Frosolono, Pharmacokinetrics of oral and transdermal triprolidine, *J Clin Pharmacol* **30** 572 (1990)

11:39. AJ Dietz, JD Carlson and CL Beck, Effect of transdermal on reducing histamine-induced wheal area, *Annals of Allergy* **57** 38 (1986)

11:40. JC Findlay, VA Place and PJ Snyder, Transdermal delivery of testosterone, *J Clin Endocrin and Metab* **64** 266 (1987)

11:41. HM Wolff, HR Hoffmann and G Cordes, Development of process and technology for adhesive-type transdermal therapeutic systems, in Transdermal controlled systemic medications, YW Chien, ed, Marcel Dekker, New York, 1987, p 365

11:42. JW Dohner, Development of processes and equipment for rate-controlled transdermal therapeutic systems, YW Chien, ed, Marcel Dekker, New York, 1987, p 349

11:43. YW Chien, The use of biocompatible polymers in rate-controlled drug delivery systems, *Pharm Technol*, **9** 50 (1985)

11:44. BW Barry, *Dermatological formulations,* Marcel Dekker, New York, 1983, pp243 and 246

Chapter 12

12:1. DL Akins, JL Meiseinheimer and RL Dobson, Efficacy of a drionic unit in the treatment of hyperhydrosis, *J Am Ac Dermatol*, **16**(4) 828 (1987)

12:2. ML Elgart and G Fuchs, Tap water iontophoresis in the treatment of hyperhydrosis, *Pharmacol and Ther*, **26**(3) 194 (1987)

12:3. JL Shen, GS Lin and WM Li, A new strategy of iontophoresis for hyperhydrosis, *J Am Acad Dermatol* **22** 239 (1990)

12:4. *Clinical Diagnosis by Laboratory Methods*, 15th ed, I Davidson and J Henry, eds,

287

Philadelphia PA: WB Saunders Co (1974) p 876

12:5. LP Gangarosa, Iontophoresis for surface local anesthesia, *JADA* **88** 125 (1974)

12:6. LP Gangarosa and AL Buettner, Four month results with iontophoretic tooth desensitization, *J Dental Res* **66** 151 (1987)

12:7. LP Gangarosa, AL Buettner, WP Baker, BK Buettner and WO Thompson, Double-blind evaluation of duration of dentin sensitivity reduction by fluoride iontophoresis, *Gen Dentistry* **37**(4) 316 (1989)

12:8. JA Hobden, JJ Reidy, RJ O'Callaghan, MS Insler and JM Hill, Ciprofloxacin iontophoresis for aminoglycoside resistant Pseudomonal keratitis, *Invest Ophthmol Vis Sci* **31**(10) 1940 (1990)

12:9. JM Glass, RL Stephen and SC Jacobsen, The quantity and distribution of radiolabeled dexamethasone delivered to tissue by iontophoresis, *I J Dermatol*, **19**(9) 519 (1980)

12:10. L Zeltzer, M Regalado, LS Nichter, D Barton, S Jennings and L Pitt, Iontophoresis versus subcutaneous injection: A comparison of two methods of local anesthesia delivery in children, *Pain* **44**(1) 73 (1991)

12:11. P Tyle, Iontophoretic devices for drug delivery, *Pharm Res* **3**(6) 318 (1986)

12:12. AK Banga and YW Chien, Iontophoretic delivery of drugs: Fundamentals, developments and biomedical applications, *J Contr Rel* **7** 1 (1988)

12:13. JB Sloan and K Soltani, Iontophoresis in dermatology, *J Am Acad Dermatol* **15**(4) 671 (1986)

12:14. AJ Singh and MS Roberts, Transdermal delivery of drugs by iontophoresis: A review, *Drug Des Del* **4** 1 (1989)

12:15. D Parasrampuria and J Parasrampuria, Percutaneous delivery of peptides and proteins using iontophoretic techniques, *J Clin Pharm Ther* **16** 7 (1991)

12:16. RL Stephen, TJ Petelenz and SC Jacobsen, Potential novel methods for insulin administration: I. Iontophoresis, *Biomed Biochim Acta* **43** 553 (1984)

12:17. B Kari, Control of blood glucose levels in alloxan-diabetic rabbits by iontophoresis of insulin, *Diabetes* **35** 217 (1986)

12:18. YW Chien, O Siddiqui, W-M Shi, P Lelawongs and J-C Lui, Direct current iontophoretic transdermal delivery of peptide and protein drugs, *J Pharm Sci* **78**(5) 376 (1989)

12:19. SB Ruddy and BW Hadzija, Iontophoretic permeability of polyethylene glycols through hairless rat skin: Application of hydrodynamic theory for hindered transport through liquid-filled pores, *Drug Des Disc* **8** 207 (1992)

12:20. LL Miller, CJ Kolaskie, GA Smith and J Rivier, Transdermal iontophoresis of gonadotropin releasing hormone (LHRH) and two analogs, *J Pharm Sci* **79**(6) 490 (1990)

12:21. NA Monteiro-Riviere, Altered epidermal morphology secondary to lidocaine iontophoresis: in-vivo and in-vitro studies in porcine skin, *Fund Appl Tox* **15** 174 (1990)

12:22. PH Dugard and RJ Scheuplein, Effects of ionic surfactants on permeability of human epidermis: An electrometric study, *J Invest Dermatol* **60** 263 (1973)

12:23. RR Burnette and D Marrero, Comparison between the iontophoretic and passive transport of thyrotropin releasing hormone across excised nude mouse skin, *J Pharm Sci* **75**(8) 738 (1986)

12:24. W Megerl, RA Westerman, B Mohner and H Handwerker, Properties of transdermal histamine iontophoresis: Differential effects of season, gender and body region, *J Invest Dermatol* **94**(3) 347 (1990)

12:25. YB Bannon, J Corish and OI Corrigan, Iontophoretic transport of model compounds from a gel matrix across a cellophane membrane, *Drug Dev Ind Pharm* **13**(14) 2617 (1987)

12:26. JB Phipps, RV Padmanabhan and GA Lattin, Transport of ionic species through skin, *Sol St Ionics* **28-30** 1778 (1988)

12:27. T Yamamoto and Y Yamamoto, Non-linear electric properties of skin in the low frequency range, *Med Biol Eng Comput* **19** 302 (1981)

288

12:28. P Lelawongs, JC Liu and YW Chien, Transdermal iontophoretic delivery of arginine-vasopressin (II): Evaluation of electrical and operational factors, *Int J Pharm* **61** 179 (1990)

12:29. T Koizumi, M Kakemi, K Katayama, H Inada, K Sudeji and M Kawasaki, Transfer of diclofenac sodium across excised guinea pig skin on high-frequency pulse iontophoresis. I. Equivalent circuit model, *Chem Pharm Bull* **38**(4) 1019 (1990)

12:30. RJ Scheuplein and IH Blank, *Physiol Rev* **51** 702 (1971)

12:31. RR Burnette and B Ongpipattanakul, Characterization of the pore transport properties and tissue alteration of excised human skin during iontophoresis, *J Pharm Sci* **77** 132 (1988)

12:32. PD Gadsby, Visualization of the barrier layer through iontophoresis of ferric ions, *Med Inst* **13**(5) 281 (1979)

12:33. MJ Pikal, Transport mechanisms in iontophoresis. I. A theoretical model for the effect of electroosmotic flow on flux enhancement in transdermal iontophoresis, *Pharm Res* **7**(2) 118 (1990)

12:34. MJ Pikal and S Shah, Transport mechanisms in iontophoresis. II. Electroosmotic flow and transference number measurements for hairless mouse skin, *Pharm Res* **7**(3) 213 (1990)

12:35. MJ Pikal and S Shah, Transport mechanisms in iontophoresis. III. An experimental study of the contributions of electroosmotic flow and permeability change in transport of low and high molecular weight solutes, *Pharm Res* **7**(3) 222 (1990)

12:36. RR Burnette and B Ongpipattanakul, Characterization of the permselective properties of excised human skin during iontophoresis, *J Pharm Sci* **76**(10) 765 (1987)

12:37. MJ Pikal and S Shah, Transport of uncharged species by iontophoresis: Electrophoretic flow, *Pharm Res* **3**(5) suppl 79 (1986)

12:38. N Harper Bellantone, S Rim, ML Francoeur and B Rasadi, Enhanced percutaneous absorption via iontophoresis I. Evaluation of an in-vitro system and transport of model compounds, *I J Pharm* **30** 63 (1986)

12:39. O Siddiqui, MS Roberts and AE Polack, Iontophoretic transport of weak electrolytes through the excised human stratum corneum, *J Pharm Pharmacol* **41** 430 (1989)

12:40. PP Sarpotdar, CR Daniels, GG Liversidge and LA Sternson, Facilitated iontophoretic delivery of thyrotropin releasing hormone (TRH) across cadaver skin by optimization of formulation variables, *Pharm Res* **6** suppl 107 (1989)

12:41. V Srinivasan and WI Higuchi, A model for iontophoresis incorporating the effect of solvent flow, *Int J Pharm* **60** 133 (1990)

12:42. LL Wearley, K Tojo and YW Chien, A numerical approach to study the effect of binding on the iontophoretic transport of a series of amino acids, *J Pharm Sci* **79**(11) 992 (1990)

12:43. T Masada, WI Higuchi, V Srinivasan, U Rohr, J Fox, C Behl and S Pons, Examination of iontophoretic transport of ionic drugs across skin: Baseline studies with four-electrode system, *I J Pharm* **49** 57 (1989)

12:44. LL Wearley, JC Liu and YW Chien, Iontophoresis-facilitated transdermal delivery of verapamil. I. In-vitro evaluation and mechanistic studies, *J Contr Rel* **8** 237 (1989)

12:45. P Glikfeld, C Cullander, RS Hinz and RH Guy, A new system for in-vitro studies of iontophoresis, *Pharm Res* **5**(7) 443 (1988)

12:46. DA Nyambi, VH Dawes and MJ Lawrence, Evaluation of a new iontophoretic system using model compounds, *J Pharm Pharmacol* **42**(s) 83P (1990)

12:47. GA Lattin, RV Padamanabhan and JB Phipps, Electronic control of iontophoretic drug delivery, *Ann NY Acad Sci* **618** 450 (1991)

12:48 US Pat 4,747,819, *Iontophoretic drug delivery*, JB Phipps and DF Untereker (May 31, 1988)

12:49 US Pat 4,752,285, *Methods and apparatus for iontophoresis application of medicaments*, TJ Petelenz, RL Stephen and SC Jacobsen (Jun 21, 1988)

12:50 US Pat 4,722,726, *Method and apparatus for iontophoretic delivery*, JE Sanderson and

SR Deriel (Feb 2, 1988)

12:51. LL Miller and GA Smith, Iontophoretic transport of acetate and carboxylate ions through hairless mouse skin. A cation exchange membrane model, *Int J Pharm* **49** 15 (1989)

12:52. PP Sarpotdar and CR Daniels, Use of polymeric buffers to facilitate iontophoretic transport of drugs, *Pharm Res* **7** suppl 185 (1990)

12:53. K Okabe, H Yamaguchi and Y Kawai, New iontophoretic transdermal administration of the beta-blocker metoprolol, *J Contr Rel* **4** 79 (1986)

12:54. T Koizumi, M Kakemi, K Katayama, H Inada, K Sudeji and M Kawasaki, Transfer of diclofenac sodium across excised guinea pig skin on high-frequency pulse iontophoresis. II. Factors affecting steady-state rate, *Chem Pharm Bull* **38**(4) 1022 (1990)

12:55. K Sudeji, K Furusawa, H Inada, K Katayama, M Kakemi and T Koizumi, Enhanced percutaneous absorption of formeterol fumarate via pulsed iontophoresis. II. Effect of polarity, pulse frequency and duty, *Yakugaku Zasshi* **109** (10) 771 (1989)

12:56. YW Chien, O Siddiqui, Y Sun, WM Shi and JC Liu, Transdermal iontophoretic delivery of therapeutic peptides/proteins I: Insulin, *Annals of NY Acad Sci* **507** 32 (1987)

12:57. V Srinivasan, WI Higuchi, SM Sims, AH Ghanem and CR Behl, Transdermal iontophoretic drug delivery: Mechanistic analysis and application to polypeptide delivery, *J Pharm Sci* **78**(5) 370 (1989)

12:58. L Wearley and YW Chien, Enhancement of the in-vitro skin permeability of azidothymidine (AZT) via iontophoresis and chemical enhancer, *Pharm Res* **7**(1) 34 (1990)

Chapter 13

13:1. G Wyszecki and WS Stilles, *Color Sciences: Concepts and Methods, Quantitative Data and Formula*, 2nd ed, John Wiley and Sons, New York, 165 (1982)

13:2. JB Dawson, DJ Barker, DJ Ellis, E. Grassam, JS Correrill, GN Fisher and JW Feather, A theoretical and experimental study of light absorption and scattering by in vivo skin, *Phys Med Biol* **25** 695 (1986)

13:3. LL Hartman, Methods for studying the skin surface, *J Soc Cosm Chem* **34** 407-418 (1983)

13:4. BL Diffey, RJ Oliver and PM Farr, A portable instrument for quantifying erythema induced by ultraviolet radiation, *Brit J Dermat* **111** 663 (1984)

13:5. PM Farr and BL Diffey, Quantitative studies on cutaneous erythema induced by ultraviolet radiation, *Brit J Dermat* **111** 673 (1984)

13:6. SW Babulak, LD Rhein, DD Scala, FA Simion and GL Grove, Quantitation of erythema in a soap chamber test using the Minolta Chroma reflectance meter: comparison of instrumental results with visual assessments, *J Soc Cosm Chem* **37** 475 (1986)

13:7. W Cui, LE Ostrander and BY Lee, In vivo reflectance of blood and tissue as a function of light wavelength, *IEEE Transact Biomed Eng* **37** 6 (1990)

13:8. P Bjerring, PH Andersen, Skin reflectance spectrophotometry, *Photoderm* **4** 167 (1987)

13:9. N Kollias, A Bager, Spectroscopic characteristics of human melanin in vivo, *J Invest Dermatol* **85** 593 (1985)

13:10. DP Conner, K Zamani, D Nix, E Millora, RG Almirez, V Shah, CC Peck, Use of reflectance spectrometry in the corticosteroid skin blanching assay, *Clin Pharmacol Ther* **47**(2) 170 (1990)

13:11. AW McKenzie, RB Stoughton, Method for comparing percutaneous absorption of steroids, *Arch Dermatol* **86** 608 (1962)

13:12. C Queille-Roussel, M Poncet, H Schaefer, Quantification of skin colour changes induced by topical corticosteroids on normal skin using the Minolta Chromameter, *8th International Symposium on Bioengineering and the Skin*, Stresa, Italy (1990)

13:13. *Perimed Literature Reference List No. 10*, Perimed, Stockholm, Sweden, (April 1990)

290

13:14. RH Guy, RC Wester, E Tur, HI Maibach, Noninvasive assessments of the percutaneous absorption of methyl nicotinate in humans, *J Pharm Sci* **72**(9) 1077 (1983)

13:15. JK Wilkin, G Fortner, LA Reinhardt, OV Flowers et al, Prostaglandins and nicotinate-provoked increase in cutaneous blood flow, *Clin Pharmacol Ther* **38**(3) 273 (1985)

13:16. PM Dowd, M Whitefield and MW Greaves, Hexyl-nicotinate-induced vasodilation in normal human skin, *Dermatologica* **174**(5) 239 (1987)

13:17. DA Perednia, What dermatologists should know about digital imaging, *J Am Acad Dermatol* **25** 89 (1991)

13:18. R Murphy, DWK Cotton, AL Wright and SS Bleehen, Computer-assisted image analysis of skin surface replicas, *Brit J Dermatol* **124** 571 (1991)

13:19. R Marks, RPR Dawber, Skin surface biopsy, an improved technique for the examination of the horny layer, *Brit J Dermatol* **84** 117 (1971)

13:20. Cunliffe and Cotterill, *The Acnes*, WB Saunders Co Ltd, London, p 294

13:21. DG Groh and AM Kligman, The Quantitative Assessment of Cyanoacrylate Follicular Biopsies by Image Analysis, Program Soc Cosm Chem Annual Scientific Meeting, **13** (1991)

13:22. GL Grove, Dermatological applications of the Magiscan image analyzing computer, *Bioengineering and the Skin*, MTP Press Ltd, Lancaster, p 176 (1979)

13:23. MJ Grove, PF Alfano and GL Grove, Image analysis of Sebutape specimens to monitor the activity of individual sebaceous glands, *Int J Bioeng Skin* **2** 142 (1986).

13:24. AM Kligman, DL Miller and KJ McGinley, Sebutape: A device for visualizing and measuring human sebaceous secretion, *J Soc Cosm Chem* **37** 369 (1986)

13:25. GP Kushla and JL Zatz, Evaluation of a noninvasive method for monitoring percutaneous absorption of lidocaine in vitro, *Pharm Res* **7** 1033 (1990)

13:26. "Noninvasive assessment of topical anesthesia in humans and comparison with in vitro flux data," presented at the American Association of Pharmaceutical Scientists Annual Meeting, Washington, DC, (November 1991)

13:27. GP Kishla and JL Zatz, Correlation of water and lidocaine flux enhancement by cationic surfactants in vitro, *J Pharm Sci*, in press

13:28. P Muller, R Keller and P Imhof, Laser Doppler flowmetry, a reliable technique for measuring pharmacologically-induced changes in cutaneous blood flow?, *Methods Find Exp Clin Pharmacol* **9**(6) 409 (June 1987)

13:29. H Fruhstorfer, O Selbmann and U Ziegenhagel, Automatic scanner for multi-point laser Doppler flux recordings on human skin, *Skin Pharmacol* **4**(2) 113 (1991)

13:30. RC Cornell and RB Stoughton, Correlation of the vasoconstriction assay and clinical activity in psoriasis, *Arch Dermatol* **121** (Jan 1985)

13:31. ME Stewart, DT Downing and JS Strauss, Sebum secretion and sebaceous lipids, *Dermatol Clinics* **1** 335 (July 1983)

13:32. JJ Leyden, KJ McGinley et al, Topical antibiotics and topical antimicrobial agents in acne therapy, *Acta Derm Venereol (Stockholm) Suppl* **89** 75 (1980)

Index

C

D

294

S

V

W

X

Z